Therapeutic Exercise for Lumbopelvic Stabilization

For Churchill Livingstone:

Commissioning Editor: Mary Law/Sarena Wolfaard
Project Development Manager: Mairi McCubbin
Project Manager: Samantha Ross
Design: Judith Wright

Therapeutic Exercise for Lumbopelvic Stabilization

A Motor Control Approach for the Treatment and Prevention of Low Back Pain

SECOND EDITION

Carolyn Richardson   BPhty(Hons) PhD

Associate Professor and Reader, Division of Physiotherapy, School of Health and Rehabilitation Science, University of Queensland, Brisbane, Australia

Paul W. Hodges   BPhty(Hons) MD(Neurosci) PhD

NHMRC Senior Research Fellow and Associate Professor, Division of Physiotherapy, School of Health and Rehabilitation Science, University of Queensland, Brisbane, Australia

Julie Hides   BPhty MPhtySt PhD

Clinical Supervisor, The University of Queensland/Mater Hospital Back Stability Clinic, Brisbane, Australia

This book has been endorsed by the MACP

MANIPULATION ASSOCIATION OF CHARTERED PHYSIOTHERAPISTS

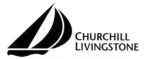

CHURCHILL LIVINGSTONE

EDINBURGH LONDON NEW YORK OXFORD PHILADELPHIA ST LOUIS SYDNEY TORONTO 2004

CHURCHILL LIVINGSTONE
An imprint of Elsevier Limited

First edition 1999
Second edition 2004

ISBN 0443 07293 0

British Library Cataloguing in Publication Data
A catalogue record for this book is available from the British Library

Library of Congress Cataloging in Publication Data
A catalog record for this book is available from the Library of Congress

Notice
Knowledge and best practice in this field are constantly changing. As new research and experience broaden our knowledge, changes in practice, treatment and drug therapy may become necessary or appropriate. Readers are advised to check the most current information provided (i) on procedures featured or (ii) by the manufacturer of each product to be administered, to verify the recommended dose or formula, the method and duration of administration, and contraindications. It is the responsibility of the practitioner, relying on their own experience and knowledge of the patient, to make diagnoses, to determine dosages and the best treatment for each individual patient, and to take all appropriate safety precautions. To the fullest extent of the law, neither the Publisher nor the author nor the MACP assume any liability for any injury and/or damage.

The Publisher

ELSEVIER
your source for books, journals and multimedia in the health sciences

www.elsevierhealth.com

The Publisher's policy is to use paper manufactured from sustainable forests

Printed in China

Contents

Preface

Over the past decade a major focus of rehabilitation has turned to exercise to improve the stability of the lumbar spine and pelvis. There are a variety of clinical and research opinions in this area and many methods have become popular in both the clinical arena and fitness industry. This book provides an overview of our interpretation of the field based on our research and clinical practice. While the first edition provided an introduction to our new models of exercise and the state of knowledge at that time, this second edition provides an updated view that integrates the burgeoning research in this field and the clinical advances.

In relation to therapeutic exercise in low back pain, we believe that the focus of exercise interventions by physiotherapists and other health professionals should be designed to establish the optimum interaction of muscles necessary to control and protect the joints, during the performance of a great variety of functional body movements.

In our first edition, we focused on the system of deep muscles that our research and clinical evidence suggest are vital in control of the lumbar segments: the multifidus, transversus abdominis, diaphragm and the pelvic floor muscles. So how has our research progressed over the last 5 years? Several key aspects have progressed. For instance long term follow-up data now indicates that the interventions described in the first edition led to reduction of low back pain recurrence rates. Our biomechanical studies have confirmed the important contribution of the deep muscle system to control of not just the lumbar spine, but also the pelvis.

Clinical studies have also confirmed the presence of muscle dysfunctions involving the deep muscle system in pelvic pain syndromes. Other developments include greater understanding of the mechanisms for control and coordination of this system and the effects of unloading, and pain and injury. Our recent research involving microgravity environments is providing the opportunity to evaluate the effects of extreme environments that are likely to have an impact on functional environments on Earth. An additional area that is continuing to expand is in the assessment of muscle control in lumbopelvic pain. In this field we have made major advances in non-invasive methods to assess this system.

As research physiotherapists in the area of therapeutic exercise for low back pain we have chosen to investigate, in the first instance, the neurophysiological mechanisms involved in joint protection of the lumbo-pelvic region and the dysfunctions which can occur. Even though many of the ideas and hypotheses presented have not yet undergone rigorous scientific scrutiny, we feel that we have an obligation in a text book on therapeutic exercise to provide details of the new ways to approach exercise prescription as well as providing hypotheses for why certain exercise techniques traditionally used by physiotherapists are likely to be very effective.

Thus the research findings plus argued hypotheses in this text have been used to give some insight into therapeutic exercise techniques which are likely to be effective and also to develop non-invasive measures which will reflect the problems in the musculoskeletal system in relation to joint protection. The principles presented can be applied to any region of the body.

One of the main aims of our past as well as our future research is to demonstrate that the prescribed therapeutic exercises are resulting in improvement in the joint protection systems, and hence demonstrate that changes in these mechanisms are closely linked to the resolution and even prevention of painful symptoms. As a final note, we also would like to emphasize the importance of using therapeutic exercise as a preventative measure and to promote a change in lifestyle, not only as a treatment after problems have occurred. This is a major focus for our ongoing work.

We hope that you find reading the second edition of this textbook thought provoking and enjoyable. We are excited that the work continues to evolve and grow in new directions. We hope that this book will be useful to clinicians, students and researchers alike, and may stimulate new ideas which will ultimately help those with lumbopelvic pain.

Acknowledgements

The authors wish to first of all acknowledge the past efforts of Gwendolen Jull whose exceptional knowledge of physiotherapy rehabilitation have made a significant contribution to this book.

With the expansion of the research, each researcher has their own group of people to thank.

Caroline and Julie extend their thanks to the primary overseas research collaborator, Professor Chris Snijders from Erasmus University in Holland, whose biomechanical models blended well with their therapeutic exercise models for low back pain. In addition it was Professor Snijders who invited them onto the Topical Team for Low Back Pain, an initiative of the European Space Agency (ESA).

Thanks also to Benny Elmann Larsen, Senior Physiologist for ESA, and Richard Linnehan, NASA astronaut, who have given Caroline and Julie the confidence to pursue the ideas on the 'Deload Model of Injury'. Dr Steve Wilson and Daniel Belavy deserve special mention with their exceptional expertise in instrument and software development for the measures used for the University of Queensland's contribution to ESA's Berlin bed rest study at the Free University in Berlin.

The collaborative research with Dr. Joseph Ng, of the Hong Kong Polytechnic University, has led to new discoveries of the dysfunctions present in the trunk muscles of low back pain patients and assisted with the development of the exercise model. It was physiotherapist, Christine Hamilton who alerted us, many years ago, of the importance of a neutral spine position for both the testing and treatment of spinal and trunk muscles.

Thanks to the staff, clinicians and students of the Joint Stability Research Unit Warren Stanton, Alison Grimaldi, Ruth Sapsford, Sally Hess, Chris Hamilton, Daniel Belavy, Nathan Stewart, Quentin Scott, Helen Fleming, Sue Roll, Sue Kelley, Jan Smith, Mark Comerford, Rowena Toppenberg, Heidi Keto and the staff at the Back Stability Clinic for their contribution to the development of the exercise model.

The editors' knowledge and expertise in real-time ultrasound imaging has only developed and evolved with the assistance of Dr David Cooper, an obstetrician and gynaecologist who specializes in ultrasound imaging. His encouragement and guidance have been invaluable. Introducing something new into a profession is never easy, and evidence of the success of the medium can be seen as it develops into being a routinely used rehabilitation and assessment tool in many physical therapy practices around the world.

A SPECIAL THANKS TO OUR FAMILIES

Caroline thanks her husband, Bren, for his never failing support with this very difficult but exciting task of writing a book and his numerous trips to Europe with her to meetings and conferences.

Julie sends special thanks to her husband, Damian, and children Emma, Jonathon and Cameron for their patience and encouragement.

Without the support of her parents, Jill and David Cooper (and provision of extensive childcare assistance) she never would have completed the 'last yards'.

PH

Paul thanks the collaborators in Australia and overseas for their contribution to this work. At the University of Queensland he thanks the team of the Human Neuroscience Unit (Michel Coppieters, Catharina Bexander, Andrew Chapman, Rebecca Mellor, Angela Chang, Sallie Cowan, Paulo Ferreira, Manuela Ferreira, Joanna Knox, Linda-Joy Lee, David McDonald, Nicola Mok, Steven Saunders, Michelle Smith, Donna Urquhart, Richard Yang) for their stimulating debate and contribution to the work presented here. In particular, thanks to Lorimer Moseley who has contributed significantly to the work dealing with pain and its effect on the motor system. This work is providing new insights into the possible reasons for development of recurrent pain.

He is also grateful to his colleagues at the Prince of Wales Medical Research Institute in Sydney (Simon Gandevia, Jane Butler, Janet Taylor) who opened his eyes to the delights of neuroscience and challenged him to test the limits of human experimentation to gain a greater understanding of the neural control of the spine. They have taught him the rigor of scientific endeavour.

Thanks particularly to the international collaborators. The team in the Biomechanics and motor control laboratory of the Department of Neuroscience at Karolinska Institute (Alf Thorstensson, Andy Cresswell, Karl Daggfeldt and Anatoli Grigorenko) have provided important guidance in biomechanics and motor control and stimulated Paul's pursuit of a second doctorate, in neuroscience. On the other side of Sweden the collaborators at the Sahlgrenska University Hospital (Allison Kaigle Holm, Sten Holm, Lars Ekstrom, Tommy Hansson) have provided an unrivalled opportunity to test the mechanisms of spinal control when the methods go beyond the limits of human experimentation.

He would also like to thank his collaborators at the University of Melbourne (Kim Bennell, Sallie Cowan, Kay Crossley) for giving him the opportunity to be involved in testing the model of motor learning, albeit in another part of the body. This research is providing a foundation for understanding the mechanisms for efficacy of exercise.

Finally, he thanks his family (Merryn, Freya, Finn and Sofia) who have provided unrelenting support, despite the fact that Paul has been away often to undertake research and present the outcomes.

SECTION 1

Introduction

Chapter 1

The time to move forward

Carolyn Richardson

INTRODUCTION

Painful musculo-skeletal health problems such as low back pain contribute significantly to morbidity in the general population and form a major part of the high costs of health care in the industrialized world. Ironically, back pain is very prevalent in the general 'health-focused' population who exercise to prevent health problems in the cardiovascular system, and it is also a major problem for those who train and compete at a high level in sports and athletic events.

Until recently, the prevention and treatment of insidious-onset mechanical low back pain have relied on the premise that the cause of mechanical low back pain is a gradual breakdown (i.e. 'wear and tear') of the joint structures and associated soft tissues over periods of time. Biomechanical and ergonomic research has successfully focused on ways of minimizing high forces on the spine and has highlighted to the community the value of such factors as safe working postures and furniture design in the prevention of low back pain.

EMPHASIS ON MOTOR CONTROL PROBLEMS AS A BASIS OF EXERCISE

The first edition of this book addressed, for the first time, the deep muscles close to the lumbar spine and pelvis, their possible function in protecting the joints from injury and their dysfunction in low back pain. From this new information, a new paradigm of exercise was devised that addressed the motor control problems in the muscles and focused on improving the mechanical support of the spinal joints through specific deep-muscle contraction exercises. This 'segmental stabilization training' technique aimed at relieving the pain that had resulted from irritation of pain-sensitive structures, subsequent to tissue injury. This initial breakthrough was possible because of astute clinical observation of patients with low back pain and through novel research approaches, which allowed the morphology and control of the deep muscles to be investigated scientifically for the first time. We also explained the clinical tests that could be used to assess the problems in the deep muscles in patients with low back pain.

This new paradigm of deep muscle function and dysfunction, and the type of exercise required for the management of low back pain, was developed with recognition of the close relationship between muscle function and the biomechanics of spinal stability. The models of the spinal stability are overviewed in detail in Chapter 2.

Widening understanding of joint protection mechanisms in relation to exercise for the prevention and treatment of low back pain

An expanded model for therapeutic exercise for the prevention and treatment of low back pain has evolved through a deeper understanding of the joint protection mechanisms from two different but essential perspectives. Chapters 2, 3 and 4 discuss, based on research findings, the role of the local muscle system in the support of the spinal segments, and its role in complex functions where the control of the spine must be matched to the demands of internal and external forces. To provide a further basis for exercise to promote the integration of the local and global muscle systems into function, another aspect of the joint protection mechanisms is introduced in this edition. This aspect is related to the role of the antigravity muscle support system.

The antigravity muscle support system and joint protection

Weightbearing mechanisms and the way load is specifically transferred through the pelvis have always been considered important concepts in the development of mechanical low back pain. The complexity of this mechanism through the bones, muscle and soft tissue has attracted the interest of many researchers. Load transfer has been studied in relation to biomechanical models dealing with the stresses across the bones of the pelvis (Dalstra and Huiskes 1995); other biomechanical models predict that muscle forces and associated soft tissues (e.g. fascias and ligaments) have a stabilizing effect on load transfer and decrease the stress on the pelvic joints.

Some models have focused more on the way muscles protect the spine for weightbearing in terms of their effect on neutral spinal curves in relation to the pelvis. The biomechanical models of Keifer et al (1997, 1998), which defined spinal stability in terms of the compressive load-bearing capacity of the spine, included pelvic rotation in the model of neutral postures. This model has contributed to our understanding of how a lordotic posture enhances the compressive loading of the spine. In addition, it demonstrated that the global muscles are sufficient to stabilize and maintain equilibrium for small sagittal movements, although the addition of the local muscles, most importantly multifidus, could decrease the forces in the global muscles and further enhance stability.

It has been the extensive biomechanical modelling and anatomical studies from Erasmus University in the Netherlands that has alerted researchers in low back pain to innovative ideas of the role of muscles and associated soft tissues in decreasing stress on the structures of the lumbopelvic region during load transfer. Snijders and colleagues (1995 (review), 1998) have carried out many studies on the important interaction between gravity, muscle forces, load transfer and the stability of the sacro-iliac joints.

Erasmus University also pioneered the load transfer concept by studying the loading patterns in terms of the effect on the posterior layer of the thoracolumbar fascia (Vleeming et al 1995) and the effects of the loading patterns on the ligaments of the pelvis, which are often painful in low back pain (Vleeming et al 1996). These models and anatomical studies highlighted the importance of particular muscles, not only the transverses abdominis and the erector spinae but also the large superficial muscles that attach to the fascia. Gluteus maximus and the contralateral latissimus dorsi are considered important in the mechanism of load transfer diagonally from arms to legs. These models have provided the impetus for strengthening programmes for patients with low back pain, involving a trunk extension–rotation action (Mooney et al 2001).

While all these models for weightbearing function of muscles are important in our understanding of the biomechanical action of muscles, it is our contention that the way in which the central and peripheral neural system links specific muscles from each segment of the kinetic chain to give an effective antigravity support system forms a basis for optimal exercise for the integration of the local and global muscles within the framework of an effective prevention and rehabilitative exercise programme for low back pain.

For an understanding of the antigravity muscle support system, it will be argued that skeletal muscles can be classified, from a neurological point of view, into weightbearing and non-weightbearing categories. This delineation of skeletal muscle function relies on the premise that weightbearing is the entity that separates muscles into two distinct functional categories. In essence, the minimization of weightbearing (deloading) promotes activity in the non-weightbearing muscles and reduces the contribution of the weightbearing muscles, while increasing weightbearing promotes activity in the weightbearing muscles and reduces the contribution of the non-weightbearing muscles. An understanding of this classification is essential both for prescribing preventative exercise for low back pain and for generating a well-balanced management approach.

The scientific significance of the delineation of skeletal muscle function into weightbearing and non-weightbearing categories came, in part, from a study of muscle function by Richardson and Bullock (1986), where the effects of gravity and weightbearing, including the gravitational load cues, were minimized in a rapid, non-weightbearing motor task. This situation of reduced weightbearing and minimal sensory input resulted in reduced use of the antigravity (one-joint) musculature and higher levels of use of the multijoint, multifunction muscles, which were facilitated in the non-weightbearing motor tasks.

More convincing scientific support for the delineation of skeletal muscle function into these two categories has been provided by our involvement in microgravity (space) research. The microgravity environment, with minimal gravitational load cues present but where body movement remains important, provides the ideal model to test the theories of the delineation of muscle function into functional categories. Results of animal and human research to date strongly support the concept that lack of information to the body about gravity differentially affects the antigravity (one-joint) muscles, which change their patterns of use, and display changes in physiology. Opposite changes occur in the multijoint, multifunction muscles, which experience increased use in the microgravity environment; this results in a lack of atrophy and indications are that they may even increase their levels of recruitment. This change in muscle physiology occurs through a process known as neuromuscular plasticity, where the physiological structure of muscles is determined by the pattern of neural impulses delivered to it.

This evidence has resulted in the change of terminology for muscles from an anatomical to a motor control perspective, into weightbearing and non-weightbearing muscle categories, to allow for a clearer understanding of their role in therapeutic exercise and in the methods used to prevent and treat low back pain. Interestingly, from a 'global' perspective, the microgravity (deloaded) environment results in problems to astronauts when they return to earth. The impairments in the antigravity joint-support mechanisms (i.e. reduced weightbearing muscle function) that develop in microgravity would result in their weightbearing joints being unprotected on their return to a gravitational environment. For this reason, astronauts could be prone to significant musculo-skeletal injuries, especially low back pain, on their return to Earth, emanating from injury to the joint structures of the lumbopelvic region. It will be argued that a similar process occurs on Earth as a result of lack of weightbearing (deloading) during many functional and recreational activities.

The argument for an emphasis on the antigravity, weightbearing muscle system in the prevention and rehabilitation strategies for low back pain is developed in four separate chapters within this text.

Chapter 5 provides more detail of how the local system operates within a framework of joint protection for weightbearing to provide stiffness and sensory input locally for the lumbopelvic region. In Chapter 6, the argument will be developed that the local muscles form part of a separate, larger antigravity muscle system, which links the joints of the entire functional kinetic chain including both the upper and lower limbs. Chapter 7 describes the impairments to the joint protective mechanisms that can develop in the antigravity muscle system with deloading (i.e. a reduction in weightbearing), while Chapter 12 describes the impairments that can develop in pelvic orientation and weightbearing function in patients with low back pain.

Although the case is put forward for the importance of the spinal stability mechanisms as well as the antigravity muscle support system in the design of therapeutic exercise for the prevention and treatment of low back pain, the impairments that occur in these systems also have a significant influence on exercise design.

EXERCISE BASED ON IMPAIRMENTS IN THE NEUROPHYSIOLOGICAL MECHANISMS OF JOINT PROTECTION

The exercise model explained in this text is based not only on the joint protective mechanisms but also on impairments in the neurophysiological mechanisms of joint protection. New perspectives of motor control impairments are included, not only for 'deloading' (Ch. 7) but also for 'injury' (Ch. 8) and 'pain' (Ch. 9). These have been added to this edition to provide essential information for improving the efficiency of the conservative treatment of low back pain as well as to provide the basis for new guidelines for the prevention of chronic, disabling spinal pain.

These effects of deloading, injury and pain on the protective muscle system have led to new mechanistic models that explain how the development of impairments in the joint protection mechanism can result in a continuous cycle of increasing disability. It will be argued that these three factors are closely linked with the impairments that develop in the joint protection mechanisms. In turn, a lack of joint protection would lead to further joint injury and pain as well as deloading of the

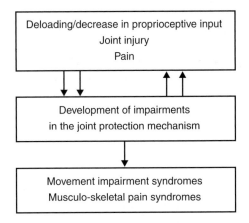

Figure 1.1 The continuous cycle of increasing disability in the joint protection system and its relationship to impairments in movement.

musculo-skeletal system. Thus a vicious cycle results, which eventually leads to progressive and increasing disability. These impairments in the joint protection mechanisms will eventually result in impaired movement patterns and musculo-skeletal pain syndromes (Fig. 1.1).

A recurring theme, which must be addressed in clinical treatment trials in the future, is that these three factors (deloading, injury, pain) may all lead to changes in motor control and motor function and that the impairments may vary considerably between individuals with similar low back pain symptoms. Therefore, patients with low back pain require individualized exercise management, based on individual clinical assessment of the impairments within the three stages of the training model.

The segmental stabilization training model

This expanded segmental stabilization training management approach is based on principles of prevention and treatment (summarized in Ch. 13) developed through our increased understanding of the complex neurophysiological processes involved in joint protection and the impairments that are involved in the development of painful symptoms.

The change in perspective that divides muscles into local, weightbearing and non-weightbearing categories rather than into groups based on motor control categories (or on anatomical descriptions), and the close relationship between local and weightbearing categories, has resulted in an expanded view of segmental stabilization exercise. While local muscles support the joints (i.e. individual segments) of the spine and pelvis, the weightbearing (usually one-joint) muscles play an important role, together with the local muscles, in linking each segment of the kinetic chain to give an effective antigravity support system. Therefore, segmental control is also required for the large joints of the girdles and limbs within a framework of antigravity weightbearing control. A more clearly defined model of exercise management of low back pain has been devised that has been expanded to include three levels of progressive segmental control.

Stage 1: local segmental control   The aim is to develop segmental control via activation and training of the local muscle system (Ch. 14). The deep local muscles, which form the most basic element of the joint protection system, are activated and exercises are given to enhance kinaesthetic awareness and muscular control.

Stage 2: closed chain segmental control   The aim is to continue to develop segmental control at individual joints through activation and training of the local muscles in conjunction with the antigravity system that links the specific weightbearing muscles from each segment of the kinetic chain to give an effective antigravity support system (Ch. 15). This step in the functional rehabilitation process is devised with a knowledge of the optimal patterns of muscle activation required for weightbearing and joint support.

Stage 3: open chain segmental control   The aim is to continue to develop segmental control at individual joints in relation to open kinetic chain movement of adjacent segments (Ch. 16). This final step directs progression so that all muscles (i.e. the local, weightbearing and non-weightbearing) are integrated into functional movement tasks in a formal way, so that compensations by more active (i.e. non-weightbearing) muscles can be detected.

THE FUTURE

Clinical screening assessments must be validated that reflect the mechanisms of joint protection and the level of impairment. Evidence must be provided that an improvement in the joint protection mechanisms correlates well with the reduction in pain and disability. From this, evidence-based treatments and prevention strategies that are based on the impairments present in an individual with pain can be expected to be developed in the near future.

In addition, new non-invasive laboratory-based assessment procedures of the antigravity, weightbearing function of muscles are currently being developed at the University of Queensland to help to understand the possible causes of low back pain. These procedures, which would be suitable for use by all health professionals, are now being investigated as part of the European Space Agency Bedrest Study, which is being undertaken at the Free University in Berlin.

SECTION 2

The joint protection mechanisms

PART 1

Introduction

Chapter **2**

Lumbopelvic stability: a functional model of the biomechanics and motor control

Paul Hodges

INTRODUCTION

Many contemporary approaches to therapeutic exercise for the spine are based on the premise that the low back pain results from, and is perpetuated by, repetitive microtrauma to the spinal structures resulting from poor control of spinal stability (Farfan 1975). Although the neurobiology of pain indicates that this simple biomechanical hypothesis is unlikely to explain the complexity of pain, there is considerable evidence to validate the biomechanical model. One factor that complicates the debate regarding the validity of 'stability exercises' is the complexity of the biomechanics and motor control of stability. A key issue is what authors mean by the term 'stability'. The aim of this chapter is to develop a clinical model of stability that can be used to guide exercise intervention. To develop the model, it is necessary to consider the general requirements for spinal stability, the muscle systems that may contribute to this control and the strategies used by the central nervous system (CNS) to meet the demands of spinal control.

BIOMECHANICAL CONSIDERATIONS OF LUMBOPELVIC CONTROL AND STABILITY

Lumbopelvic stability is often regarded to be a static principle. For instance, exercise interventions that aim to improve stability commonly involve training patients to maintain a static trunk posture during function. However, this is an oversimplified notion of stability. Instead, stability and control should be thought of as a dynamic process of controlling static position when appropriate in the functional context, but allowing the trunk to move with control in other situations. Any intervention that focuses solely on one extreme of this spectrum is unlikely to lead to an optimal functional outcome. It is important to consider a functional definition of stability and then to consider the elements that may contribute to its control.

Spinal stability is commonly modelled in the context of Euler mechanics. In this context, stability is considered in terms of buckling from compressive forces (Crisco and Panjabi 1991, Gardner-Morse et al 1995, Cholewicki and McGill 1996). In this highly developed model, it is considered that the spine is inherently unstable to compressive forces. In line with this hypothesis, in vitro studies have indicated that collapse of the lumbar spine (with all of the passive elements removed) occurs with compressive loading of as little as 90 N. In view of this, the model argues that antagonistic muscle activity is required to maintain the lumbar spine in a mechanically stable equilibrium and prevent buckling (Crisco and Panjabi 1991, Gardner-Morse et al 1995, Cholewicki and McGill 1996). Although it is clear that this model explains a component of lumbopelvic stability and control, it can be criticized from several perspectives. First, it likens the spine to a mast of a yacht, which must be maintained upright without buckling; clearly, this cannot explain the breadth of human functional requirements. Second, it does not emphasize the control of movement. For instance, as the spine is moved from flexion to extension, a controlled sequence of intervertebral rotation and translation is required (Bogduk et al 1995). This component of stability requires a fine-tuned system to coordinate stability and movement. Several authors have considered the requirement for control during movement. Panjabi (1992a,b) has recognized that around the neutral position, where the spine exhibits least stiffness, the requirement for spinal control is increased. Towards the end of range, increasing support is provided by the passive elements.

An additional consideration is that lumbopelvic stability must be considered at several interdependent levels: intervertebral control, control of lumbopelvic orientation and the control of whole-body equilibrium (Hodges and Jull 2003) (Fig. 2.1). At the most general level, as the trunk forms a large proportion of the mass of the body, trunk movement is important for the control of postural equilibrium with respect to imposed forces (Oddsson 1988). If the equilibrium of the body is disturbed by external (e.g. unexpected movement of the support surface) or internal (e.g. by reactive forces from limb movement) forces, movement of the trunk occurs to move the centre of mass (COM) over the new base of support or to alter the orientation of the body (e.g. Keshner et al 1989). It is important to consider this function of the trunk as the demands for control of equilibrium may conflict with the requirements for control of spinal orientation or intervertebral motion. For instance, trunk alignment cannot be maintained if movement of the trunk is required to move the COM over a new base of support (Huang et al 2001). The next level in the hierarchy of spinal control is the control of orientation of the spine and pelvis. At this level, it is important to consider the control of the curvature and posture of the spine. It is at this level that control of buckling is most critical. In function, a complex array of internal and external forces, including gravity, are imposed on the body. For instance, in a simple task such as rapid flexion of the arm, the reactive moments from the movement generate a flexion moment at the trunk, while at the same time the forward position of the arm moves the COM of the body forward, again causing the spine to flex (Bouisset and Zattara 1981, Hodges et al 1999). If the goal is to maintain upright posture, these perturbations must be overcome. Similarly, when a weight-lifter raises a mass from the floor, buckling of the spine must be prevented by muscle activity (Cholewicki et al 1991).

At the most basic level of spinal control is the control of intervertebral translation and rotation; however, this cannot be completely separated from the control of spinal orientation (Panjabi et al 1989). That is, buckling can occur at the intervertebral level and changes in spinal orientation involve intervertebral motion. However, separate attention must be paid to control of translations and rotations. For instance, during an arc of movement it is important to control the coordination between translation and rotation between segments (Bogduk et al 1995). It has been shown that if the spine is modelled with all segments crossed by muscle, but with one vertebrae with no muscle attachment, then the spine is as

(a)   (b)   (c)

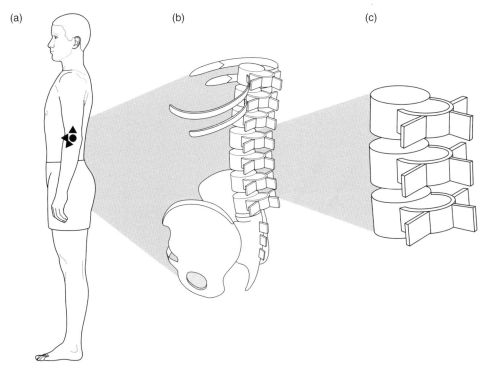

Figure 2.1
Lumbopelvic
stability at
interdependent
levels. (a) Control of
whole-body
equilibrium;
(b) control of
lumbopelvic
orientation;
(c) intervertebral
control.

stable as having no muscle at all (Crisco and Panjabi 1991). Consequently, segmental control is an essential component for spinal stability, and this control is particularly relevant in the context of low back pain as it is the control of this element that appears to be compromised in this population.

The same principles of control of orientation and intervertebral motion also apply to the pelvis. At one level, there is the need to control orientation of the pelvis around the three orthogonal axes. However, there is also the requirement to control the relationship between segments of the pelvis. In upright positions, the sacro-iliac joints are subjected to considerable shear force as the mass of the upper body must be transferred to the lower limbs via the ilia (Snijders et al 1993, 1995). The body has two mechanisms to overcome this; one mechanism depends on the wedge shape of the sacro-iliac joints ('form closure'), and the other involves compression of the sacro-iliac joints via muscle contraction ('force closure') (Snijders et al 1993, 1995).

In summary, a composite model is required that considers the spectrum of demands for stability; this will include control of buckling forces and control during movement, as well as the multiple levels of control, from the control of whole-body equilibrium to the control of intervertebral motion. As yet, no single biomechanical model considers each of these elements, and any criteria that aim to optimize stability based on these separate models is unlikely to be adequate. In a clinical context, it is important to consider all elements, although evidence suggests that emphasis should be placed on control of intervertebral motion, at least initially. The next layer of complexity is to consider how these multiple demands of stability may be controlled.

CONCEPTUAL MODEL OF CONTROL OF LUMBOPELVIC STABILITY

Panjabi (1992a,b) introduced an innovative model of the spinal stabilization system, which serves as an appropriate model for understanding the maintenance of spinal stability, the entity of instability and the clinical paradigm for the assessment and treatment of the muscle dysfunction in the patient with low back pain. The model incorporates a passive subsystem, an active subsystem and a neural control subsystem (Fig. 2.2). The first consideration is that passive structures of the spine and pelvis

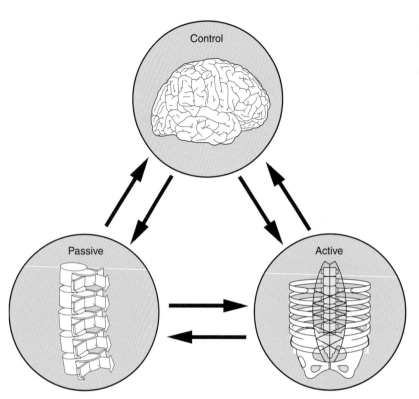

Figure 2.2 The three systems that contribute to lumbopelvic stability. (Adapted from Panjabi 1992a.)

contribute, to some extent, to the control of all of the elements of stability described in the previous section. This passive subsystem incorporates the osseous and articular structures and the spinal ligaments, all of which contribute to the control of spinal movement and stability. While being integral components of the spinal stabilization system, the passive elements offer most restraint towards the end of the range of movement, but they do not provide substantial support around the neutral position, where the spine exhibits least stiffness (Panjabi 1992b).

The active subsystem refers to the force-generating capacity of the muscles themselves, which provides the mechanical ability to stabilize the spinal segment. However, the muscle system is only as good as the system that drives it, the control subsystem. This latter system must sense the requirements of stability and plan strategies to meet those demands. This model recognizes that the neural control subsystem must coordinate muscle activity in advance of predictable challenges to stability – and coordinate responses to afferent feedback from unpredictable challenges. The system must activate muscles at the right time, by the right amount, in the correct sequence and then turn muscles off appropriately. Based on this model, Panjabi contended that the three subsystems are interdependent components of the spinal stabilization system with one capable of compensating for deficits in another (Panjabi 1992a). From the purely biomechanical perspective, back pain may occur as a consequence of deficits in control of the spinal segment when abnormally large segmental motions cause compression/stretch on neural structures or abnormal deformation of ligaments and pain-sensitive structures. These deficits may potentially be caused by a dysfunction in any of the three systems, which cannot be compensated for by the other systems. Instability will be considered in greater detail later in this chapter.

MUSCLE SYSTEM CONSIDERATIONS FOR LUMBOPELVIC CONTROL

As described by Panjabi (1992b), the active subsystem, or muscles, provides the mechanism by which the control system may modulate the stability of the spine. Consideration of the need to modulate stability is important. Many biomechanical models argue for optimal stability of the spine. In this context, it may be considered that stability would be optimal if stiffness was maximized and no lumbopelvic movement was allowed. However, in reality, the muscle system modulates or changes stiffness to match the demands of internal and external forces. Why do we not just stiffen the spine? The answer lies in the fact that movement is important for optimal spinal health. Movement is required to assist in the dissipation of forces and to minimize energy expenditure. For example, energy expenditure in gait is increased if pelvic motion is reduced (Perry 1992). If it is important to match the demands for stability, which muscles are involved? A large number of muscles cross the spine and may contribute to modulation of lumbopelvic stability. All of these muscles can contribute to stability to some extent. Although considerable effort has been placed on identification of the muscles that contribute the 'most' to stability, this is the wrong question. With consideration of the complexity of stability described above, it can be seen that no single muscle could provide the greatest contribution to all elements of stability. Consider the complexity of muscles required to ensure the dextrous movements of the hand, which contains multiple layers of muscle, to fine-tune the control motion of individual segments of the fingers. Estimation of which muscle(s) provides the greatest force for finger flexion hardly encapsulates the requirements for fine-tuned control. Instead, it is important to consider the differential control of the separate elements of the stability. Several classification systems have been developed that ascribe different muscles to the control of individual elements of stability. These are described in the next section.

Muscular control of segmental motion and spinal orientation

The first suggestion that some muscles surrounding the spine are primarily concerned with control of intersegmental motion is ascribed to Leonardo da Vinci (Crisco and Panjabi 1991). In describing muscles of the neck, he suggested that the more central muscles stabilized the spinal segment (i.e. provided intersegmental control of the neck) while

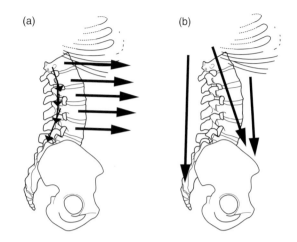

Figure 2.3 Muscles of the lumbopelvic region: (a) local and (b) global.

the more lateral muscles acted as guy ropes supporting the vertebrae, as they would the mast of a ship, and were more concerned with bending the neck (i.e. the control of neck orientation). It has been realized over succeeding years that the way in which muscles support and stabilize the spine is far more intricate than this simple model. Nevertheless, it is pertinent to address this issue of local (central) and global (guy ropes) muscles systems in an attempt to understand muscle function in relation to the stability of the spine.

Bergmark (1989) categorized the trunk muscles into local and global muscle systems based on architectural properties (Fig. 2.3). The local muscle system included deep muscles and the deep portions of some muscles that have their origin or insertion on the lumbar vertebrae. These muscles control the stiffness and intervertebral relationship of the spinal segments and the posture of lumbar segments. Although this system of muscles is essential for stability, it is not sufficient for stability as the muscles are ineffective for control of spinal orientation. The lumbar multifidus muscle, with its vertebrae-to-vertebrae attachments (Macintosh and Bogduk 1986), is a prime example of a muscle of the local system. The smaller intersegmental muscles, such as the intertransversarii and interspinales, may not predominate as mechanical stabilizers but have a proprioceptive role instead (Bogduk 1997). In the abdominal group, Bergmark (1989) suggested that the posterior fibres of the obliquus internus abdominis, which insert into the thoracolumbar fascia, form part of the local system. However, the significance of this insertion is uncertain, as it is only present in a minority of individuals (Bogduk and MacIntosh 1984). The deepest muscle, the transversus abdominis, with its direct attachments to the lumbar vertebrae through the thoracolumbar fascia and the decussations with its opposite in the midline, can also be considered a local muscle of the abdominal muscle group.

The global muscle system encompasses the large, superficial muscles of the trunk that do not have direct attachment to the vertebrae and cross multiple segments. These muscles are the torque generators for spinal motion and act like guy ropes to control spinal orientation, balance the external loads applied to the trunk and transfer load from the thorax to the pelvis (Bergmark 1989). In this way, the large variations in external loads that occur with normal daily function are accommodated by the global muscles so that the resulting load on the lumbar spine and its segments is continually minimized. Consequently, this system is critical for lumbopelvic stability but cannot fine-tune the control of intervertebral motion. Notably, data from a biomechanical in vivo model indicate that, although the large muscles linking the pelvis to the rib cage provided a significant amount of stiffness to the spinal column, activity of the local muscle system was vital in providing stability of the spinal segments (Cholewicki et al 1997). Even when forces generated by the large global muscles were substantial, the spine was unstable if there was no activity in the local muscle system. A small increase in the level of activity of the muscles of the local system could prevent spinal instability. Muscles that may be considered as part of the global system are the obliquus internus abdominis, the obliquus externus abdominis, the rectus abdominis, the lateral fibres of the quadratus lumborum and portions of the erector spinae.

Although this system is likely an oversimplification of the complex control of spinal stability, it provides a useful model to consider clinically. An important consideration is that evidence suggests that it is the local system which is most impaired in low back pain, although both systems are necessary to meet the demands of spinal stability. Therefore, while modelling studies may argue that the global

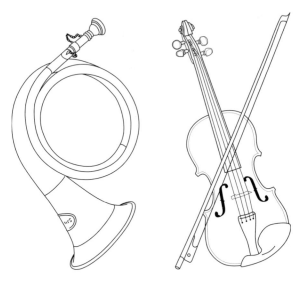

Figure 2.4   The coordination between the local and global muscles of the trunk is analogous to the coordination of musical instruments in an orchestra. Like the trunk muscles, all instruments contribute to the final output, but the contribution of each is specialized and all are needed for optimal function.

muscles provide the optimal control of buckling forces (McGill et al 1996), training those muscles is unlikely to resolve the deficits in muscle control. To put this in perspective, it can be useful to consider the spine as an orchestra. At one extreme we have loud instruments that give volume with ease, such as a tuba (Fig. 2.4). This is akin to the superficial muscles, which efficiently provide control of buckling forces and stiffen the spine. At the other extreme, we have the instruments that contribute to the finer elements of melody, such as a violin or flute. This is similar to the contribution of the deep segmental muscles, which provide minimal contribution to the control of buckling forces but provide an efficient mechanism to fine-tune the control of intervertebral motion and the segments of the pelvis. Neither system alone can provide optimal spinal control, and both elements must be coordinated to meet the demands for spinal health. This does not appear to be the case in low back pain. We will return to this topic in Chapter 10. A final consideration is that local muscle control is required over the spectrum of functional demands from light tasks such as reaching or moving while sitting to weight-lifting tasks. This is particularly notable as the requirement for strong global muscle activity is likely to be minimal in light activities, yet the muscles of the local system are needed for safe function at the segmental level.

Limitations of the global system

In the previous section, it was argued that the global muscles cannot contribute to the control of intervertebral motion. This is not completely correct as the global system can influence intervertebral motion as a result of compressive forces exerted by co-activation of antagonist global muscles. While compression can assist in the control of shear and rotation forces, this is associated with a 'cost'.

First, global co-activation increases the compressive load on lumbar segments (Gardner-Morse and Stokes 1998). The superficial trunk muscles generate torque at the trunk. This torque must be overcome by antagonist activation in order to keep the spine upright, and this co-activation results in a compressive load on the spine (Lavender et al 1992, Mirka and Marras 1993, Thelen et al 1995, Gardner-Morse and Stokes 1998). Excessive compression, which results in increased intradiscal pressure and loading through the posterior elements of the spine, has long been considered to be a risk factor for spinal degeneration and pain (Nachemson and Morris 1964). If greater demand is placed on the superficial muscle system, the loading may be increased. While increased co-contraction is expected during lifting activities and with increased trunk acceleration (Marras and Mirka 1990) and unpredictability (van Dieen and de Looze 1999), increased co-contraction of the global muscles has been detected in patients who develop low back pain compared with normal pain-free subjects (Radebold et al 2000). Excessive global muscle co-contraction during light functional tasks may even be indicative of inappropriate trunk muscle control in patients with back pain (Radebold et al 2000). These clinical findings support the hypothesis of Cholewicki et al (1997), who studied the stabilizing function of the trunk flexors and extensors around a neutral spine posture. Their hypothesis was that a dysfunction in the passive stabilizing system may be indicated by increased levels of trunk muscle co-activation. This hypothesis challenges many current exercise programmes for low back pain that incorporate high levels of trunk muscle co-activation.

Second, global muscles can only provide a non-specific contribution to spinal control. Panjabi et al (1989) argued that a major advantage of the multifidus muscle was that its segmental organization provides an ideal mechanism for the nervous system to control individual segments. This is not possible with the global muscles.

Third, global muscles have a limited ability to control shear forces. This has been argued biomechanically (Bogduk 1997) and from in vivo studies. For example, if shear forces are imposed on the spine, there is no change in activity of the global muscles, implying that deeper local muscles must control this element (Raschke and Chaffn 1996). A similar situation may exist in the sacro-iliac joints. As mentioned above, stability of the sacro-iliac joints is dependent on their compression (Snijders et al 1995). Although it is argued that this compression force is, to a large extent, provided by the large global muscles working in discrete synergies (e.g. the contraction of gluteus maximus with the diagonally opposed latissimus dorsi), this is likely to be ineffective in light tasks in which these muscles are relatively inactive. Instead, horizontal forces produced by the local abdominal muscles (e.g. transversus abdominis) will compress and stabilize the sacro-iliac joints (Snijders et al 1995).

Fourth, antagonist global muscle co-activation results in a restriction of spinal motion, that is in 'rigidity' of the spine. It is known that in healthy subjects the CNS uses movement rather than simple stiffening of the spine to overcome challenges to stability (Hodges et al 1999, 2000a) (Fig. 2.5) and reduce energy expenditure (Perry 1992). A strategy of trunk stiffening, although requiring less-complex neural control, may compromise optimal spinal function.

Finally, trunk muscles are involved in functions other than spinal control and movement (Hodges and Gandevia 2000a). As the superficial abdominal muscles depress the rib cage and are involved in forced expiration (DeTroyer and Estenne 1988), increased activity of these muscles in individuals with pain may lead to compromised respiratory function, for example restricted movement of the chest wall. In contrast, local muscles have limited effect on rib cage motion (DeTroyer and Estenne 1988). Therefore, reliance on global muscles for

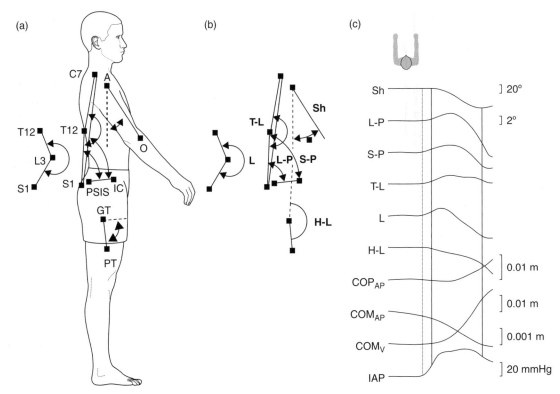

Figure 2.5 Postural responses use movement rather than simply making the spine rigid. The placement of markers to measure trunk motion and the angles that are measured are shown in (a) and (b), respectively. (c) The onset of arm movement is shown with a solid vertical line. The data indicate that when the arm is flexed rapidly at the shoulder (downward motion in (c)), the spine moves in the opposite direction initially and this spinal motion starts before the onset of movement. AP, anteroposterior; C, cervical; COM, centre of mass; COP, centre of pressure; H–L, hip–lumbar angle (angle between the thigh and lumbar spine); L, lumbar; PSIS, posterior superior iliac spine; S, sacral; Sh, shoulder; T, thoracic.

control may be problematic from a systemic point of view. In contrast, local muscles allow controlled spinal motion and have the ability to control individual segments, with minimal effect on the rib cage, thus minimizing conflict with respiration.

MOTOR CONTROL MECHANISMS FOR LUMBOPELVIC CONTROL

The challenge is immense for the CNS to move and control the spine, despite constant changes in internal and external forces. The CNS must continually interpret the status of stability, plan mech-anisms to overcome predictable challenges and rapidly initiate activity in response to unexpected challenges. It must interpret the afferent input from the peripheral mechanoreceptors, and other sensory systems, compare these requirements against an 'internal model of body dynamics' and then generate a coordinated response of the trunk muscles so that the muscle activity occurs at the right time, at the right amount and so on. To complicate this issue further, muscle activity must be coordinated to maintain control of the spine within the hierarchy of interdependent levels: control of intervertebral translation and rotation, control of spinal posture/ orientation, and control of body with respect to the environment. Notably, under the effects of gravity, the CNS must integrate the control of external forces for weightbearing and control of COM. The specific characteristics of that control of are considered in more detail in Chapters 5 and 6. In addition, unlike the muscles of the limb, trunk muscles perform a variety of homeostatic functions as well as

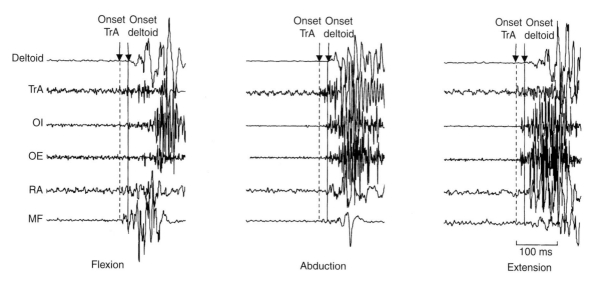

Figure 2.6 Electromyographic activity of the abdominal (rectus abdominis (RA), obliquus externus abdominis (OE), obliquus internus abdominis (OI) and transversus abdominis (TrA)), superficial multifidus (MF) and deltoid muscles for shoulder flexion, abduction and extension in a representative subject. The time of alignment of the traces at the onset of electromyographic activity of the deltoid is noted, and the onset of activity of the TrA is shown by the dashed line. Note the onset of activity of the TrA prior to that of the deltoid and the other trunk muscles, and the consistent period between the onset of activity of the TrA and deltoid. Also note the change in sequence of activity onset of the RA, EO, IO, and MF as a function of limb-movement direction. (Reproduced with permission from Hodges and Richardson 1997b, p. 364.)

movement and control of the trunk, including respiration and continence. This section will consider the strategies used by the CNS to undertake this control.

Feedforward control of lumbopelvic stability

Lumbopelvic stability is controlled in advance of imposed forces (i.e. feedforward) when the perturbation to the trunk is predictable. For instance, activity of the trunk muscles occurs in advance of the muscle responsible for movement of the lower (Hodges and Richardson 1997a) and upper (Belen'kii et al 1967, Bouisset and Zattara 1981, Aruin and Latash 1995, Hodges and Richardson 1997b) limbs and prior to loading when a mass is added to the trunk in a predictable manner (Cresswell et al 1994) (Fig. 2.6). In this type of task, the CNS predicts the effect that this movement will have on the body and plans a sequence of muscle activity to overcome this perturbation. This prediction involves an 'internal system of body dynamics', which is an abstract construct built up

over a lifetime of movement experience and holding information of the interaction between internal and external force (Gahery and Massion 1981, Gurfinkel 1994). An important feature of this feedforward control of the spine is that it provides insight into the differential strategies used by the CNS to control each of the elements of stability and how these may be integrated. Consistent with the architectural properties of the trunk muscles described above, the temporal and spatial parameters of activity of the superficial or global trunk muscles is linked to the direction of forces acting on the spine (i.e. superficial trunk muscle activity is earlier and of larger amplitude when their activity opposes the direction of reactive forces), which is consistent with the control of orientation of the spine (Aruin and Latash 1995, Hodges and Richardson 1997c, Hodges et al 1999). In association with limb movements, this activity has been shown also to be consistent with the control of the disturbance to equilibrium and to move the COM in a manner consistent with the maintenance of upright stance (Aruin and Latash 1995, Hodges et al 1999). In contrast, activity of the deep intrinsic

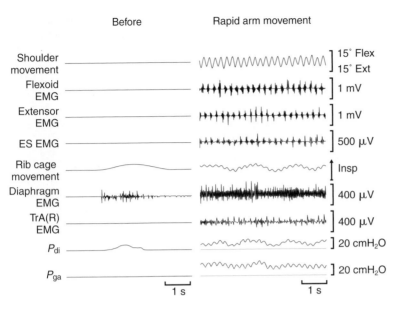

Figure 2.7 Activity of the trunk muscles measured with electromyography (EMG) during repetitive arm movement. Standing subjects rapidly and repetitively moved their arm. Activity of transversus abdominis (TrA) and the diaphragm occurred tonically throughout the movement, while activity of the erector spinae (ES) muscles occurred phasically with each movement of the arm. P_{ga}, intra-abdominal pressure; P_{di}, transdiaphragm pressure. (Adapted from Hodges and Gandevia 2000a.)

muscles (both transversus abdominis and multifidus) is independent of the direction of reactive forces (Hodges and Richardson 1997c, Moseley et al 2002). This is consistent with the architectural properties of these muscles to provide a general increase in intervertebral control. Therefore, the data suggest that the CNS uses feedforward non-direction specific activity of the intrinsic local muscles to control intervertebral motion, and it uses tuned direction-specific responses of the superficial global muscles to control spinal orientation (Hodges et al 1999). Recent data suggest that the CNS uses discrete strategies to control each factor. When the preparation for movement is manipulated or subjects perform an attention-demanding task, the latency for limb movement and the postural activity of the superficial muscles is delayed, but there is no change in the latency of the deep muscle response: transversus abdominis (Hodges and Richardson 1999b) and deep fibres of multifidus (Moseley et al 2003). This suggests that the deep muscle response is more rudimentary and may be controlled by a more basic mechanism by the CNS. Importantly, these responses have been shown to be linked to the speed of limb movement (Hodges and Richardson 1997c) and the mass of the limb (Hodges and Richardson 1997b,c), suggesting that the CNS predicts the amplitude of the reactive forces and adjusts the feedforward responses accordingly.

Repetitive limb movements may also provide an example of open loop control. However, as the movement is ongoing, it is not possible to exclude the contribution of afferent input to the organization of the trunk muscle activity, and studies have suggested that spinal mechanisms dependent on afferent feedback may be important for this control (Zedka and Prochazka 1997). Although the mechanism for control of repetitive movement is not completely understood, there is evidence of differential activity of the deep and superficial muscles that is consistent with the different roles of these muscles. For instance, tonic activity of the intrinsic spinal muscles occurs in association with repetitive upper limb movement (transversus abdominis (Hodges and Gandevia 2000a), multifidus (Moseley et al 2002); Fig. 2.7), repetitive lower limb movement during gait (Hodges and Saunders 2001) and repetitive trunk movement (Cresswell et al 1992a). In contrast, superficial muscle activity occurs in a phasic manner linked to the direction of limb movement (Hodges and Gandevia 2000a).

Feedback control of lumbopelvic stability

When the spine is perturbed unpredictably, the nervous system must respond rapidly. At the more basic end of the spectrum, feedback-mediated control may operate at a reflex level. These

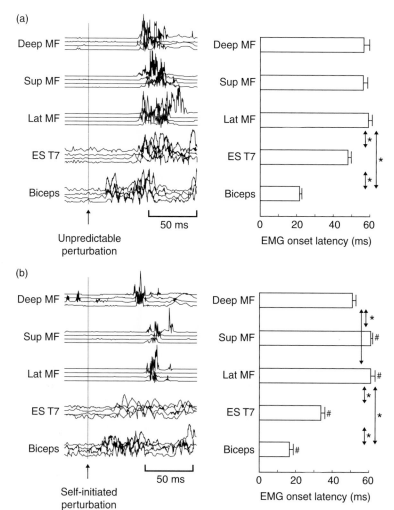

Figure 2.8 Response of the multifidus (MF) muscles to unexpected and self-initiated trunk loading. Data are shown for four repetitions of catching a load in a bucket held in front of the body. The onset of the perturbation is shown by the vertical line. The mean data for the group are shown in the right panel. Note that the activity of deep, superficial (sup) and lateral (lat) fibres of multifidus are active with the same latency when the loading is unexpected, but are active at different latencies when they initiate the loading themselves. ES, erector spinae; EMG, electromyography. (Adapted from Moseley et al 2003.)

responses may include monosynaptic stretch reflexes, which involve stretch of a muscle spindle generating an afferent impulse from the receptor region of the spindles to excite the alpha motoneurons in the same muscle, resulting in contraction. Short-latency reflexes have been identified in the paraspinal muscles when subjects catch an unexpected mass in their hands (King et al 1988, Wilder et al 1996, Moseley et al 2003), and responses have been recorded in paraspinal (Dimitrijevic et al 1980, Zedka et al 1999a) and abdominal (Kondo et al 1986, Myriknas et al 2000, Beith and Harrison 2001) muscles in response to a mechanical tap to the muscle. These reflex responses activate the paraspinal muscles en masse, with no differentiation between deep and superficial components

(Moseley et al 2003) (Fig. 2.8). Simple responses are inflexible and represent a basic mechanism for the motor system to correct an error, for example to resist an imposed stretch. However, there appears to be some integration. For instance, reflex changes may occur in other related muscles, including contralateral muscles (Beith and Harrison 2001); activity of transversus abdominis occurs prior to that of the paraspinal muscles when the trunk is unexpectedly flexed by addition of a mass to the front of the trunk (Cresswell et al 1994). Furthermore, activity of transversus abdominis and the paraspinal muscles occurs at the same time as the trunk is perturbed when a mass is added to the upper limbs during arm movement (Hodges et al 2001a). This latter finding suggests that afferent input

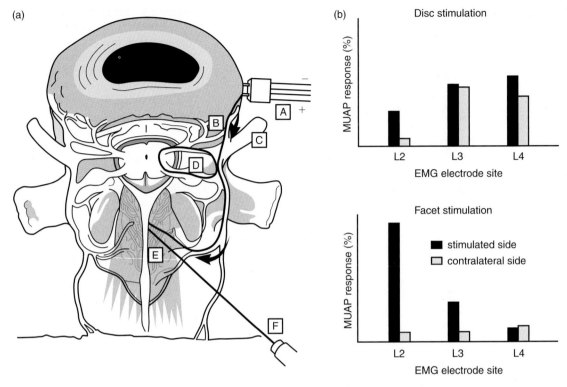

Figure 2.9 Response of the multifidus muscles to electrical stimulation of the intervertebral disk and facet joints in pigs. (a) The experimental procedure. Responses in multifidus muscle recorded with an intramuscular electrode (F) were identified with short latency after the stimulus (A). (b) The group data produced. MUAP, motor unit action potential amplitude. (Adapted from Indahl et al 1995.)

from distant segments may be involved in initiation of the trunk muscle response. When the predictability of the perturbation is increased and higher centre input may influence the response, the paraspinal muscles are differentially active, with earlier activity of deep multifidus (Moseley et al 2003) (Fig. 2.8). This also occurs when paraspinal muscle activity is reduced when load is removed from the trunk by removal of a load from the upper limbs (Hodges et al 2002a). This unloading response is commonly argued to be be caused by removal of the support for muscle contraction from spindle afferent input (Angel et al 1965, Nitz and Peck 1986).

Other basic responses have been identified using electrical and/or mechanical stimulation of afferents in the ligaments, annulus, facet joint capsule and sacro-iliac joint in pigs (Fig. 2.9), cats and humans (Indahl et al 1995, 1997, 1999, Solomonow et al 1998, 1999). In general, activity of multifidus was initiated with short latency, on both sides and over multiple spinal segments in response to the stimulus. The nature of the response was affected by the site of stimulation on the annulus (Holm et al 2002) and the sacro-iliac joint (Indahl et al 1999) and could be modified by injection of analgesic or saline into the facet joint capsule (Indahl et al 1997). These reflexes provide a strategy for mechanical stimulation of the spinal structures to influence trunk muscle activity in a reflex manner. Alternatively, the response may modulate descending drive to the muscles.

The long-loop reflexes are more complex than simple stretch reflexes and involve information processing at higher levels of the CNS, including transcortical mechanisms. These responses have a longer latency than the simple stretch reflex, are more flexible and can be modified voluntarily

(Marsden et al 1977). Because of their flexibility, these responses are thought to have a greater role in error correction. For instance, when the support surface on which a person is standing is rapidly moved, a complex interplay of several body segments, including response of trunk muscles, is initiated in order to maintain the equilibrium of the body (Horak and Nashner 1986, Keshner and Allum 1990). Two main strategies have been identified, which involve either ankle movement ('ankle strategy') or hip movement ('hip strategy'), depending on the context and the support surface characteristics (Horak and Nashner 1986). Trunk movement, and thus activation of the superficial trunk muscles, is a critical component of these strategies, particularly the hip strategy.

Contribution of muscle stiffness to lumbopelvic stability

A third type of control strategy is related to both feedback and feedforward control and involves modulation of the 'tone' in specific muscles to provide an underlying degree of stability to the joints. This activity increases the stiffness of muscles that surround the joints (Bergmark 1989, Gardner-Morse et al 1995). Muscle stiffness is the property of muscles to act as springs (i.e. the ratio of length change to force change) and has viscoelastic- and activity-related components. Muscle stiffness provides control of forces applied to a joint and contributes to control before even the shortest reflex response can be initiated (Johansson et al 1991a), and it has been argued that postural stability may be controlled by modulation of stiffness of the ankle muscles (Winter et al 1998). Similarly, stability of the trunk may be controlled by stiffness of the spinal muscles. Importantly, the activity-related component of muscle stiffness is modulated by feedback from spindle and ligament afferents (Johansson et al 1991a) (Fig. 2.10). It is the stretch reflex and the control of the gamma motoneurons that control the sensitivity of the sensory component of the muscle spindles in this system. In addition, the reflex activity of multifidus muscle in response to stimulation of mechanoreceptors in the lumbar disc and ligaments (Indahl et al 1995, 1997, 1999) and supraspinous ligament in humans (Solomonow et al 1998) may contribute to stiffness control.

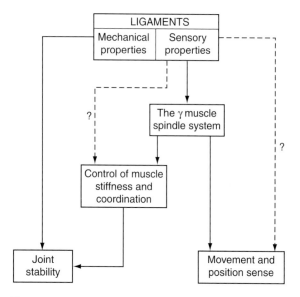

Figure 2.10   Mechanisms by which ligaments may contribute to the regulation of joint stability and proprioception. (Reproduced with permission from Johansson et al 1991a, p. 174.)

Integrated control of lumbopelvic stability and movement

It is important to consider that all the processes described above may act concurrently and the outcome of feedforward processes may be moulded by later feedback-mediated processes. In general, feedforward- and feedback-mediated responses closely match the demands of the task and are scaled to the amplitude of the perturbing forces and the context of the perturbation. As such, muscle activity directed to the control of stability represents a finely tuned component of human movement.

FUNCTIONAL MODEL OF INSTABILITY

There is considerable debate regarding what constitutes instability; it has been variously defined as a loss of joint stiffness (Pope and Panjabi 1985, Gardner-Morse et al 1995), an increase in mobility and abnormal spinal motion (Frymoyer et al 1990) and changes in the ratios of segmental rotations and translations (Weiler et al 1990). Traditionally, instability has been more aligned with the presence of abnormal motion at the end-point of the range, even though instability has long been associated

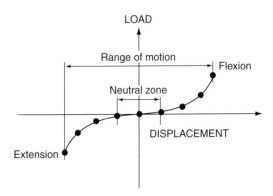

Figure 2.11 The load–deformation behaviour of the spinal segment highlighting the region known as the neutral zone. (Reproduced with permission from Panjabi, 1994.)

with degenerative disease where the segment may exhibit lesser total motion. In contrast, Panjabi (1992b) hypothesized that control of intersegmental motion around the neutral zone is a major parameter of spinal instability involved in the mechanism of clinical instability. The load–deformation behaviour of the spinal segment is non-linear and is highly flexible in the vicinity of the neutral position. This is the region known as the neutral zone (Panjabi 1992b) (Fig. 2.11). Motion occurs in this region of the physiological intervertebral motion against minimal internal resistance, with the ligamentous structures providing restraint in the elastic zone to limit end range of motion. The neutral zone presents a specific problem for the spinal stability mechanism, and there is evidence supporting its contribution to clinical instability. Injuring the spine in vitro, by dividing ligaments or the disc or by removing the posterior spinal elements, results in potentially multidirectional instabilities and an increase in both the neutral zone and the physiological range of motion (Panjabi et al 1989, Abumi et al 1990). In a study subjecting porcine cervical spines to high-speed trauma, the neutral zone was found to increase to a greater extent than the range of motion, and also to be the first indicator of the onset of injury (Oxland and Panjabi 1992). In a pivotal study that suggested a link between excessive neutral zone motion and pain, the effect of external fixation of the cervical segment was evaluated (Panjabi 1992a). This technique is used clinically to evaluate the effect of fixation on the likely control of

spinal pain as a prognostic indicator for treatment by spinal fusion. When the technique was applied to cadaveric cervical spine specimens, the motion parameter that decreased the most was the neutral zone (71% compared with a 38% decrease in the total range of motion) (Panjabi 1992a). This evidence of the sensitivity of, and increase in the neutral zone relating to, spinal instability has led to a new definition of clinical instability where instability occurs when the stabilizing system cannot maintain the intervertebral neutral zone in physiological limits.

While the concept of the neutral zone was developed from studying passive structures, it is the contribution of active muscle contraction or muscle tone in relation to the control of the neutral zone that links this theory to the real-life situation. The ligaments and other passive structures can only provide support towards the end of the range. Instability within this broader definition, which encompasses three interrelated systems, may, therefore, relate also to insufficiency of the muscle system (Panjabi 1992a). Decreased muscle stiffness resulting from fatigue, degenerative changes or injury may lead to spinal instability (Gardner-Morse et al 1995). Furthermore, damage to spinal structures may result from insufficient muscle control to maintain stability at spinal postural control and/or control at the intersegmental level (Gardner-Morse et al 1995). Conversely, the muscle system also has the potential to compensate for instability by increasing the stiffness of the lumbar spine and decreasing the size of the neutral zone (Panjabi 1992a, Gardner-Morse et al 1995, Cholewicki and McGill 1996).

This link between muscle function and spinal stiffness and the neutral zone provides the basis of the possible conservative management, through therapeutic exercise, of spinal instability.

CLINICAL APPLICATION

It is well recognized that the osseoligamentous spine is inherently unstable and that it requires a combination of muscle forces and muscle stiffness (with different combinations of muscles) to make it a secure and stable structure in vivo (Crisco et al 1992). From anatomical and biomechanical studies, some guidelines can be gained for management approaches to enhance the stabilizing role of the muscle system of the lumbopelvic region. Such principles can help in devising appropriate preventive and rehabilitative exercises for patients with low back pain.

Basically, there are two broad approaches for improving the spinal-protection role of the muscles that can be gleaned from anatomical and biomechanical studies on lumbopelvic stabilization. The first utilizes the principle of minimizing forces applied to the lumbar spine during functional activities. The second is to ensure that the muscle system is coordinated appropriately to optimize control of each of the elements of lumbopelvic control.

Minimizing forces applied to the spine

There are several different ways to minimize the forces applied to the lumbar spine during everyday and work-related activities. The study and practice of ergonomics has increased knowledge and helped to establish suitable working postures, lifting techniques and furniture design, which are essential in decreasing joint forces potentially harmful to spinal structures. Although not specifically addressed here, the value in addressing ergonomic principles in protecting the spine from injury cannot be overstated. The other principle involved in reducing forces placed on the lumbar spine deals with strength and endurance training of the global muscles to enhance their torque-producing role during high-level functions such as heavy lifting.

However, global muscle function can cause potentially harmful effects if there is excessive activity. Methods of treatment aimed at decreasing any unnecessary activity in these muscles will assist in minimizing harmful forces. Logically, this could only be safely pursued if the protective function of the deep local muscles was being re-established at the same time.

The presence of an operational deep local muscle system

It is possible that, even if the global muscle system is working appropriately, the local system may not be operating well enough to control intersegmental motion (Gardner-Morse et al 1995) (Fig. 2.12). A deficit in segmental control while global muscle activity was near maximal was uniquely captured

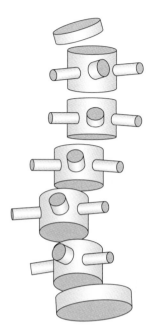

Figure 2.12   Lack of spinal intersegmental control. (Adapted from Gardner-Morse et al 1995.)

in vivo in a lifting study done by Cholewicki and McGill (1992).

It has been realized from the more recent biomechanical studies that the local muscle system is important in providing support and control to the individual vertebral segments, whether functional tasks are light (walking) or heavy (lifting) in nature. The picture emerging is of local muscles, particularly transversus abdominis, being required to contract continually, at low levels, no matter what functional activity is being undertaken. The functional supportive role of these muscles may depend not only on the development of force in the muscle but also on the neuromuscular control and coordination of that force. Panjabi (1992a,b), in his model of spinal stabilization, stressed that the neural control of these supporting muscles will be closely linked with development of appropriate tension. Poor stabilization will ensue if the forces developed are 'too small, too large, too early or too late'. Gardner-Morse et al (1995) also acknowledged that, while various programmes for the prevention of injury and rehabilitation have been aimed at minimizing spinal forces, the possible 'destabilizing effects of poor neuromuscular coordination' have not been taken into account. Thus, the local muscle system and its control have been brought forward as possibly the most important factor in providing continuous spinal support. For these reasons, it can be argued that specific testing and training of these muscles are required for patients with low back pain.

This line of thought regarding neuromuscular control and local muscle function encourages practitioners to note particularly the patient's mechanism of injury. The history of onset of low back pain may give the practitioner some insight into the origin of muscle problems as well as insight into the challenges likely to be faced in rehabilitation. Low back pain with insidious onset or associated with a trivial incident is more likely to be linked to gradual tissue breakdown that has occurred over a period of time. The term coined by Gardner-Morse et al (1995) for this type of back pain is 'self-injury', where the spine has not been adequately 'self-stabilized'. Inherent poor muscle control in the local muscle system, as well as decreased strength and endurance of the global system, could play a pivotal role in the development of such back pain over time. The potentially harmful effects of 'deloading' are considered in Chapter 7. The other extreme in the spectrum of low back pain is one where direct overload to the muscles or substantial trauma to the spine has precipitated an acute injury. Pain and injury resulting from this trauma are likely to affect muscle control, commonly the deep local muscle most significantly (see Chs 8 and 9). In this case, changes in motor control resulting from the pain and injury may contribute to the recurrence of low back pain.

PART 2

Specific joint protection of the spinal segments

PART CONTENTS

Chapter 3

Abdominal mechanism and support of the lumbar spine and pelvis

Paul Hodges

INTRODUCTION

It has long been argued that the anterolateral abdominal muscles and the muscles that form the roof (diaphragm), floor (pelvic floor muscles) and posterolateral (quadratus lumborum and psoas) aspects of the abdominal cavity contribute to the control of the lumbar spine and pelvis. There is ongoing debate regarding the relative contribution of these muscles to stability and the mechanisms by which they may mechanically control spinal and pelvic motion. This section reviews key anatomical considerations, the mechanisms by which these muscles provide mechanical stability to the region, the complex strategies used by the central nervous system to control integrated activity of the multiple muscle layers and optimize spinal control, and factors that complicate this control that have relevance to clinical management of patients with low back and pelvic pain.

ANATOMY OF THE MUSCLES OF THE ANTEROLATERAL ABDOMINAL WALL AND ABDOMINAL CAVITY

Transversus abdominis

Transversus abdominis (TrA), the deepest of the abdominal muscles, arises from the thoracolumbar fascia between the iliac crest and the twelfth rib at the lateral raphe, the internal aspects of the lower six costal cartilages, where it interdigitates with the diaphragm, the lateral third of the inguinal ligament and the anterior two-thirds of the inner lip of the iliac crest (Fig. 3.1). The medial attachment of the muscle is a complex and variable bilaminar aponeurosis. The lower fibres arise from the inguinal ligament and pass down and medially, blending with fibres of the obliquus internus abdominis to form the conjoint tendon, which attaches to the pubic crest behind the superficial inguinal ring. The remaining fibres pass medially, where they decussate and blend with the linea alba (Hollinshead and Jenkins 1981, Williams et al 1989). Above the umbilicus, the aponeurotic fibres of TrA pass either upward or downward and pass posterior to the rectus abdominis (Fig. 3.2). The downturned fibres attach to the upturned fibres of the opposite TrA or the posterior lamina

of the contralateral obliquus internus abdominis aponeurosis. In contrast, below the umbilicus, both layers are inclined downwards, with the anterior portion passing in front of therectus abdominis and the posterior portion passing behind (Askar 1977, Rizk 1980). Proceeding from the umbilicus to the pubic crest, the fibres of the posterior layer are progressively transferred to pass anterior to the rectus abdominis (Rizk 1980). Because of the decussation in the midline, the TrA can be considered to be a digastric muscle, attaching to either the contralateral TrA or the obliquus internus abdominis (Askar 1977, Rizk 1980).

The posterior attachment of the TrA to the lumbar vertebrae is via the thoracolumbar fascia (Fig. 3.3).

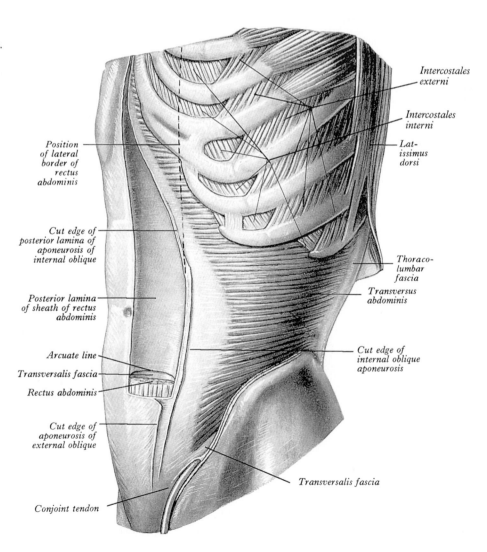

Figure 3.1 The transversus abdominis. (Reproduced with permission from Williams et al 1989, p. 599.)

Position of lateral border of rectus abdominis

Cut edge of posterior lamina of aponeurosis of internal oblique

Posterior lamina of sheath of rectus abdominis

Arcuate line

Transversalis fascia

Rectus abdominis

Cut edge of aponeurosis of external oblique

Conjoint tendon

Intercostales externi

Intercostales interni

Latissimus dorsi

Thoracolumbar fascia

Transversus abdominis

Cut edge of internal oblique aponeurosis

Transversalis fascia

The thoracolumbar fascia comprises three layers that are fused at the lateral border of the erector spinae (i.e. the lateral raphe). The anterior layer arises from the anterior surface of the transverse process of the lumbar vertebrae and passes as a thin fibrous layer over the anterior surface of quadratus lumborum (Bogduk and MacIntosh 1984).

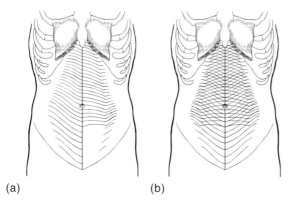

(a)   (b)

Figure 3.2   The transversus abdominis anterior attachment. There are two layers of the aponeurosis. (a) The superomedial fibres on the right are continuous with the inferomedial fibres on the left. (b) The completed pattern of the two layers. (Adapted from Askar 1977 p. 318.)

The middle layer is a thick strong aponeurotic structure passing transversely from the length and tips of the lumbar transverse processes and inter-transverse ligaments.

Anatomically, TrA can be divided into three regions that have distinct morphological differences (Urquhart et al 2001). Fibres of the upper region that are rostral to the inferior border of the rib cage have the most transverse orientation but have the shortest fibre length and are thinner than the other regions of the muscle. The fibres that pass between the rib cage and iliac crest are those with the only direct attachment to the thoracolumbar fascia. These fibres are oriented slightly inferomedially and have the longest fibre length. The lower fibres from the iliac crest and inguinal ligament generally extend inferiorly to two-thirds of the distance between the iliac crest and pubic symphysis, are the most inferomedially oriented and are thickest. Because of these anatomical variations, the function is likely to vary between regions.

When the TrA contracts bilaterally, it reduces the circumference of the abdominal wall and flattens the abdominal wall in the lower region to increase the intra-abdominal pressure (IAP) and tension in the thoracolumbar and anterior fascias. Of the

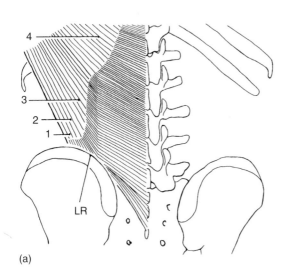

(a)

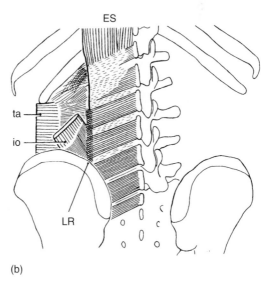

(b)

Figure 3.3   Thoracolumbar fascia. The superficial (a) and deep (b) lamina of the posterior layer. The superficial lamina can be divided into four major components, as described in the text. Both laminae have an extensive attachment to the lateral raphe (LR), which also serves as an attachment for the transversus abdominis (ta) and the obliquus internus abdominis (io). ES, erector spinae. (Reproduced with permission from Bogduk 1997, pp. 116–117.)

abdominal muscles, activity of TrA has the closest relationship to the modulation of IAP (Cresswell et al 1992a, 1994, Cresswell 1993). Because of its fibre orientation, TrA has a limited ability to generate trunk motion, although it is active during rotation efforts (Hemborg 1983, Cresswell et al 1993, Urquhart et al 2002). Therefore, TrA is considered to have its major effects on lumbopelvic stability via increases in IAP and fascial tension and via compression of the sacro-iliac joints and, potentially, the pubic symphysis (Cresswell et al 1992a, Snijders et al 1995, Hodges 1999). These mechanisms are described in detail below. Two issues are important to consider. First, unless activity of the diaphragm and pelvic floor muscles accompanies that of TrA, contraction of TrA will simply displace the abdominal contents with minimal effect on the IAP and fascial tension; second, TrA also contributes to control of abdominal contents and respiration, and these functions must be coordinated. These issues are addressed below.

Obliquus internus abdominis

Obliquus internus abdominis forms the middle layer of the lateral abdominal wall, with a muscular attachment to the lateral two-thirds of the inguinal ligament, the anterior two-thirds of the iliac crest and the lateral raphe of the thoracolumbar fascia in a band 2–3 cm wide, attaching to fibres of the deep lamina arising from the L3 spinous process (Bogduk and MacIntosh 1984, Williams et al 1989) (Fig. 3.4). The posterior iliac fibres pass superiorly to attach to the inferior border of the lower three or four ribs and are continuous with the internal intercostal muscles. The fibres from the inguinal ligament run inferomedially to attach to the pubic crest as the conjoint tendon with TrA. The intermediate fibres diverge from the origin, ending in a bilaminar aponeurosis with the upper fibres of the aponeurosis attaching to the outer surface of the seventh to ninth costal cartilages. The lower fibres of this intermediate region pass horizontally in parallel with the fibres of TrA (Hollinshead and Jenkins 1981, Williams et al 1989). The anterior layer of the obliquus internus abdominis aponeurosis passes superomedially towards the linea alba and lies anterior to the rectus abdominis. The position of the obliquus internus

abdominis aponeurosis relative to that of obliquus externus abdominis varies depending on its position relative to the umbilicus (Rizk 1980). The posterior layer of the fascia passes posterior to the rectus abdominis and has a similar arrangement to that of the TrA. The anterior fibres are continuous with the contralateral obliquus externus abdominis, while the posterior fibres are continuous with the TrA (Askar 1977, Rizk 1980).

Similar to the TrA, the obliquus internus abdominis contributes to the support of the abdominal contents and modulation of IAP (Agostoni and Campbell 1970). However, because of the fibre orientation this will be coupled with the production of a trunk flexion moment (Floyd and Silver 1950, Williams et al 1989, McGill and Norman 1993), ipsilateral trunk rotation (Partridge and Walters 1959, Williams et al 1989, Cresswell et al 1992a) and ipsilateral lateral flexion (Carman et al 1972). In addition, the lower fibres of obliquus internus abdominis can compress the sacro-iliac joint and contribute to the force closure mechanism (Snijders et al 1995). In a small proportion of individuals, the posterior fibres of the obliquus internus abdominis insert into the lateral raphe of the thoracolumbar fascia (Bogduk and MacIntosh 1984), which can transmit force to the thoracolumbar fascia.

Obliquus externus abdominis

Obliquus externus abdominis is the most superficial of the lateral abdominal muscles (Fig. 3.5). It arises via eight digitations from the external surface of the lower eight ribs (Williams et al 1989). The upper five segments interdigitate with serratus anterior. The muscle fibres of obliquus externus abdominis descend in various directions, with the most inferior fibres directed almost vertically down to insert on the anterior part of the iliac crest, The middle and upper fibres descend downwards and forwards to the anterior aponeurosis, interlacing with the aponeurosis of the opposite muscle to form the linea alba. The inferior regions of the aponeurosis are thickened and form the inguinal ligament.

Although obliquus externus may contribute to the modulation of IAP, its mechanical advantage is inferior to that of TrA. The major functions attributed to this muscle are a trunk flexion (Floyd and Silver 1950, Williams et al 1989, McGill and Norman

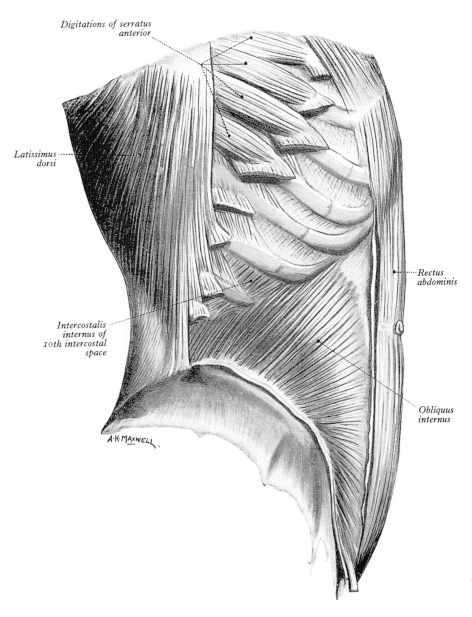

Digitations of serratus anterior

Latissimus dorsi

Intercostalis internus of 10th intercostal space

Rectus abdominis

Obliquus internus

A·K·MAXWELL.

Figure 3.4 The attachments and fibre orientation of the obliquus internus abdominis. (Reproduced with permission from Williams et al 1989, p. 598.)

1993), contralateral trunk rotation (Partridge and Walters 1959, Williams et al 1989, Cresswell et al 1992a) and ipsilateral lateral flexion (Carman et al 1972). The rib cage attachment of this muscle provides a strong mechanical advantage to reduce the lateral and vertical dimensions of the rib cage to generate expiration (DeTroyer and Estenne 1988). The obliquus externus abdominis has no attachment to the thoracolumbar fascia (Bogduk and MacIntosh 1984).

Rectus abdominis

Rectus abdominis extends the length of the anterior abdominal wall from the crest of the pubis and ligaments on the anterior symphysis pubis to the inferior rib cage in three portions, which attach to the fifth, sixth and seventh ribs, respectively (Williams et al 1989) (Fig. 3.6). The right and left muscles are separate by the linea alba. The muscle is crossed by three fibrous bands and is enclosed

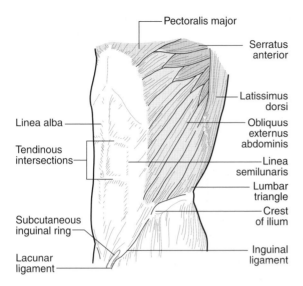

Figure 3.5 The attachments and fibre orientation of obliquus externus abdominis. (Reproduced from Williams et al 1989.)

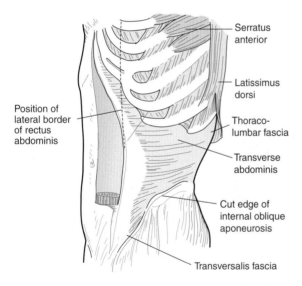

Figure 3.6 The attachments and fibre orientation of rectus abdominis. (Reproduced from Williams et al 1989.)

in the sheath formed from the aponeuroses of the obliqui and TrA (Rizk 1980).

Rectus abdominis is a major flexor of the trunk and has minimal contribution to rotation and lateral flexion (Williams et al 1989). It has a minimal ability to modulate IAP (Cresswell et al 1992a, Daggfeldt and Thorstensson 1991).

Diaphragm

The diaphragm is a thin dome-shaped muscle that separates the thorax from the abdomen. The mid region of the muscle is tendinous (central tendon) and is surrounded by muscular fibres that attach to the internal surface of the rib cage and the vertebral bodies (Williams et al 1989) (Fig. 3.7). Fibres arising from the vertebrae constitute the lumbar portion of the muscle and attach to the anterior surface of the upper lumbar vertebrae by the crurae and the lumbosacral arches. The right crus is larger and longer than the left and attaches to the anterior surface of the upper three lumbar vertebrae and the intervertebral discs. The left crus attaches to the upper two lumbar levels. Inferiorly, the crurae are continuous with the anterior longitudinal ligament in the lower lumbar region. Superiorly, the crurae meet in the midline forming an arch over the aorta. The medial lumbosacral arches traverse from the crurae and lateral vertebral bodies to the transverse process of the first and sometimes the second lumbar vertebrae (medial lumbocostal arch) over the psoas muscles. The lateral lumbocostal arches traverse over quadratus lumborum from the transverse process of the first lumbar vertebrae to the tip and lower margin of the twelfth rib.

Fibres of the costal portion of the diaphragm arise from the inner surface of the costal cartilages and adjacent regions of the lower six ribs and interdigitate with the fibres of TrA. Anteriorly, the fibres that arise from the posterior aspect of the xiphoid process form the sternal portion. Three major structures pass through the diaphragm: the aorta passes between the crurae and vertebral bodies, the oesophagus passes through an elliptical opening in the muscular portion anterior to the aorta, and the vena cava passes through the central tendon (Fig. 3.7).

The major function of the diaphragm is inspiration (Agostoni and Sant'Ambrogio 1970). During inspiration, contraction of the muscular portion of the muscle draws the central tendon down and forward, increasing the vertical dimensions of thorax and leading to reduction of intrapleural pressure and inspiration (Agostoni and Sant'Ambrogio 1970). During this descent, the dome shape of the central region remains largely unaltered and

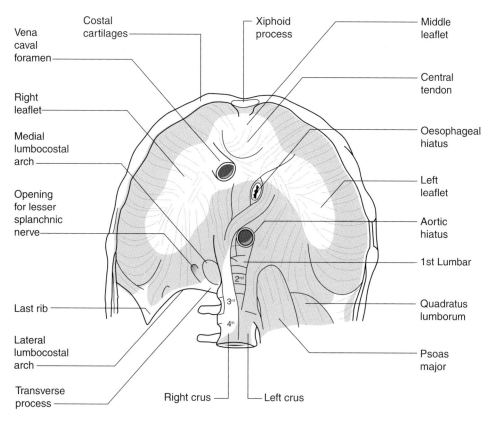

Figure 3.7   The attachments and fibre orientation of the diaphragm. (Adapted from Williams et al 1989.)

its descent is permitted by caudal motion of the abdominal viscera, which is allowed by the elasticity of the abdominal muscles (Williams et al 1989). If the descent of abdominal viscera, and therefore the domes, is restricted by abdominal muscle activity, the contraction of the costal fibres of the diaphragm, which are largely vertical in orientation, pull up the lower ribs. Because of the bucket handle action of the rib cage, this increases the transverse dimension of the rib cage (Mead 1979). Thus the interrelationship between changes in vertical and transverse dimensions of the thorax depend on the activity of the abdominal muscles (DeTroyer and Estenne 1988). During expiration, the diaphragm relaxes and the elasticity of the rib cage and lung reduces the dimensions of the thorax (DeTroyer and Estenne 1988).

In terms of spinal control, the largest contribution from the diaphragm is likely to be through its role as a major contributor to IAP (Hodges et al 1997a). Furthermore, its activity is required to prevent displacement of the abdominal viscera so that activity of TrA increases tension in the thoracolumbar fascia (Hodges et al 1997a). If shortening of the circumferential TrA is unrestricted by the abdominal contents, it will continue to shorten with minimal change in tension (McGill and Norman 1993).

Pelvic floor muscles

There is considerable disagreement regarding the nomenclature of the muscles of the pelvic floor (Williams et al 1989). In general, it is considered that the pelvic diaphragm comprises a group of muscles that include the pubococcygeus, iliococcygeus and ischiococcygeus (Fig. 3.8). Iliococcygeus arises from the ischial spine and the posterior tendinous arch of the pelvic fascia and is attached to the coccyx and the anococcygeal raphe, which,

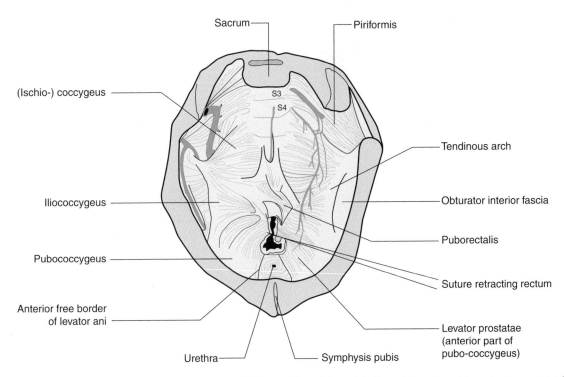

Figure 3.8 The attachments and fibre orientation of the muscles of the pelvic floor. (Reproduced from Anderson 1983.)

as its name suggests, is a thin fibrous structure running from the anus to the coccyx. Pubococcygeus arises from the back of the pubis and the anterior portion of the obturator fascia and is directed backwards so that the major part of the muscle attaches to the coccyx and the distal segments of the sacrum. The muscle sits beside the anal canal. Between the vertebral termination and anus, the pubococcygeal muscles come together to form a fibromuscular layer at the join between the iliococcygei. This region may be largely fibrous and has led many authors to argue that pubococcygeus does not have a direct vertebral attachment. The medial fibres attach to corresponding fibres from the opposite side to form a sling for the rectum called the puborectalis. Isciococcygeus arises from the spine of the iscium and sacrospinous ligament and inserts into the margin of the coccyx and the lower segments of the sacrum.

The iliococcygeus and pubococcygeus constrict the lower end of the rectum and vagina and elevate and invert the lower end of the rectum to assist with faecal continence (Williams et al 1989). Ischiococcygeus pulls forward (counternutate the

sacrum) and supports the coccyx. All muscles of the pelvic floor support the pelvic viscera and this is critical during forced expiration and for modulation of IAP (Deindl et al 1993). It is via this latter mechanism that the pelvic floor muscles contribute most to spinal control, although the muscle may also influence the sacro-iliac joints via the coccyx attachment.

Psoas major

Psoas major forms part of the posterior aspect of the abdominal cavity and can be loosely divided into two portions (Bogduk et al 1992a): the posterior fibres that arise from the anterior surface and bases of the transverse processes of all the lumbar vertebrae and an anterior portion that attaches to the inferior and superior edges of the vertebral bodies, tendinous arches that extend between the direct body attachments and intervertebral discs of the last thoracic and all lumbar vertebrae (Williams et al 1989) (Fig. 3.9). These fibres attach to an intramuscular tendon and pass across the brim of the pelvis, beneath the inguinal ligament and in front of the capsule of the hip to end in a

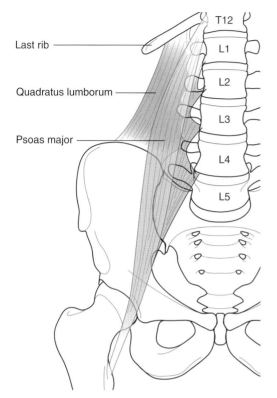

Last rib

Quadratus lumborum

Psoas major

T12
L1
L2
L3
L4
L5

Figure 3.9 The attachments and fibre orientation of psoas and quadratus lumborum muscles. (Reproduced from Williams et al 1989.)

tendon that receives the fibres of iliacus to attach to the lesser trochanter. In the upper lumbar regions, the psoas passes under the medial lumbocostal arch of the diaphragm.

There has been considerable debate regarding the function of psoas major. Although it has been variously argued to have functions associated with hip flexion, lumbar flexion and lateral flexion, more recently attention has been directed to differential functions of the posterior and anterior portions. In general, it is argued that the posterior fibres have a role in intervertebral compression, whereas the anterior fibres generate compression and movement of the spine and hip (Bogduk et al 1992a). This has led to the proposal that the posterior fibres contribute to segmental control of the spine (Gibbons 2001), although part of the posterior aspect of the abdominal wall psoas has minimal contribution to IAP generation (Williams et al 1989).

Quadratus lumborum

Like psoas major, quadratus lumborum is generally regarded to have two major components (Williams et al 1989). The lateral portion of the muscle arises from the iliolumbar ligament and adjacent iliac crest to insert onto the lower border of the twelfth rib (Fig. 3.9). The medial portion arises from the iliac crest to attach by four small tendons to the apices of the transverse processes of the upper lumbar vertebrae. Other fibres, anterior to the superomedially directed fibres, pass superolaterally from the lower three to four transverse processes to the lower margin of the twelfth rib. Quadratus lumborum passes through the lateral lumbocostal arch of the diaphragm.

Quadratus lumborum is a lateral flexor of the trunk (Andersson et al 1996); it can elevate the pelvis or depress the thorax depending on the relative flexibility of each component (Williams et al 1989). In addition, it pulls down on the twelfth rib and is active during inspiration to stabilize the attachment of the posterior costal portion of the diaphragm (Williams et al 1989). The medial fibres, in particular, have been argued to provide an important contribution to the control of spinal buckling (McGill et al 1996). Although not a strong trunk extensor, unlike the paraspinal muscles it does not exhibit silence at the end range of trunk flexion (Andersson et al 1996).

BIOMECHANICAL CONTRIBUTION TO LUMBOPELVIC CONTROL

As discussed in Chapter 2, there has been considerable discussion of the relative contribution of the trunk muscles to lumbopelvic stability (Cholewicki and Van Vliet 2002, McGill 2002a,b). A key factor to reiterate is that all muscles contribute to stability. However, the neural system is unlikely to use all muscles all of the time, and activity of specific muscles is likely to be utilized for specific functions. This section will outline how the muscles of the abdominal mechanism may contribute to the multiple elements of stability.

Superficial abdominal muscles

The superficial or global abdominal muscles (obliquus internus abdominis, obliquus externus abdominis and rectus abdominis) make a critical contribution to spinal stability and, as mentioned above, muscles such as obliquus externus abdominis provide a powerful contribution to the control of buckling forces (Gardner-Morse and Stokes 1998, McGill 2002a,b). In general, the contribution of the superficial muscles to lumbopelvic movement and stability is predictable, based on the moment arm and direction of force provided by the muscles. That is, flexors generate flexion torque and oppose extension. In many situations, activity of the superficial muscles is phasically and specifically matched to the direction of internal and external forces. For instance, if the surface on which a person is sitting is rapidly moved forwards, a rapid burst of abdominal muscle activity is initiated to restore the upright position of the trunk (Keshner and Allum 1990, Forssberg and Hirschfeld 1994, Henry et al 1998). However, in many situations, particularly tasks that involve high load or tasks that are unpredictable, muscles on either side of the trunk are co-activated to stiffen the trunk (van Dieen and de Looze 1999). For instance, abdominal muscles are co-active with the extensors during lifting (Cholewicki et al 1991); they are active bilaterally during forced rotation (Zetterberg et al 1987, McGill et al 1996) and to control the pelvis during leg lifts (Richardson et al 1990). Although co-contraction has been observed in numerous tasks and is commonly included in models of spinal control, most functions involve finely tuned activity of discrete muscles (Hodges et al 1999, Radebold et al 2000).

Predictably, activity of rectus abdominis controls trunk extension; obliquus externus abdominis contributes to the control of ipsilateral rotation and to contralateral lateral flexion and extension, and obliquus internus abdominis contributes to the control of contralateral rotation and contralateral lateral flexion and extension. The lower fibres of obliquus internus abdominis, which are transversly and inferomedially oriented, may also contribute to the control of the sacro-iliac joints (see below) (Snijders et al 1995).

Transversus abdominis

There has been considerable debate regarding the contribution of TrA to control of the lumbar spine and pelvis. This has been largely caused by its biomechanical complexity. As the muscle has mainly transversely oriented muscle fibres, it has a limited ability to flex, extend or laterally flex the spine (Williams et al 1989). Although it has been shown to be active during rotation of the trunk (Hemborg 1983, Cresswell et al 1993, Urquhart et al 2002), it has a limited moment arm to contribute to rotary torque. Regardless of this fact, several authors have modelled the contribution of TrA to lumbar stability from the perspective of control of spinal buckling (McGill 2002a,b). Not surprisingly, its contribution to this element of control is not large. Interestingly, although its contribution was small, it was the most efficient at generating an effect (McGill 2002a,b). Alternatively, it has been argued that TrA may primarily act via modulation of IAP, fascial tension and compression of the sacro-iliac joints (Cresswell et al 1992a, Snijders et al 1995, Hodges 1999). Here we review the evidence for each of these mechanisms and their specific contribution to lumbopelvic stability.

Intra-abdominal pressure

IAP is increased in many everyday tasks such as lifting, running and walking (Bartelink 1957, Grillner et al 1978, Kumar 1980) and since the 1920s it has been argued that it contributes to trunk control. The initial hypothesis argued that the abdominal cavity functions as a pressurized 'balloon' in front of the spine, with a force up on the diaphragm and down on the pelvic floor to extend the trunk (Fig. 3.10) (Bartelink 1957, Morris et al 1962, Grillner et al 1978). It was proposed that the extension moment from IAP would reduce the demand for back extensor activity and decrease the compressive load on the lumbar spine (Bartelink 1957, Troup et al 1983, Thomson 1988). Although this proposal was supported by initial models (Thomson 1988) and experimental data (Wedin et al 1987, McGill and Sharratt 1990), more recently this hypothesis has been questioned by arguments that early models overestimated factors such as the surface area of the diaphragm and the moment arm of IAP (McGill and Norman 1987, 1993). Furthermore, it has been argued that the extensor torque produced by IAP may be offset by the flexion moment generated by the abdominal

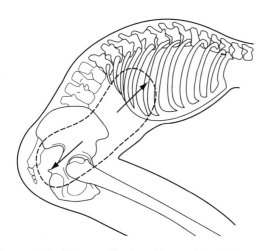

Figure 3.10 The contribution of intra-abdominal pressure to the production of an extensor movement by exerting a distracting force between the diaphragm and the pelvic floor. (Adapted from Bartelink 1957, p. 722.)

muscles (Nachemson et al 1986, McGill and Norman 1987).

Until recently, no studies had measured whether IAP can generate an extension moment in vivo. This has been difficult to assess because, when IAP is increased voluntarily by abdominal muscle activity, it is impossible to disentangle whether any change is caused by the increased IAP or by trunk muscle activity (Cholewicki et al 1999a). Recently, we have directly measured this effect in vivo in humans (Hodges et al 2001b). In this study, IAP was increased involuntarily by electrical stimulation of the phrenic nerves in the neck. The evoked contraction of the diaphragm increased IAP, but without concomitant abdominal or back extensor muscle activity (Fig. 3.11). This IAP increase was associated with a small but consistent extension moment. Therefore, if IAP is increased by contraction of the

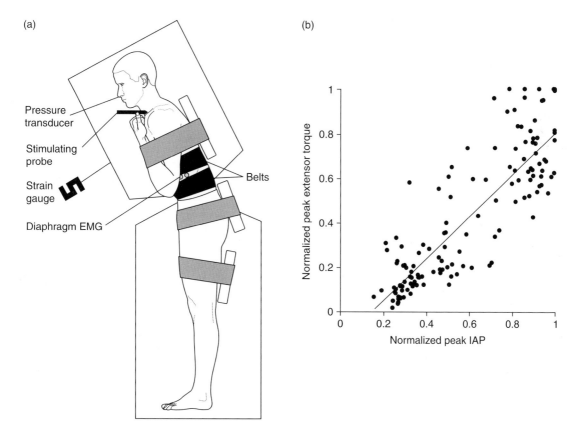

Figure 3.11 When intra-abdominal pressure (IAP) is increased by electrical stimulation of the phrenic nerves to evoke contraction of the diaphragm (a), but not the abdominal muscles, the pressure increase is associated with a small but consistent extension moment (b). EMG, electromyography. (Adapted from Hodges et al 2001b.)

diaphragm, pelvic floor muscles and the transversely orientated muscle fibres of TrA (and to a lesser extent obliquus internus abdominis), which produce IAP with no or minimal concurrent flexor moment (Cresswell et al 1992a, Daggfeldt and Thorstensson 1997), the IAP rise may extend the spine. This has been confirmed in pigs with electrical stimulation of the diaphragm and TrA (Hodges et al 2003a,b). According to the model of Daggfeldt and Thorstensson (1991), fibres of the abdominal muscles with an inclination to the vertical of greater than 55 degrees can contribute to unloading. The possibility that situations may occur where these muscles are recruited preferentially has not been considered in many biomechanical studies (Nachemson et al 1986, McGill and Norman 1987, Cholewicki et al 1999a,b); activity of these muscles has been shown to occur in conjunction with tasks in which IAP was elevated (Cresswell et al 1992a, Cresswell and Thorstensson 1994, Hodges and Richardson 1997a–c, Hodges et al 1997a, 1999, Hodges and Gandevia 2000a) and correlated better than the other abdominal muscles with the modulation of IAP amplitude during movement tasks (Cresswell et al 1992a, Hodges et al 1999). Furthermore, previous data have suggested that TrA is the most active of the abdominal muscles in back extension efforts (Cresswell et al 1992a). However, it must be considered that contractions of the TrA, diaphragm and pelvic floor muscles do not occur alone during functional tasks, and activity will be present in the other abdominal muscles (Cresswell et al 1992a, Hodges and Richardson 1997b, Hodges et al 1999). Therefore, any net effect of the extensor torque depends on the specific abdominal muscles responsible for the pressure increase in real-life situations, but this is likely to be small in many situations. Instead, the concurrent flexion and extension moments may increase spinal stiffness, similar to co-contraction of flexor and extensor muscles (Cholewicki et al 1999a,b).

Alternatively, IAP may directly increase spinal stiffness (Hodges and Richardson 1997c). Recently, we have shown that increasing IAP in humans tonically by tetanic contraction of the diaphragm results in increased stiffness of the spine (measured from the force–displacement response with a motor placed over the L4 spinous process) (Hodges et al

2001c). In pigs, intervertebral stiffness (measured directly from the intervertebral kinematics in response to movement of L4 using markers inserted into the spinous processes of the L3 and L4 vertebrae) was increased in association with diaphragm and TrA contraction (Hodges et al 2003a) (Fig. 3.12). However, this was only with certain specific directions of force in association with diaphragm contraction. Notably, the mechanical effect of TrA contraction on spinal stiffness only occurred with bilateral contraction of the muscle and was reduced in one direction if the fascial attachments were cut (see below).

Fascial tension

Tension in the thoracolumbar fascia has long been considered to contribute to spinal stability (Fairbank and O'Brien 1980, Gracovetsky et al 1985). However, there has been considerable debate regarding the extent of its contribution and the specific parameters of spinal control that may be influenced. Of the abdominal muscles, TrA is likely to have the greatest influence on the tension of the thoracolumbar fascia as a result of its extensive attachment. The attachment of TrA to the entire lateral raphe allows this muscle to exert tension on the middle and posterior layers of the thoracolumbar fascia in the middle and lower regions of the fascia (Bogduk and MacIntosh 1984) (Fig. 3.3). In contrast, the attachment of the posterior fibres of the obliquus internus abdominis is restricted to the portion of the lateral raphe connected to the L3–L5 spinous processes (Bogduk and MacIntosh 1984). Furthermore, when the fibres of the obliquus internus abdominis are tractioned, no visible displacement of the deep lamina of the posterior layer is produced (Vleeming et al 1995).

Observations of lumbar extension produced by bilateral lateral tension of the thoracolumbar fascia in cadavers (Fairbank and O'Brien 1980) and theoretical evaluations of thoracolumbar fascia anatomy (Farfan 1973) led to the proposal that the TrA could produce an extensor torque owing to the oblique orientation of the fibres of the fascia (Gracovetsky et al 1985). It has been suggested that the orientation of the fibres of the posterior layer of the thoracolumbar fascia may assist in the production of an extensor moment by converting

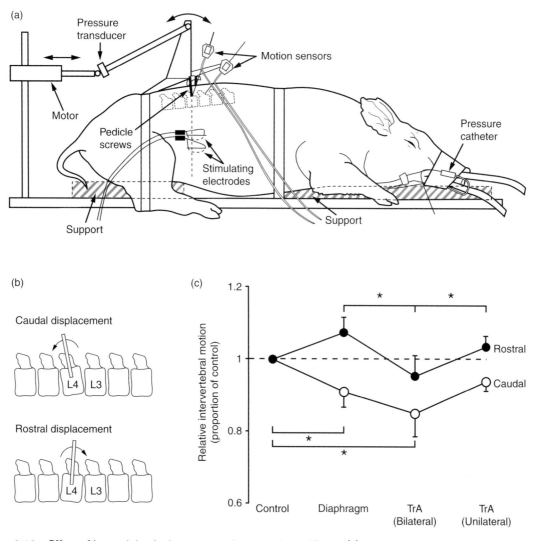

Figure 3.12 Effect of intra-abdominal pressure on intervertebral stiffness. (a) Intra-abdominal pressure was increased by electrically evoked contraction of transversus abdominis or the diaphragm in pigs. (b) Intervertebral stiffness was investigated by measurement of relative motion between the L3 and L4 vertebrae when the L4 vertebra was moved by a motor. Increased stiffness would be indicated if the intervertebral motion was reduced. (c) Intervertebral motion was reduced (i.e. stiffness was increased) by contraction of the diaphragm and by bilateral, but not unilateral contraction of transversus abdominis. (Adapted from Hodges et al 2003a.)

lateral tension to longitudinal tension (Fig. 3.13) (Gracovetsky et al 1977, 1985). At any point along the lateral raphe, there is a fibre of the superficial lamina passing caudomedially and a fibre of the deep lamina passing caudolaterally towards the spine; these form a series of triangles, each subtending two levels (Gracovetsky et al 1985). Because of the obliquity of the attachment, the force exerted at the basal angle would have a horizontal and a vertical vector. With bilateral tension, the sum of the horizontal vectors is zero, while the vertical vectors produce opposite movement approximating the spinous processes (or preventing separation of the spinous processes) and resulting in trunk extension (Gracovetsky et al 1977, 1985). This would provide a mechanism for TrA to contribute to control of

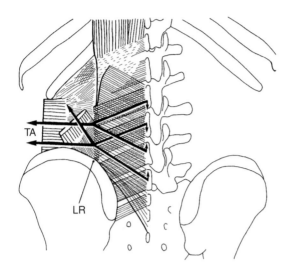

Figure 3.13 The mechanics of the thoracolumbar fascia. From any point in the lateral raphe (LR), lateral tension in the posterior layer of thoracolumbar fascia is transmitted upwards through the deep lamina of the posterior layer, and downwards through the superficial layer. Because of the obliquity of these lines of tension, a small downward vector is generated at the midline attachment of the deep lamina, and a small upward vector is generated at the midline attachment of the superficial lamina. These mutually opposite vectors tend to approximate or oppose the separation of the L2 and L4, and L3 and L5 spinous processes. Lateral tension on the fascia can be exerted by the transversus abdominis (TA), and to a lesser extent by the few fibres of the internal oblique muscle when they attach to the lateral raphe. (Reproduced with permission from Bogduk 1997, p. 123.)

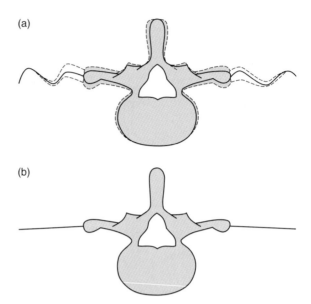

Figure 3.14 Control of intersegmental motion via lateral tension in the thoracolumbar fascia. Motion of the vertebrae is associated with changes in the length of the fascia (a). This motion can be restricted by preventing lengthening of the fascia. As the tensile stress in the fascia is increased the amount of rotation and translation can be limited.

spinal orientation. However, more recent studies have suggested that the effect of this mechanism is minimal (Macintosh et al 1987, McGill and Norman 1988) when realistic fibre angles and muscle tension are used; when tension of the thoracolumbar fascia was replicated in a cadaver, no approximation of the spinous processes (i.e. extension) was observed (Tesh et al 1987). However, the small amount of compression produced by this mechanism may contribute to the control of shear forces.

Alternatively, tension in the thoracolumbar fascia may contribute to the control of intersegmental motion via production of lateral tension to restrict vertebral displacement (Hodges and Richardson 1997c, Hodges et al 2003a,b) (Fig. 3.14). This mechanism is dependent on the bilateral contraction of TrA and is likely to be greatest in the mid lumbar levels, which have a direct attachment of TrA to the transverse processes. The thoracolumbar fascia has also been suggested to contribute to the control of coronal plane motion via the convergence of the fibres of the middle layer of the fascia onto the transverse processes of the lumbar vertebrae (Tesh et al 1987). It was proposed that approximation of the transverse processes would occur in a similar manner to that proposed for the production of trunk extension, involving conversion of a lateral force into a longitudinal force (Fig. 3.15). The vertical vector producing an approximation of the transverse processes has a large mechanical advantage because of the distance from the centre of rotation of the lateral flexion (Tesh et al 1987). The ability of this mechanism to control the spine in the coronal plane was assessed by placing cadavers in a laterally flexed position and measuring the force required to maintain this position as the tension in the fascia was increased by inflating a balloon in the abdominal cavity (Tesh et al 1987).

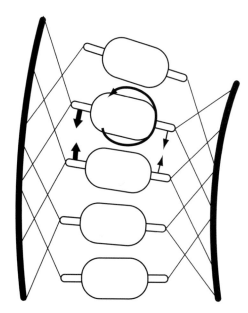

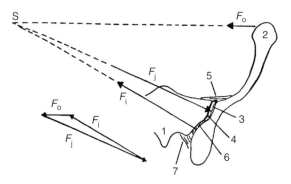

Figure 3.15 Stabilization of the lumbar spine in the coronal plane via tension in the middle layer of the thoracolumbar fascia. The oblique orientation of the fibres of the middle layer allows lateral tension of the fascia to produce a vertical vector acting to approximate the adjacent vertebrae. When the spine is laterally flexed, the magnitude of the resultant vertical vector is greater on the convex side, potentially contributing to the return of the spine to the neutral position. (Adapted from Tesh et al 1987, p. 504.)

Figure 3.16 Cross-section of the pelvis at the level of the sacro-iliac joints. The application of force by the transversus abdominis and oblique abdominal muscles (F_o), in combination with stiff dorsal sacro-iliac ligaments (F_l), compresses the sacro-iliac joints (F_j). Because the lever arms of the muscle and ligament force are different, the joint reaction force is much greater than the muscle force. 1, Sacrum; 2, iliac bone; 3, joint cartilage; 4, joint space; 5, ventral sacroiliac ligament; 6, interosseous sacro-iliac ligaments; 7, dorsal sacro-iliac ligaments. (Reproduced with permission from Snijders et al 1995, p. 423.)

The balloon was prevented from exerting pressure against the diaphragm and pelvic floor, which would simulate an increase in IAP. The maximum lateral flexion moment acting to straighten the spine as a result of this procedure was 14.5 mN. Therefore, up to 40% of trunk stability in the coronal plane may be produced by tension of the middle layer of the thoracolumbar fascia (Tesh et al 1987).

In a recent study, we electrically stimulated contraction of TrA in pigs and showed that when tension was developed in the middle layer of the thoracolumbar fascia, without an associated increase in IAP, there was no significant effect of contraction on intervertebral stiffness (Hodges et al 2003a). However, the importance of the fascial system was highlighted by the finding that when the fascial attachments were cut, an increase in IAP had the potential to decrease spinal stiffness in specific directions of movement.

In summary, this suggests that it is the interaction between pressure and fascial tension that is critical for spinal stability. A final consideration is that numerous authors have argued that fascial tension can be further increased by contraction of the erector spinae muscles in the envelope formed by the middle and posterior layers of the thoracolumbar fascia (Gracovetsky 1990).

Pelvic stability

As outlined in Chapter 2, the mechanism of stability of the sacro-iliac joint is dependent on compression between the ilia and the sacrum (i.e. force closure) in addition to the shape and structure of the joint surfaces (i.e. form closure) (Snijders et al 1995). The anterior attachment of the TrA (and the obliquus internus abdominis) to the iliac crest ideally places this muscle to act on the ilia to produce compression of the sacro-iliac joints anteriorly. Because of the lever arm of the ilia, the force generated by the TrA is amplified by a factor of four (Fig. 3.16), thus contributing effectively to the stability mechanism of this joint (Snijders et al 1995). The ability of TrA to stiffen the sacro-iliac joints has recently been confirmed in vivo, where the laxity of the sacro-iliac joints was measured using ultrasound to detect motion of the sacrum and ilium as a measure of the transmission of vibration across the sacro-iliac joints (Buyruk et al 1999). When subjects performed a specific voluntary contraction of TrA, the laxity of the sacro-iliac joint was reduced (Richardson et al 2002). Furthermore, this reduction was greater than during a bracing contraction of the other oblique abdominal muscles. However, it is not possible to exclude changes in activity of other muscles, such as the pelvic floor muscles, which may reduce the laxity of the joint via counternutation of the sacrum (Snijders et al 1995). Regardless, these data provide convincing evidence of the effect of TrA for control of the sacro-iliac joints. The importance of this effect in controlling shear forces at the sacro-iliac joints in weightbearing positions is revisited in Chapter 5.

Summary

In summary, these data suggest that TrA has a limited ability to control the orientation of the lumbar spine but has a significant function in the control of intervertebral motion and intersegmental control of the pelvis. While further investigation is required, it appears that a combination of IAP and fascial tension are responsible for the effect of contraction of this muscle on the spine. These data provide convincing evidence that TrA makes an important contribution to stability and control of motion of the segments of the spine and pelvis. Consequently, interventions that aim to improve the control of this muscle are likely to influence, specifically, the fine-tuning of intervertebral motion.

Diaphragm and pelvic floor

As mentioned above, the contributions of the diaphragm and pelvic floor muscles to spinal control are primarily through their role in the generation of IAP and the restriction of movement of the abdominal viscera, so that the hoop-like geometry of the abdominal muscles can be maintained and tension can be developed in the thoracolumbar fascia (Cresswell et al 1992b, Hodges et al 1997a,

Hodges 1999, Hodges and Gandevia 2000a,b). The contribution of these elements to stability is outlined above. Notably, electrical stimulation of the diaphragm in humans and in pigs has shown that contraction of this muscle can generate a minor extension moment (Hodges et al 2001b); however, more importantly, it can increase spinal stiffness to posteroanterior force in humans (Hodges et al 2001c) and increase the intervertebral stiffness of the spine to imposed lumbar motion in pigs (Hodges et al 2003a). An additional consideration is the potential for the lumbar fibres of the diaphragm to contribute to control of the upper lumbar spine via the direct attachment of the muscle to the spine (Hodges et al 2001c, Shirley et al 2003). This has been supported by the observation that the effect of electrically evoked contraction of the diaphragm on spinal stiffness is greater at the upper lumbar levels than on the lower region (Hodges et al 2001c, Shirley et al 2003).

Although no studies have directly assessed the effect of pelvic floor muscle activity on spinal stiffness, it may be reasonable to assume that its effect will be similar to that of the diaphragm. An additional consideration is the role of the pelvic floor muscles on the control of the sacrum and coccyx. In general, contraction of these muscles will counternutate the sacrum, which places the sacro-iliac joints out of the closed packed position (Snijders et al 1995). Therefore, while the pelvic floor muscles may support these structures, they may also destabilize. This highlights the necessity to coordinate the activity of all muscles of the system. Hyperactivity of the pelvic floor muscles would requires additional consideration.

Muscles of the posterior abdominal wall

Although the posterior muscles of the abdominal wall have only a limited role in the development of IAP, they have been argued variously to have significant effects on the control of the spine (Bogduk et al 1992a, McGill et al 1996).

Psoas

Psoas has been considered extensively in the clinical literature in back pain. To many, the muscle is regarded as one that has a tendency to over-activity and tightness, and clinical techniques have been developed to stretch the muscle and reduce its activity (Janda 1978, 1986, Travell and Simons 1983). More recently, the argument that this muscle is really two separate muscles has been presented. Bogduk et al (1992a) argued that the posterior fibres, which arise from the transverse processes, have a limited capacity to move the spine or hip but generate compression at the lumbar segments. In contrast, the anterior fibres make a larger contribution to movement. Therefore, the posterior fibres could have a mechanical contribution to the control of intervertebral motion (Gibbons 2001). This proposal requires further investigation.

Quadratus lumborum

The lateral portion of quadratus lumborum, which spans the lumbar spine, belongs to the global system and is primarily involved in lateral bending. In contrast, the medial portion, which attaches directly to the lumbar vertebral transverse processes, is capable of providing segmental stability via its segmental attachments (McGill et al 1996), although it is unlikely to make a substantial contribution to lateral flexion (Bogduk 1997). McGill et al (1996) provided evidence that the quadratus lumborum plays a significant role in the stability of the spine. Muscle activity was measured during a symmetrical bucket-holding task. Activity increased with increasing spinal compression provided through progressive axial loading. Further evidence for the general stabilizing role of the quadratus lumborum was provided by Andersson et al (1996), who found that, unlike with the erector spinae (Kippers and Parker 1985), there was no electrical silence of the muscle in full forward flexion. These data clearly support the idea that this muscle is a powerful contributor to control of buckling forces. Interestingly, in patients with back pain, overactivity, tightness and trigger points are often reported by clinicians (Travell and Simons 1983, Janda 1996). Treatment is focused on decreasing activity in the quadratus lumborum rather than increasing it with exercise. The medial portion of the quadratus lumborum may, in the future, be shown to be functionally separate from the lateral part of the muscle and contribute directly to the segmental support of the spine.

MOTOR CONTROL OF THE ABDOMINAL MECHANISM FOR LUMBOPELVIC CONTROL

Chapter 2 described, in general terms, the strategies used by the neural system to control the multiple elements of stability. It was argued that different strategies and different muscles are used to control lumbopelvic orientation and intersegmental control. This section will describe the role played by specific muscles of the abdominal cavity for these functions.

Global abdominal muscles

As mentioned in Chapter 2, feedforward- and feedback-mediated controls of the global muscles are linked to the demands for control of spinal orientation. In general, the strategies take two forms: either discrete activity matched to the demands of the task or co-activation to stiffen the spine generally. Limb movement tasks provide a window of opportunity to investigate the characteristics of the feedforward strategies planned by the neural system (Belen'kii et al 1967, Bouisset and Zattara 1981, Massion 1992). In general, activity of rectus abdominis, obliquus externus and internus abdominis have been shown to occur earlier and with greater amplitude during extension of the shoulder or hip, which is appropriate to control the extension moment generated at the trunk (Cresswell et al 1992a, Aruin and Latash 1995, Hodges and Richardson 1997b,c, Hodges et al 1999) (Fig. 3.17). Activity of these muscles was also matched to control of motion in the frontal and transverse planes (Hodges and Richardson 1997c, Hodges et al 2000a). Similarly, in feedback-mediated responses, activity of the global abdominal muscles was earlier with forward translation of the support surface in sitting when the trunk was caused to extend (Forssberg and Hirschfeld 1994, Hodges et al 2003c). Furthermore, activity of the global abdominal muscles was reduced when an extension load was removed from the trunk (Radebold et al 2000). In that task, activity of the abdominal muscles must be reduced to maintain the trunk in an upright position.

When the predictability of the perturbation is reduced, co-activity of the global abdominal and

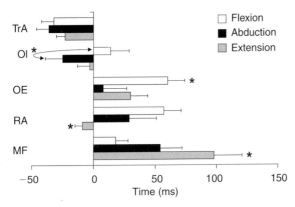

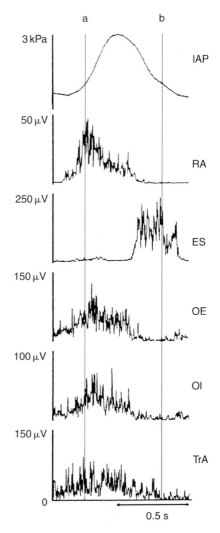

Figure 3.17 Mean time of onset of electromyographic activity of the abdominal (rectus abdominis (RA), obliquus externus abdominis (OE), obliquus internus abdominis (OI) and transversus abdominis (TrA)) and superficial multifidus (MF) muscles relative to the onset of deltoid activity for all subjects ($n = 15$) for shoulder flexion, abduction and extension. All bars are aligned to the onset of deltoid activity at zero. The end of each bar indicates the group mean time of onset of the activity of the muscles of the trunk. Standard errors of the mean are indicated. Note the significantly different onsets in activity of OI, OE, RA and MF between movement directions and the non-significant variation in the latency between the onset of deltoid and TrA activities. *$p < 0.05$. (Reproduced with permission from Hodges and Richardson 1997b, p. 365.)

Figure 3.18 Mean recordings of intra-abdominal pressure (IAP) and abdominal (rectus abdominis (RA), obliquus externus abdominis (OE), obliquus internus abdominis (OI) and transversus abdominis (TrA)) and erector spinae (ES) electromyographic activity during four consecutive oscillations between flexion and extension. Note the constant (but variable) activation of the TrA and the direction-specific activation of the other trunk muscles. (Reproduced with permission from Cresswell et al 1992a, p. 413.)

back extensors muscles has been identified. Examples include lifting a box with unpredictable or uneven mass (van Dieen and de Looze 1999). Several other factors are also associated with co-activity of the global abdominal and posterior muscles. For instance, in situations in which compressive loading is high, such as lifting (Cholewicki et al 1991) or forceful trunk movement such as rotation (Zetterberg et al 1987), co-activation is required to deal with buckling forces. This is the optimal function of the global muscle system. A key factor to note is that these data suggest that co-activation is an appropriate strategy for situations with high load and high unpredictability (Cholewicki et al 1991), but it is our contention that this strategy is not ideal in lighter tasks. This issue will be addressed in detail in Chapters 9 and 10. An additional consideration is that, because the global muscles move the trunk in multiple planes, activity of the abdominal muscles is often required to counteract unwanted torques and maintain orientation. For instance, when the oblique muscles rotate the trunk, activity of contralateral muscles is required to overcome other unwanted torques (Zetterberg et al 1987). The results of many studies concur with these findings. For example, activity

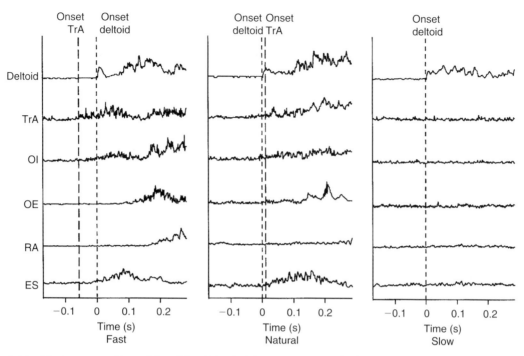

Figure 3.19   Electromyographic activity of the abdominal (rectus abdominis (RA), obliquus externus abdominis (OE), obliquus internus abdominis (OI) and transversus abdominis (TrA)), superficial multifidus (MF) and deltoid muscles rectified and averaged over 10 repetitions of shoulder flexion at three different speeds of movement: fast (~300°/s), natural (~150°/s) and slow (~30°/s). The time of alignment of the traces is the onset of deltoid activity at zero; the onset of activity of the TrA is shown. The figure demonstrates the delay in the onset of activity of each of the trunk muscles relative to that of the deltoid, with natural compared with fast movement, and the absence of trunk muscle activity compared with slow movement. ES, erector spinae. (Reproduced with permission from Hodges and Richardson 1997c, p. 1224.)

of the global abdominal muscles has been shown to be linked with trunk movement demands during gait (Hodges and Saunders 2001), and if there is an unexpected addition of a load to the trunk (Cresswell et al 1994).

Local abdominal muscles

In contrast to the global muscles, activity of TrA is generally independent of the direction of force applied to the trunk. As mentioned in Chapter 2, the timing and amplitude of this muscle does not differ between directions of limb movement and, therefore, directions of force acting on the trunk (Hodges and Richardson 1997a,b, Hodges et al 1999, 2000a) (Fig. 3.17). For this reason, non-direction-specific feedforward activity of TrA is not consistent with a contribution to the control of orientation of the trunk (the demand for which differs between directions of movement) but is consistent with the proposed contribution of TrA to general intervertebral control (Hodges 1999). Data from other tasks provide supporting evidence. For instance, activity of TrA was shown to occur tonically during repeated trunk flexion and extension efforts (Cresswell et al 1992a) (Fig. 3.18) and during gait (Hodges and Saunders 2001). In response to unexpected perturbations to the trunk, TrA activity was initiated with short latency during tasks that extended or flexed the spine (Cresswell et al 1994, Hodges et al 2001a).

Although the activity of TrA is independent of the direction of force acting on the spine, its activity is linked to the demands for control of spinal stability. For instance, a threshold velocity of arm movement can be seen below which a response of TrA does not occur (Hodges and Richardson 1997c) (Fig. 3.19), and during repetitive arm movements

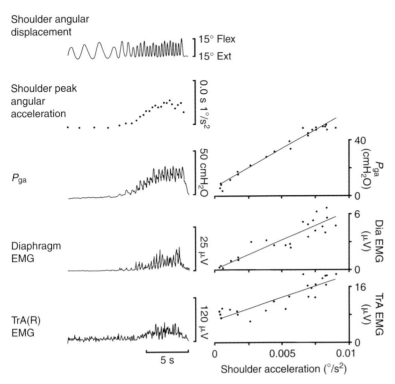

Figure 3.20 The amplitude of activity of transversus abdominis (TrA) and the diaphragm (Dia), and the associated increase in intra-abdominal pressure (P_{ga}) is linearly related with the peak shoulder acceleration (and, therefore, the amplitude of reactive moment) during repetitive arm movement. (Adapted from Hodges and Gandevia 2000a.)

the amplitude of TrA activity could be correlated with the peak acceleration of the limb (Hodges and Gandevia 2000a) (Fig. 3.20). Furthermore, movement of the more massive lower limb was associated with an earlier burst of activity of this muscle (Hodges and Richardson 1997a) (Fig. 3.21). One factor to consider is that the response of TrA may also be delayed or reduced if the stability of the spine is increased. For instance, if TrA activity is already increased by respiratory tasks, the postural response is delayed (Hodges et al 1997b). This is consistent with other studies that indicate changes in postural responses in tasks in which background activity is increased (Stokes et al 2000). Therefore, the response of TrA is matched to the demands of movement, at least in terms of the amplitude of forces acting on the spine. It is plausible that if the nervous system interprets that stability of the spine is already achieved, although potentially inappropriately, by excessive contraction of the global muscles to stiffen the spine, a local muscle response may not be initiated. This may explain some of the findings in patients with low back pain (see Ch. 10).

As mentioned previously, there are several similarities between the TrA and the obliquus internus abdominis. Anatomically, the fibres are similarly oriented in the lower region of the abdominal wall (Williams et al 1989, Urquhart et al 2001). Consequently, obliquus internus may contribute to similar functions as TrA. It is notable that, unlike TrA, the activity of obliquus internus differs between directions of force acting on the spine and thus functions in a manner consistent with control of orientation (Hodges and Richardson 1997c, Hodges et al 1999). One criticism is that this activity has been recorded from the mid region of the muscle, which has a greater moment arm for torque production. However, recent recordings from the lower region of the muscle have similar differential activation to TrA (D. M. Urquhart and P. W. Hodges, unpublished observations). Additional issues to consider are that, while the lower region may contribute to sacro-iliac joint control, this region has no attachment to the thoracolumbar fascia and has only a minor mechanical advantage to increase IAP (Bogduk and MacIntosh

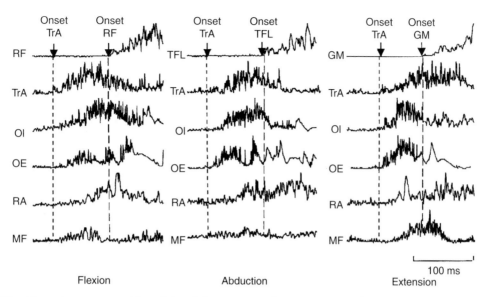

Figure 3.21 Mean electromyographic activity of the abdominal (rectus abdominis (RA), obliquus externus abdominis (OE), obliquus internus abdominis (OI) and transversus abdominis (TrA)), superficial multifidus (MF) muscles and the prime movers of hip flexion (rectus femoris (RF)), abduction (tensor fascia latae (TFL)) and extension (gluteus maximus (GM)) averaged over 10 repetitions for hip flexion, abduction and extension. The time of alignment of the traces at the onset of activity of the prime mover is noted, and the onset of activity of the TrA is shown. The figure demonstrates the onset of activity of the TrA prior to that of the prime mover and the other trunk muscles. (Reproduced with permission from Hodges and Richardson 1997a, p. 139.)

1984). Further studies are required to clarify the contribution of this muscle to intervertebral control.

Diaphragm and pelvic floor muscles

There is increasing evidence that the diaphragm and pelvic floor muscles contribute to the postural response of the trunk muscles and are active in a manner that is consistent with the control of intervertebral motion rather than the control of spinal orientation. Feedforward activity of the diaphragm has been observed in advance of upper limb movements with a latency that was similar to that of TrA (Hodges et al 1997a) (Fig. 3.22). Notably, these responses were found during inspiration and expiration and were confirmed by ultrasound measurement of muscle shortening in advance of the movement of the limb. In addition, tonic activity of the diaphragm has been observed during repetitive limb movements (Hodges and Gandevia 2000a,b). The integration of the postural and respiratory functions of the diaphragm is discussed below. Recent

studies have also investigated the activity of the diaphragm in response to support-surface translation. These studies indicate short-latency activity of the diaphragm with movement of the support surface, and the spatial and temporal aspects of this activity did not differ between directions of movement (Hodges et al 2003c). Other studies have reported non-respiratory activity of the diaphragm during arm cycling tasks (Sinderby et al 1992).

In terms of the pelvic floor muscles, activity has been recorded with surface electrodes in advance of limb movement and that is not dependent on the direction of limb movement; in addition, tonic activity was shown to occur during repetitive arm movement tasks (Hodges et al 2002c). Additional studies have investigated the relationship between the activity of TrA and the pelvic floor muscles. This question arose from the clinical observation that activity of TrA often accompanies pelvic floor muscles and that pelvic floor muscle activity accompanies TrA activity. Two studies have investigated these questions. In the first study, recordings of activity of the abdominal muscles were made

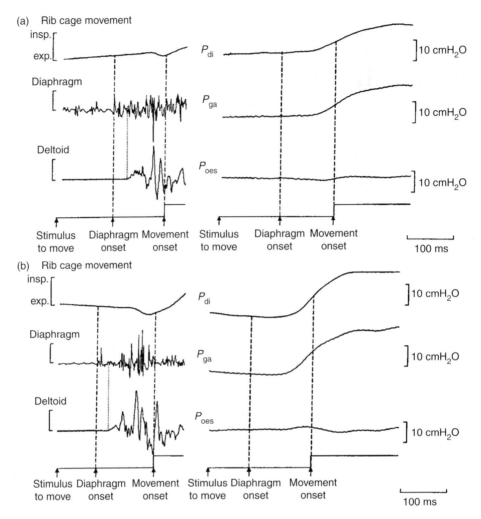

Figure 3.22 Representative single recordings of the electromyographic activity of the costal diaphragm and deltoid, rib-cage motion, intra-abdominal pressure (P_{ga}), intrathoracic pressure (P_{oes}) and transdiaphragmatic pressure (P_{di}) with rapid shoulder flexion occurring during inspiration (a) and expiration (b). The onset of diaphragm activity and the initiation of movement of the limb are denoted by the dashed lines, and the onset of deltoid activity is denoted by the dotted line. The time scale is identical in the left- and right-hand panels. The figure demonstrates the onset of increase in P_{ga} and P_{di} prior to the initiation of movement of the limb, thus providing evidence that the feedforward contraction of the TrA and the diaphragm is associated with a mechanical response that precedes the onset of movement. The figure also shows the onset of an increase in costal diaphragm activity prior to that of the deltoid, providing evidence of a contribution of the diaphragm to the preparatory spinal stability mechanism. (Reproduced with permission from Hodges et al 1997a, p. 542.)

during maximal and submaximal contractions of the pelvic floor muscles (Sapsford et al 2001). The key observations were, first, that maximal contraction of the pelvic floor muscles was associated with activity of all abdominal muscles; second, that submaximal activity of the pelvic floor muscles was associated with a more isolated contraction of TrA (Fig. 3.23);

and, third, that the specificity of the response was better when the lumbar spine and pelvis were in a neutral position rather than in posterior pelvic tilt. This has been confirmed in recent studies in which activity of the abdominal muscles was judged with ultrasound imaging (Critchley 2002). In a second study, activity of the pelvic floor muscles was

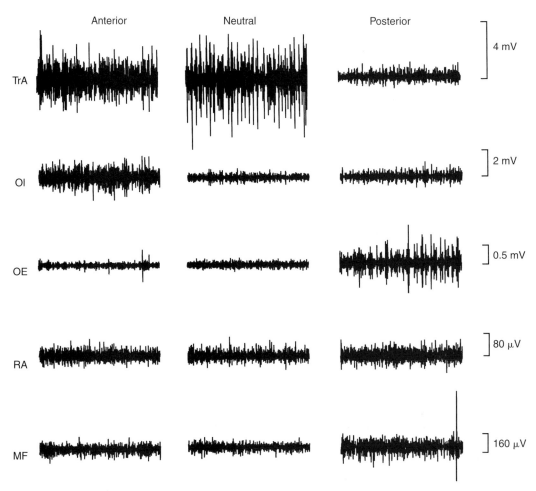

Figure 3.23   Representative raw electromyogram of each of the abdominal muscles and the superficial multifidus (MF) during the performance of a submaximal pelvic floor contraction in supine crook lying. Contractions were performed in three conditions: anterior (anterior pelvic tilt with padding placed under the lumbar curve to maintain the position); neutral (with the spine and pelvis in a neutral position); posterior (posterior pelvic tilt with padding under the sacrum to maintain the position). Note the relatively isolated activity in the transversus abdominis (TrA) with pelvic floor muscle contraction in the neutral position, and the additional activation of other abdominal muscles in the anterior and posterior conditions. OE, obliquus externus abdominis; OI, obliquus internus abdominis; RA, rectus abdominis.

increased in association with gentle contraction of the abdominal muscles (Sapsford and Hodges 2001). This latter finding has potential implications for the management of incontinence, but further studies of clinical populations are required.

Posterior muscles

In contrast to the other muscles that surround the abdominal cavity, few studies have directly recorded from the posterior abdominal muscles. A major factor has been the difficulty in making recordings from these muscles owing to their placement. Several studies have made recordings with intramuscular electrodes; however, these have largely been confined to studies of activity of these muscles during static postures and during exercise manoeuvres (Andersson et al 1995, 1996, McGill et al 1996). In general, these studies indicate that quadratus lumborum is a lateral flexor

(Andersson et al 1995) and psoas is a flexor or lateral flexor of the trunk (Andersson et al 1996, McGill et al 1996); however, the studies throw little light on the role played by these muscles in lumbopelvic stability. One study does report activity of quadratus lumborum during compressive loading, which is consistent with the hypothesis that this muscle is associated with the control of buckling under compressive forces (McGill et al 1996). Further studies are required to investigate whether the fibres of these muscles that attach to the lumbar vertebrae are controlled in a manner that is consistent with the control of intervertebral stability. Studies are currently underway to investigate the control of the posterior and anterior fibres of psoas during a range of postural tasks.

THE CHALLENGE TO COORDINATE MULTIPLE FUNCTIONS

A key issue to consider in the rehabilitation of muscle function in people with low back pain is that many of the muscles of the trunk that appear critical for the control of intervertebral motion are also involved in homeostatic functions such as respiration and continence (Hodges 1999). In addition, these muscles must support the abdominal contents in upright positions (DeTroyer 1983). Although strategies exist to coordinate these often conflicting functions in the normal situation, this may not be true when the demand for one of these functions is increased, for instance if respiratory demand is increased by exercise or disease. This section considers the strategies for coordination of these multiple functions and situations in which the coordination may be compromised.

Abdominal support

One function attributed to the abdominal muscles is support of the abdominal contents. Based on the circumferential arrangement of TrA, this muscle is considered to have the most appropriate mechanical efficiency to perform this role (DeTroyer et al 1990). Concurrently, activity of TrA (Strohl et al 1981) and the other abdominal muscles (Floyd and Silver 1950, Campbell and Green 1955, Carman et al 1972) is commonly reported in standing. However, this activity can be abolished easily with minor

adjustment to posture or by voluntary effort (Campbell 1952, Agostoni and Campbell 1970, Hodges et al 1997b). Increased activity of TrA as patients are progressively tilted from supine to standing are consistent with the role of this activity in visceral support (Campbell 1952, DeTroyer 1983, Goldman et al 1987). As this activity is tonic, this is consistent with the function of this muscle for lumbopelvic stability and is unlikely to present a conflicting demand.

Respiration

Normal quiet respiration involves cyclical activity of the diaphragm, parasternal intercostal and scalene muscles during inspiration, with expiration generated passively by the elastic recoil of the lung and chest wall (DeTroyer and Estenne 1988). However, when the demand for respiration is increased and the rate and depth of expiration is increased, abdominal muscles are phasically activated during the expiratory phase (Campbell 1952). If respiration is increased involuntarily (e.g. hypercapnoea) TrA is recruited at lower minute ventilation than the other abdominal muscles (DeTroyer et al 1990, Abe et al 1996, Hodges et al 1997b). Recent data indicate that this may vary between regions of the abdominal wall, with activity of the mid region of TrA recruited with lower respiratory demand (D. M. Urquhart and P. W. Hodges, unpublished observations). Therefore, both TrA and the diaphragm have important respiratory functions that must be coordinated with the contribution to lumbopelvic stability. Recent studies of repetitive limb movements confirm that when the arm is moved repetitively to challenge the stability of the spine, tonic activity of the diaphragm and TrA is sustained but is modulated with respiration to meet respiratory demands (Hodges and Gandevia 2000a,b) (Fig. 2.7). In a mechanical sense, the diaphragm and TrA co-contract tonically; yet during inspiration, diaphragm activity is increased and shortens (concentric), and TrA decreases its activity and lengthens (eccentric) (Fig. 3.24). The converse pattern occurs during expiration (Hodges and Gandevia 2000a,b). Recent data confirm that this coordination also occurs during natural repetitive movements such as locomotion (Hodges and Saunders 2001). This coordination occurs as if

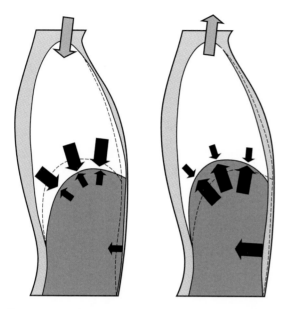

Figure 3.24 Coordination of eccentric and concentric activity of transversus abdominis and the diaphragm for breathing during tasks in which stability is maintained by tonic activity of these muscles. During inspiration, the diaphragm contracts concentrically, whereas transversus lengthens and contracts eccentrically. The converse pattern occurs during expiration. In this manner, tonic activity can be maintained with respiration.

there is summation of the respiratory and postural drives to these muscles, which may occur at the motoneuron, providing a mechanism for the CNS to coordinate these functions. More recently, we have shown that pelvic floor muscle activity is also modulated during respiration. This occurs during inspiration in association with the increased IAP caused by diaphragm contraction and during both inspiration and expiration when respiration is increased (Hodges et al 2002c). Notably, this activity is coordinated with the activity associated with lumbopelvic stability.

However, when respiratory drive is increased by respiratory disease (Hodges et al 2000b) or by breathing with an increased dead space to induce hypercapnoea (Hodges and Saunders 2001, Hodges et al 2003c), the coordination between respiratory and stability functions of TrA and the diaphragm is reduced (Fig. 3.25). This compromise involves reduced tonic activity of the diaphragm and TrA, and a reduction in phasic bursts of activity of these

muscles with each movement. Notably, this reduction in activity was associated with reduced mechanical response, and a smaller increase in IAP was measured in association with the repetitive arm movement (Hodges and Saunders 2001). Recent data indicate that response of TrA, the diaphragm and pelvic floor muscles is reduced in response to support-surface translation when subjects breathed with an increased dead space (Hodges et al 2003c). This impaired contribution of the local muscles to lumbopelvic stability was associated with increased activity of obliquus externus abdominis and rectus abdominis (Hodges et al 2003c). Similarly, McGill et al (1995) have shown that the load on the spine from muscle activity was increased when lifting tasks were performed during increased respiratory demand. The normal fine-tuning of interverbral motion is likely to be reduced in this situation. The potential long-term effects of this change are discussed in Chapter 10. A novel recent finding is that the postural function of TrA was reduced during the inspiratory pause in speech when talking while walking (P. W. Hodges et al, unpublished observations).

Respiratory movements of the rib cage and abdomen also generate a cyclical disturbance to stability of the trunk and to body equilibrium (Gurfinkel et al 1971). However, most studies have failed to identify a cyclical disturbance to the centre of pressure at the ground with respiration (Gurfinkel et al 1971, Bouisset and Duchene 1994). This is because of small-amplitude cyclical movements of the lumbar spine, pelvis and lower limb that are time-locked to respiration and that match and counteract the disturbance to postural stability (Gurfinkel et al 1971, Hodges et al 2002b). Importantly, this postural compensation does not occur when people have low back pain (Gagey 1986, Grimstone and Hodges 2003).

Continence

In contrast to the potential conflicting demands of respiratory and stability functions of the local muscles, in general the demands for continence are consistent with the demands for spinal control (Hodges 1999). That is, tonic activity is required for both functions. Whether this occurs in people with continence problems has not been established,

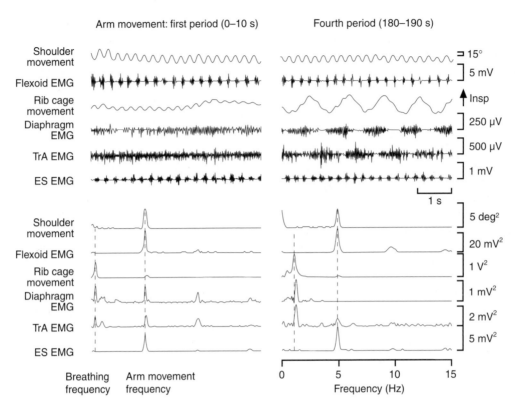

Figure 3.25 Repetitive arm movement is normally associated with tonic activity of the diaphragm and transversus abdominis (TrA) as well as phasic modulation of these muscles in association with breathing and arm movement, which is observable in the raw data (upper panel) and frequency spectra (lower panels). When the arm is moved repetitively after breathing with an increased dead space for 180 seconds to induced hypercapnoea, the tonic activity and the phasic activity with each arm movement is reduced in these muscles. ES, erector spinae; EMG, electromyography. (Adapted from Hodges et al 2001d.)

although reduced activity in association with coughing have been reported (Deindl et al 1993, 1994).

Other considerations for task conflict

As mentioned above, the trunk muscles contribute to control of intervertebral motion, trunk orientation and whole-body equilibrium, as well as performing coordinated movements of the trunk. Theoretically, this coordination may also compromise the accuracy of stability. For instance, when body equilibrium is disturbed, movement of the trunk is required to maintain the position of the centre of mass over the base of support, and this demand may be inconsistent with the demand to maintain stability (Oddsson 1989, Hodges et al 1999, Oddsson et al 1999, Huang et al 2001). Although trunk muscle activity has been found to be consistent with both

tasks in specific situations (Hodges et al 1999), this may not be the case in all situations. For instance, if the support surface is moved when a mass is being lifted, conflict between postural and movement tasks may arise (Oddsson et al 1999, Huang et al 2001). In this situation, postural control has been shown to be compromised.

CLINICAL APPLICATION

The contribution of the individual elements of the abdominal mechanism to lumbopelvic stability has significant implications for planning clinical strategies for rehabilitation of the patient with low back pain. An important consideration is that, although all muscles contribute to lumbopelvic stability, the biomechanical and motor control evidence supports the proposal that local and global muscles of the abdominal cavity contribute to different elements of control. Specific assessment of all elements of the system are required to investigate fully the extent of dysfunction in the trunk muscles. This will be readdressed in Chapter 10, after consideration of the specific nature of the control dysfunction identified in low back pain.

Consideration of the functional anatomy and control of trunk muscles indicates that rehabilitation approaches that involve trunk torque are unlikely to restore the control of TrA, as this muscle is not a torque producer. Furthermore, the data suggest that fascial tension, IAP and sacroiliac joint compression are important. Therefore, bilateral contraction of TrA is required to optimize spinal control. As identified in the porcine studies, unilateral contraction of TrA is unlikely to impact on spinal intervertebral control (Hodges et al 2003a). Similarly, the effect of TrA on the spine and pelvis is dependent on integrated activity of the diaphragm and pelvic floor muscles.

When considering the strategies used by the neural system to control the muscle of the abdominal wall, it is important to address the issues of tonic activity and early activity of TrA and the pelvic floor in particular. However, attention to the superficial global muscles must address the requirement to match the demands of spinal control, being co-active as required and phasic when appropriate. If excessive co-activation of global muscles is present, this clearly must be addressed.

A final issue to consider is that any factor which compromises the accuracy of control of any of the components necessary to coordinate respiratory and continence functions with stability may require attention. For instance, it is critical for patients to develop coordination of the stability and respiratory functions of these muscles, and people with respiratory disease may have greater difficulty in achieving this control. Additional consideration of timing of treatment around medication may be important. These issues will be considered again in Chapter 10.

Chapter **4**

Paraspinal mechanism and support of the lumbar spine

Julie Hides

INTRODUCTION

The muscles of the lumbar region that contribute to the local stabilizing system of the spine are:

- intersegmental muscles:
  - intertransversarii
  - interspinales.
- lumbar muscles:
  - lumbar multifidus
  - longissimus thoracis pars lumborum
  - iliocostalis lumborum pars lumborum.
- quadratus lumborum (medial fibres).

INTERSEGMENTAL MUSCLES

The intertransversarii and interspinales are small segmental muscles connecting the transverse processes and spinous processes, respectively, of two adjacent lumbar vertebrae (Bogduk 1997). Their small size and location close to the centre of rotation of the segment indicate that they would have little torque-producing capability. They have a segmental nerve supply (Bogduk et al 1982) and are highly rich in muscle spindles (Nitz and Peck 1986). McGill (2002b) proposed that these muscles are actually length transducers and position sensors, and Bogduk (1997) also proposed that these muscles may have a predominant proprioceptive role. As such, they could influence kinaesthetic sense in the lumbar region and, therefore, affect patterns of muscle activity. At this time, it is not possible to undertake an evaluation of this functional role, and therefore detection of any impairment in their function in patients with low back pain is, likewise, not possible.

THE LUMBAR MUSCLES

Anatomy

Lumbar multifidus

Lumbar multifidus is the most medial of the lumbar muscles and of the three lumbar muscles has the unique arrangement of predominantly vertebra-to-vertebra attachments within the lumbar and between the lumbar and sacral vertebrae (Macintosh et al 1986). The muscle has five separate bands, each consisting of a series of fascicles that stem from spinous processes and laminae of the lumbar vertebrae (Fig. 4.1a). In each band, the deepest and shortest fascicle arises from the vertebral lamina. The lamina fibres insert into the mamillary processes of the vertebra two levels caudad, with the L5 fibres inserting onto an area of the sacrum above the first dorsal sacral foramen. The other fascicles arise from the spinous process and are longer than the laminar fibres (Macintosh et al 1986). Each lumbar vertebra gives rise to one group of fascicles that overlap those of the other levels. The fascicles from a given spinous process insert onto mamillary processes of the lumbar or sacral vertebrae three, four or five levels inferiorly. The longest fascicles, from L1, L2 and L3, have some attachment to the posterior superior iliac spine (Fig. 4.1b). Some of the deepest multifidus fibres attach to the capsules of the zygapophyseal joints (Lewin et al 1962, Macintosh et al 1986). The lumbar zygapophyseal joints are covered by the multifidus on all sides, except ventrally where the joints are in direct contact with the ligamentum flavum (Lewin et al 1962). This close relationship can be demonstrated using ultrasound imaging (Fig. 4.2). The ligaments that form the capsule of the zygapophyseal joints are rich in proprioceptive organs (Pacinian and Ruffini corpuscles) (Cavanaugh et al 1996, McLain and Pickar 1998). The attachment of the lumbar multifidus to the zygapophyseal joint capsules keeps the capsule taut and free from impingement between the articular cartilages (Lewin et al 1962, Macintosh et al 1986).

Longissimus thoracis pars lumborum

Longissimus thoracis pars lumborum lies lateral to the lumbar multifidus and consists of five fascicles that arise from the medial end of the transverse processes and connect the lumbar vertebrae to the ilium (Fig. 4.3). The fascicle from L5 inserts onto the medial aspect of the posterior inferior iliac spine, while the fascicles from L1–L4 form tendons at their caudal end that converge like a common tendon to form the lumbar intermuscular aponeurosis. This attaches to a narrow area on the ilium lateral to the insertion of the L5 fascicle (Bogduk 1997).

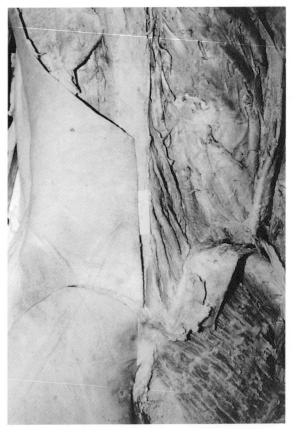

(a)

Figure 4.1   The fascicles of the lumbar multifidus. (a) Anatomical dissection of the five fascicles. (b) i, the laminar fibres at every level; ii–vi, the longer fascicles from the caudal edge and tubercles of the spinous processes at levels L1–L5. (Reproduced with permission from Bogduk 1997, p. 106.)

Iliocostalis lumborum pars lumborum

The iliocostalis lumborum pars lumborum is the most lateral of the lumbar back muscle group. It has four fascicles that arise from the tips of the transverse processes of L1–L4, and an area extending on to the middle layer of the thoracolumbar fascia (Bogduk 1997). The four fascicles insert onto the iliac crest, with the L4 fascicle deepest and the L1 fascicle most dorsal (Fig. 4.4). There is no muscle fascicle of the iliocostalis lumborum from L5 to the ilium in the adult. Any muscle fibres present at birth are replaced by collagen during growth and maturation to help to form the iliolumbar ligament (Bogduk 1997).

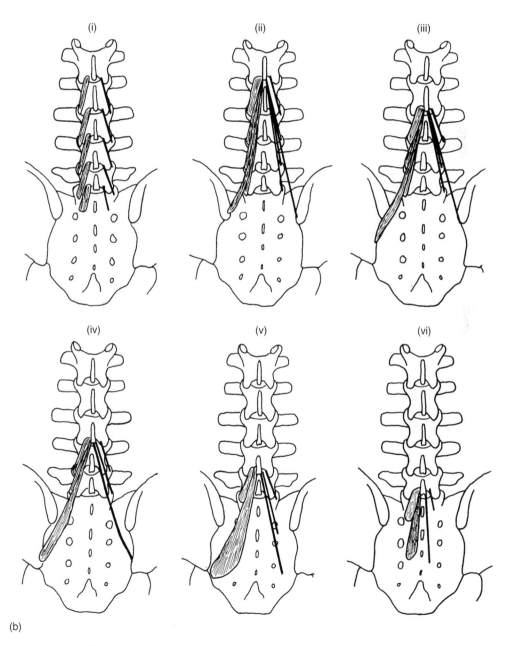

(b)

Figure 4.1 *(continued)*.

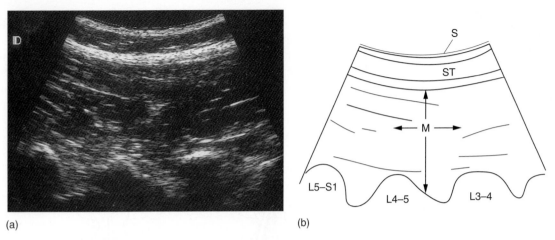

(a)　　　　　　　　　　　　　　　　　　(b)

Figure 4.2 The multifidus. (a) Ultrasound image in parasagittal section, showing the intimate relationship between the deep multifidus and the zygapophyseal joints. (b) The tissues visible: S, skin; ST, subcutaneous tissue; M, multifidus muscle; L5–S1, L4–L5 and L3–L4, zygapophyseal joints.

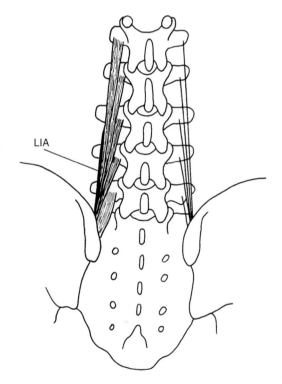

Figure 4.3 Longissimus thoracis pars lumborum. (Reproduced with permission from Bogduk 1997, p. 109.)

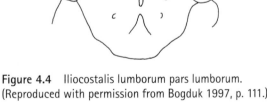

Figure 4.4 Iliocostalis lumborum pars lumborum. (Reproduced with permission from Bogduk 1997, p. 111.)

Function

The back muscles are primarily extensors of the spine when acting bilaterally, but the lumbar longissimus and iliocostalis can also assist in lateral flexion when acting unilaterally. None of the muscles is a primary contributor to axial rotation, but activity in this movement may reflect their stabilizing counter to the flexion moment produced by the oblique abdominals (Bogduk 1997, Macintosh and Bogduk 1986a or b). In trunk flexion, the multifidus and lumbar longissimus and iliocostalis control the anterior rotation and anterior translation. On return to upright, the multifidus induces posterior sagittal rotation, assisted by the lumbar erector spinae, which also control the posterior sagittal translation (Bogduk 1997). Nevertheless, it is the thoracic components of the erector spinae that produce the majority of torque to extend the thoracic cage on the pelvis. The multifidus contributes only 20% of the total extensor moment calculated at the L4 and L5 vertebral levels; the lumbar erector spinae contributes 30%, while the thoracic components of the erector spinae contribute 50% (Bogduk et al 1992b). Even though the multifidus is the largest muscle at the lumbosacral junction, it is at a mechanical disadvantage to produce extension of the thoracic cage on the pelvis.

All three of the lumbar muscles contribute to the support and control of the orientation of the lumbar spine and the support or stabilization of the lumbar segments. The importance of their supporting function may be reflected in the distribution of muscle fibre type. In contrast to most human muscles, which have a relatively even type I and type II fibre distribution, several postmortem studies have revealed that the lumbar multifidus and the lumbar and thoracic components of the erector spinae muscles have a high proportion of type I fibres (Johnson et al 1973, Fidler et al 1975, Jowett et al 1975, Sirca and Kostevc 1985, Thorstensson and Carlson 1987, Jorgensen et al 1993). These paravertebral muscles are also characterised by a large type I fibre cross-sectional area relative to other human extremity muscles and abdominal muscles (with the exception of the transversus abdominis) (Jorgensen et al 1993). The presence of both a larger percentage of type I fibres and a larger type I fibre size compared with type II fast twitch fibres supports the hypothesised tonic role of these muscles. The proportion of type I fibres in the thoracic erector spinae muscles has been reported to be as high as 70% (Sirca and Kostevc 1985), while that in the lumbar erector spinae muscles varies in the range 58–69% (Fidler et al 1975, Sirca and Kostevc 1985, Mattila et al 1986, Jorgensen et al 1993). When comparing the composition of the multifidus with the lumbar erector spinae muscles, a larger

percentage of type I fibres, in the range 8–13%, has been reported in the multifidus compared with the lumbar longissimus (Sirca and Kostevc 1985, Verbout et al 1989). The exception was in the study by Jorgensen et al (1993), who found similar percentages of type I fibres in the multifidus and the lumbar longissimus.

The histochemical composition, capillarization and muscle enzyme activities of the lumbar multifidus and lumbar longissimus and iliocostalis muscles have been studied in vivo (Jorgensen et al 1993). Multifidus muscle fibres have a large capillary network, with approximately four to five capillaries in contact with each muscle cell. The concentration of oxidative enzymes in all lumbar muscles is large and the endurance capacity high. This histochemical composition of the paravertebral muscles, with a high composition of type I fibres, indicates the tonic holding function, and thus supportive function, of these muscles.

Our particular concern with regard to the patient with low back pain is the ability to rehabilitate the muscles that have the greatest potential to provide and substitute active support to the individual spinal segment that, from injury, has some passive insufficiency. What will be argued here, on the basis of morphological and biomechanical studies as well as studies monitoring the activity of the back muscles, is that the lumbar multifidus, especially the deep fibres, has better capabilities for segmental support and control and lesser capabilities for torque production. The lumbar longissimus and iliocostalis, by comparison, have better capabilities for torque production and control of spinal orientation but may not have as much specificity for function for one vertebral segment as does the lumbar multifidus. Furthermore, the more consistent activity of the lumbar multifidus in low-load functional activities may reflect its supporting function.

Morphology

The unique segmental arrangement of the multifidus fascicles in the lumbar region indicates that it has the capacity for fine control of movements of individual lumbar vertebrae. This is reflected in its segmental innervation. Each fascicle of the lumbar multifidus and the zygapophyseal joint of that level is innervated by the medial branch of the dorsal

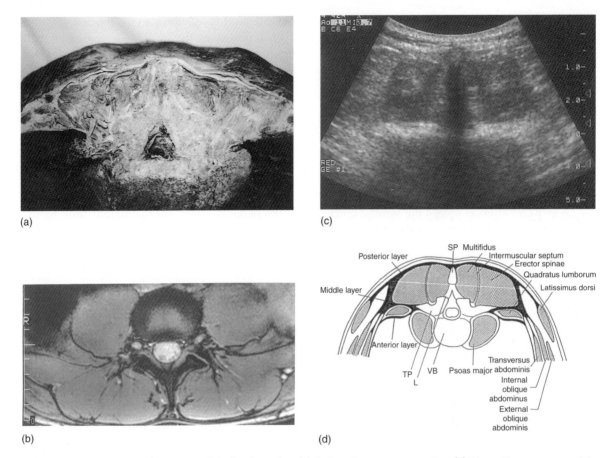

Figure 4.5 Cross-sectional anatomy of the lumbar spine. (a) Cadaveric transverse section. (b) Magnetic resonance axial image of the lumbar spine. (c) Ultrasound axial image of the lumbar spine. (d) Schematic drawing of a transverse section showing the multifidus and erector spinae muscle (separated by an intermuscular septum), other muscles surrounding the spine and the layers of the thoracolumbar fascia (posterior, middle and anterior). L, lamina; SP, spinous process; TP, transverse process; VB, vertebral body. (Reproduced with permission from Porterfield and DeRosa 1991, p. 56.)

ramus (Lewin et al 1962, Macintosh et al 1986, Bogduk 1997). Each nerve innervates only the fascicles that arise from the spinous process or lamina of the vertebra with the same segmental number as the nerve (Macintosh et al 1986), illustrating the direct relationship between a particular segment and its multifidus muscle. This suggests that the segmental multifidus can adjust or control a particular segment to match the applied load (Aspden 1992). The lumbar longissimus and iliocostalis do not show this tight segmental nerve–muscle relationship, suggesting a slightly more general relationship to the spinal segments. The lumbar longissimus is supplied by the intermediate branches of the L1–L4 dorsal rami, which form an intersegmental

plexus in the muscle, although its fibres from L5 are innervated by the corresponding nerve (Bogduk et al 1982). The lumbar portion of iliocostalis is supplied by the lateral divisions of the L1–L4 dorsal rami, which run caudally, dorsally and laterally through the muscle (Bogduk et al 1982).

The cross-sectional anatomy of the lumbar spine is shown in Figure 4.5, including the normal appearance on magnetic resonance imaging (MRI) and real-time ultrasound imaging. What is of interest in the cross-sectional area of the lumbar back muscles is that multifidus muscle bulk increases on progression caudally from L2 to S1 (Amonoo-Kuofi 1983, Ecleshymer and Schoemaker 1970) (Fig. 4.6). We have recently measured the multifidus

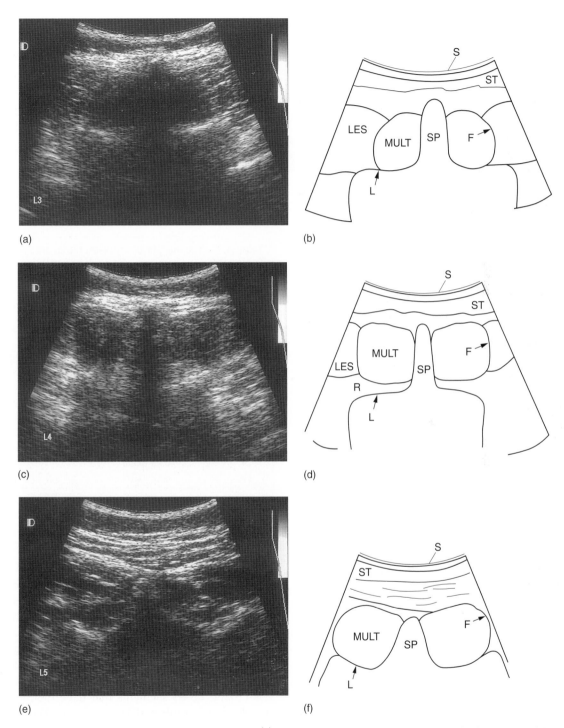

Figure 4.6 The multifidus muscle in a normal subject. (a) Ultrasound axial image appearance at the level of the third vertebra. (b) The tissues visible in (a). (c) Ultrasound axial image at the level of the fourth vertebra. (d) The tissues visible in (c). (e) Ultrasound axial image at the level of the fifth vertebra. (f) The tissues visible in (e). (g) Ultrasound axial image at the level of the first sacral vertebra. (h) The tissues visible in (g). S, skin; ST, subcutaneous tissue; SP, spinous process; L, lamina; MULT, multifidus; F, fascia; LES, lumbar erector spinae muscle; R, reflection.

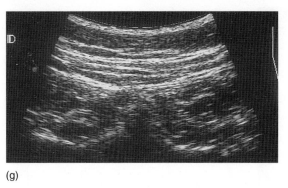

(g)

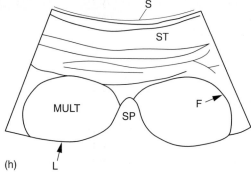

(h)

Figure 4.6 *(continued).*

Table 4.1 Average age, height and weight for 40 subjects without a history of low back pain

Variable	Males	Females	Total
No.	13	27	40
Height			
mean cm	181.85	164.85	170.37
SD	5.49	5.59	9.75
Weight			
mean kg	82.92	60.11	67.52
SD	16.49	6.27	15.06
Age			
mean years	28.92	28.11	28.37
SD	5.75	5.83	5.74

SD, standard deviation.

Table 4.2 The multifidus cross-sectional areas for the different lumbosacral vertebral levels in 40 subjects without a history of low back pain

Vertebral level	Cross-sectional area (mean cm^2 (SE))	Confidence interval
Female		
L2	2.1 (0.13)	1.85–2.35
L3	3.35 (0.17)	3.0–3.7
L4	4.78 (0.2)	4.37–5.18
L5	6.38 (0.18)	6.01–6.75
Male		
L2	3.01 (0.18)	2.65–3.38
L3	4.31 (0.25)	3.81–4.82
L4	6.27 (0.29)	5.68–6.85
L5	6.79 (0.27)	6.25–7.32

SE, standard error.
J. Hides et al, unpublished data.

cross-sectional area at five vertebral levels in subjects without a history of low back pain. Table 4.1 shows the average age, height and weight of the 13 male and 27 female subjects measured. Table 4.2 shows the multifidus cross-sectional areas for the different lumbosacral vertebral levels (J. Hides et al 2003, unpublished data). It was found that males have significantly larger multifidus muscles than females at all vertebral levels (Hides et al 1992, S. Kelley et al 2003, unpublished data) and that the cross-sectional area of the multifidus is significantly different for each vertebral level (Hides et al 1995, S. Kelley et al 2003, unpublished data). In subjects without a history of low back pain, multifidus cross-sectional area is symmetrical between sides (Hides et al 1994). The multifidus is the largest muscle spanning the lumbosacral junction (Macintosh

et al 1986). In contrast, the cross-sectional area of the lumbar longissimus and iliocostalis decreases on progression caudally. The large size of the multifidus muscle at the lumbosacral junction, compared with the adjacent lumbar erector spinae muscles, also suggests that it is the muscle most capable of providing support at this level. Notably, it is the L4–L5 and L5–S1 segments that have the highest incidence of pathology in low back pain. The multifidus has a close relationship to the zygapophyseal joints (Fig. 4.2) and by controlling the sliding movement of the zygapophyseal joints in the craniocaudal direction it controls the distribution of stresses and loading on the vertebral triad. It is considered that the multifidus is the only muscle the primary function of which is to protect the vertebral triad (Lewin et al 1962).

Biomechanical factors

Control of the neutral zone

Several studies have investigated the lumbar muscles' capacity to increase the spinal segmental stiffness and, in particular, the control of neutral zone motion in line with Panjabi's (1992b) hypothesis of clinical instability. Studies have been done on various combinations of muscles to investigate their influence on these parameters. Kaigle et al (1995) developed an in vivo animal model of lumbar segmental instability. Passive stabilizing structures (disc, zygapophyseal joints and ligaments) were transected and the effects of active musculature on spinal kinematics were examined in 33 pigs. Muscles surrounding the spine, including the multifidus, the lumbar portions of erector spinae, quadratus lumborum and psoas major and minor, were examined. The injured segments were subjected to muscle stimulation using wire electrodes. Results showed that increased, combined muscle activation stabilised the injured motion segment by reducing aberrant patterns of motion in the neutral zone.

Goel et al (1993) used a combined finite-element and optimization approach to study the effects of the actions of the interspinales and intertransversarii, the lumbar multifidus and the quadratus lumborum. The introduction of muscle forces led to a decrease in displacements in the sagittal plane, anteroposterior translation and anterior rotation. It was shown that these muscles imparted stability to the ligamentous system. The load bearing of the zygapophyseal joints was found to increase, indicating that these joints play a significant role in transmitting loads in a normal intact spine. Muscle dysfunction (simulated by decreasing the computed force in the muscles) destabilised the motion segment. This led to a shift of loads to the disc and ligaments and decreased the role of the zygapophyseal joints in transmitting loads (Goel and Gilbertson 1995).

Panjabi et al (1989), in an in vitro study of intact and sequentially injured fresh lumbar spinal units, more specifically simulated the effect of intersegmental muscle forces on spinal instability. Simulated forces represented the multifidus (deep, shorter fascicles), interspinales and rotatores muscles. The segments were subjected to three-dimensional loads with increasing muscle forces. This study, like the one by Goel et al (1993), examined the effect of the segmental muscles without the influence of the larger lumbar longissimus and iliocostalis. Panjabi et al (1989) concluded that the intersegmental nature of the deep multifidus fibres gave a tremendous advantage to the neuromuscular system for controlling the stability of the lumbar segment.

Wilke et al (1995) investigated the influence of five different muscle groups on the monosegmental motion of the L4–L5 segment. The muscles examined were the multifidus (caudal and cranial directions), lumbar longissimus, lumbar iliocostalis and psoas major. Seven human lumbosacral spines were tested on a spine tester that allowed simulation of muscle forces. The combined muscle action of the muscles tested was found to decrease the total range of motion and neutral zone motion of the L4–L5 segment. The total neutral zone motion in flexion and extension was decreased by 83%. In lateral flexion, the total range of motion was decreased by 55% and the neutral zone by 76%. Under axial rotation, the total range was reduced by 35%, but there was no significant change in neutral zone motion. Muscle forces were found to stiffen the motion segment. The strongest influence was created by the lumbar multifidus, which was responsible for more than two-thirds of the increase in segmental stiffness. The multifidus action was responsible for a significant decrease in the range of motion of all movements except rotation. These results supported those obtained by Steffen et al (1994) in another in vitro study, who also found that the influence of lumbar multifidus decreased the neutral zone in flexion and extension.

The lateral stabilizing potential of the lumbar intersegmental and polysegmental muscles has also been investigated by Crisco and Panjabi (1991). They found that the polysegmental fascicles of multifidus and lumbar longissmus and iliocostalis fascicles were more efficient in this direction than were the short deep multifidus fascicles and intertransversarii and interspinales muscles. It can be surmised that the role of the multifidus in lumbar spine stabilization is complex. The multifidus is capable of controlling the neutral zone in the sagittal plane with its deeper, intersegmental fibres, but it requires the assistance of the lumbar longissimus and iliocostalis in the lumbar muscles' contribution to the control of neutral zone motion in the frontal plane.

Some biomechanical studies have investigated the effects of co-activation of muscles on spinal stability. A recent study investigating co-activation of the multifidus and the psoas showed that the stability of the L4–L5 segment was enhanced in lateral flexion and rotation but it was destabilised in flexion (Quint et al 1998). It was concluded that the importance of the neural control strategy of the stabilization of the spine cannot be overemphasized. The neural controller must not only select the appropriate muscles to stimulate but also decide on their appropriate activation level (Quint et al 1998).

The deep multifidus fibres in particular are placed close to the centres of rotation of spinal movements and connect adjacent vertebrae at appropriate angles. McGill (1991) confirmed the role of lumbar multifidus in a three-dimensional study of lumbar spine mechanics and concluded that the unchanging geometry of the multifidus through a range of postures indicated that the purpose of this muscle is finely to adjust vertebrae with small movements rather than to function as a prime mover. This study showed that the multifidus could function in this way in any physiological posture.

Control of the lordosis

It has been well accepted in the area of biomechanics and ergonomics that the spinal curves are an efficient way for the body to deal with forces of gravity. When the spinal curves are maintained, this is the most energy-efficient position for the body to stay upright against the forces of gravity and to withstand further forces that are applied to the spine. For the lumbar region, it has been proposed that the multifidus can contribute to stability of the spine via control of the lordosis, allowing equal distribution of forces (Aspden 1992).

Contraction of the polysegmental multifidus fascicles can restore the lumbar lordosis. Recent studies have confirmed this finding; the compressive load-bearing capacity of the passive thoracolumbar spine was significantly enhanced by pelvic rotation caused by minimal muscle forces in the sagittal plane (Keifer et al 1997). When local muscles were examined in the model, multifidus was found to contribute 80% of the required activity (Keifer et al 1998).

To maintain the spinal curves requires a balance between and integration of local, mono-articular and global muscles. This relationship has been examined in biomechanical studies (Keifer et al 1997, 1998). The studies used a finite element model (passive osseoligamentous spine) with optimization of the muscles (active and passive components of muscle force). In the first study, Keifer et al (1997) loaded the spine using compressive axial forces. They showed that the thoracolumbar spine translated into hypermobility under axial loads less than physiological loads without the muscles (indicated by displacement of the T1 vertebra). Addition of local and global muscles into the model increased the ability of the spine to withstand compressive forces without buckling. Pelvic rotation (anterior tilt) stiffened the spine, and only 2 degrees of anterior rotation allowed the spine to carry axial compression of up to 400 N, with only 7 mm of anterior displacement of T1. There was less anterior displacement of T1 with local and global muscles incorporated into the model than with global muscles alone, highlighting the importance of integration of the two muscle systems. In the second study, Keifer et al (1998) investigated the synergy of the spine in neutral positions. Using the same model, they displaced T1 40 mm anteriorly and 20 mm posteriorly. Results showed that the global muscles and passive structures are sufficient to stabilize the spine for very small displacements. However, the system is far more efficient with inclusion of the local muscles. Activation of the local muscles decreased muscle forces in the global system, provided stiffness, increased stability and increased compression. Considering the contribution of the local muscles, 80% was provided by multifidus, with some contribution by iliocostalis. Another finding was that the position of the thoracolumbar junction is important. If T12 was held back, then the upper lumbar spine was forced into flexion, and the synergy was disturbed. This had a resultant marked effect on the distribution of intersegmental rotations and lessened the capacity of the passive system to carry sagittal moments.

Tensioning the thoracolumbar fascia

Muscles enhance spinal stability by increasing the stiffness of the spinal segment. It has already been shown that the multifidus acts to stiffen the motion segment (Wilke et al 1995). From a mechanical perspective, the bending stiffness of the spine will also be influenced by other factors. One structure that can contribute to lumbar stabilization by increasing the bending stiffness of the spine is the thoracolumbar fascia. The thoracolumbar fascia is a strong tissue with a well-developed lattice of collagen fibres, suggesting that its function may be that of an extensor muscle retinaculum (Bogduk and Macintosh 1984). In addition, the fascia does contain both Ruffini and Pacinian corpuscles together with diffuse innervation (Yahia et al 1988). It is important to recognize that it is a musculofascial system that protects the lumbosacral region, and the influence of the muscles on tensioning fascias is vitally important. The transversus abdominis (plus or minus the internal oblique muscle) may tension the thoracolumbar fascia (see Ch. 3). In addition, the thoracolumbar fascia constrains the radial expansion of the three lumbar back muscles (Aspden 1992). It has been proposed that contraction of these muscles exerts a pushing force on the fascia (Farfan 1973). The influence of the multifidus and the lumbar longissimus and ilicocostalis on the thoracolumbar fascia was investigated by Gracovetsky et al (1977) using a mathematical model. It was proposed that the thoracolumbar fascia could serve to brace the back muscles because it surrounded them. The authors called this the 'hydraulic amplifier mechanism'. While this mechanism has been dismissed on the grounds that it is unlikely to generate extensor forces (McGill 2002b), it is more than likely that the thoracolumbar fascia, through its muscular attachments, contributes to increased lumbar stiffness and lumbar stabilization. It may well also have a proprioceptive role.

Control of shear forces

Shear forces are those that cause two vertebrae to slide with respect to one another (Bogduk 1997). During flexion of the lumbar spine, a forward or anterior shear is exerted on the intervertebral joint. Particular attention has been given to these shear forces, which are induced by bending and lifting tasks (Cholewicki et al 1991, Porterfield and DeRosa 1991). The control of anterior shear forces is essential for the protection of the intervertebral joint, especially at the lower lumbar levels where these forces are greatest. This control is provided not only by the passive elements and articular configuration of the vertebral column but also by the muscle system.

Traditionally, the lumbar extensor muscles have been assigned this role. When contracting bilaterally, on the one hand, the lumbar longissimus and the lumbar iliocostalis can draw their vertebra of origin posteriorly, owing to their posterior and caudal direction, and hence oppose the anterior shear. On the other hand, contraction of the multifidus fascicles produces posterior sagittal rotation of the vertebra of origin rather than posterior translation. It is likely that during activities such as forward bending and lifting the induced forces are controlled by the lumbar erector spinae muscles and the multifidus together. McGill et al (2000) propose that, for lifting, the lumbar longissimus and lumbar iliocostalis lose their oblique line of action if the lumbar spine flexes and, as a result, the lumbar spine is unable to resist damaging shear forces. This would highlight the importance of the neutral spine position and may show how the lumbar longissimus, lumbar iliocostalis and multifidus could work together, as one of the known roles of the multifidus is adjustment and control of lumbar lordosis.

However, the control of shear forces appears to be a far more complex issue. A model of back muscles that mapped the actions of individual fascicles (Bogduk et al 1992a) showed that shear forces can be induced by these muscles on maximal exertion. From L1 to L4, the net result was a posterior shear force. However, the net balance was an anterior shear force at the L5 level. This would suggest that various muscles in addition to the back extensors may be involved in the control of anterior shear forces during lifting and bending tasks. Interestingly, Farfan (1975) proposed that anterior shear forces were resisted more by the zygapophyseal joints, with countering forces in the reverse direction being provided by the abdominal musculature.

The back muscles in posture and movement

It is possible that there are different primary functions for the different fascicles of multifidus. The longer fascicles, which originate from the spinous processes, have a mechanical advantage over the shorter, deeper fibres. The longer fascicles may contribute more to extensor torque, while the shorter deeper fibres, which have little leverage for torque production, may be more involved in a tonic stabilizing role. There is evidence to suggest this from electromyographic (EMG) studies, where tonic activation of the deeper fibres has been examined during the maintenance of upright postures and during active trunk movements. EMG analysis has allowed the function of the multifidus to be studied in vivo. Many classic studies have been performed using in-dwelling electrodes to access the activation of the deeper fascicles, which are likely to be involved in a stabilizing role. A tonic or almost continuous level of activation of the multifidus has been demonstrated in many of these studies of upright postures and primary active movements. Moseley et al (2002) studied the response of the multifidus during perturbation produced by movement of a limb in response to a stimulus. Results confirmed that the deep fibres of the multifidus behave differently from the superficial fibres and the lumbar erector spinae muscles. During both flexion and extension of the arm, the onset of EMG in the deep multifidus occurred prior to arm movement and at the same time as deltoid. In contrast, the other muscles behaved differently during flexion and extension, suggesting that, while most of the posterior trunk muscles appear to counteract perturbation of global spinal orientation, the deep multifidus may be more involved in segmental stabilization (Moseley et al 2002). Furthermore, during repetitive upper limb movement, tonic activity of the deep multifidus was observed, in line with its role in stabilization of the spine (Moseley et al 2002). There is evidence

that the multifidus muscle is continuously active in upright postures, compared with relaxed recumbent positions. Along with the lumbar longissimus and iliocostalis, the multifidus provides antigravity support to the spine with almost continuous activity (Asmussen and Klausen 1962). The multifidus is probably active in all antigravity activity (Morris et al 1962, Donisch and Basmajian 1972, Valencia and Munro 1985) and is tonically active during walking (Morris et al 1962). In the standing position, slight to moderate activity of the multifidus has been demonstrated (Jonsson 1970, Donisch and Basmajian 1972, Valencia and Munro 1985), exemplifying its tonic postural role. In fact, maintaining a neutral spine may be the one element that is crucial to maintain this tonic activation. Evidence has been provided by a neurophysiological in vivo study where lumbar spines of cats were placed into moderate sustained flexion and intramuscular EMG of the multifidus was recorded (Williams et al 2000). Prolonged flexion of the lumbar spine resulted in tension–relaxation and laxity of its visco-elastic structures, loss of protective reflexive muscular activity within 3 minutes followed by EMG spasms in the multifidus and other posterior muscles. Although performed on cats, this study holds implications for humans and would lend support to proponents of the importance of the neutral spine concept.

Results of studies performed in the sitting position have varied. It has been reported that the multifidus was inactive in relaxed sitting as well as when subjects were instructed to 'sit upright' (Valencia and Munro 1985). In contrast, Donisch and Basmajian (1972) reported that the multifidus was active in straight unsupported sitting, which accords with a tonic antigravity function. The difference in results between the two studies may relate to the way in which subjects assumed an upright sitting posture, and this becomes an important point in the clinical re-education of upright postural position.

Activation of the multifidus has been examined in forward trunk flexion and extension from the flexed position, trunk extension in the prone position and trunk rotation. An argument can be presented that the function of this activity appears to include primarily one of stabilization. As the spine bends forward from the standing position, there is an increase in multifidus activity (Floyd and Silver 1951, Morris et al 1962, Pauly 1966, Valencia and Munro 1985). At a certain point during flexion, the activity of the back muscles ceases; this is known as the 'critical point' (Floyd and Silver 1951, Morris et al 1962, Kippers and Parker 1984, 1985). The EMG activity of the lumbar erector spinae ceases at about 90% of lumbar spine flexion. The critical point for the multifidus is not such a characteristic feature as it is for the erector spinae muscles. Although a decrease in activity is evident, EMGs of the multifidus show silence infrequently, in contrast to those for the lumbar longissimus and iliocostalis (Valencia and Munro 1985).

Extension of the trunk from the flexed position predictably evokes high levels of multifidus activity (Floyd and Silver 1951, Morris et al 1962, Pauly 1966, Donisch and Basmajian 1972). Marked activity of the multifidus also occurs when the trunk is extended or hyperextended in the prone position (Pauly 1966, Jonsson 1970, Donisch and Basmajian 1972, Valencia and Munro 1985). Even though, as has been mentioned, activity in the multifidus is marked in extension, the majority of the actual trunk extension torque (80% at the L4 and L5 vertebral levels) is provided by the thoracic components of the erector spinae muscles (Bogduk et al 1992b). The multifidus has been shown to be active bilaterally in both ipsilateral and contralateral rotation of the trunk in sitting and standing (Morris et al 1962, Pauly 1966, Jonsson 1970, Donisch and Basmajian 1972). For this reason, it has been suggested that the multifidus acts as a stabilizer rather than as a prime mover during rotation (Valencia and Munro 1985).

As a general observation in movement studies, Donisch and Basmajian (1972) reported that activity of the multifidus was related to its proposed action for only 50% of the time. Pauly (1966) also showed almost continuous activity during the majority of the different directional activities tested. These findings can be interpreted as evidence for a stabilizing role of the multifidus rather than a primary role in torque production only.

The other important role of the multifidus in posture and movement is a proprioceptive one. In studies on humans, the importance of the multifidus as a muscle that provides feedback on spinal position has been highlighted. Solomonow et al (1998) have proposed the existence of a feedback system from the spinal ligaments to the multifidus. Certainly, the supraspinous and interspinous ligaments contain free nerve endings, Ruffini corpuscles and Pacinian corpuscles (Yahia et al 1988, Jiang et al 1995). Position–reposition tasks have been used for evaluating the position sense of the spine, and it has been shown that young healthy individuals are capable of repositioning the pelvis and back (absolute error of approximately 2 degrees) both during standing and sitting (Brumagne et al 1999a,b). Both exercise-induced fatigue and mechanical low back pain have a deleterious effect on lumbosacral positioning accuracy (Brumagne et al 2000). It is thought that the degraded position sense results from altered multifidus muscle spindle afference and central processing of this sensory input, and that deficits in the spinal reflex system might also contribute.

Summary

The lumbar multifidus, lumbar longissimus and iliocostalis play an important role in lumbar spine stability. Because of its unique morphology and segmental innervation, the multifidus would appear to be a muscle well suited to this role of segmental support and control. Biomechanical research has confirmed this important role. The biomechanical study by Wilke et al (1995), which included both the multifidus and the erector spinae muscles in the model, found that the multifidus had the strongest influence on lumbar segmental stability. The morphology of the multifidus, our clinical findings of a dysfunction in the segmental multifidus (Hides et al 1994, 1996b) and work such as that by Wilke et al (1995) all provide a basis for focusing specifically on the lumbar multifidus in patients with low back pain.

QUADRATUS LUMBORUM (MEDIAL FIBRES)

The quadratus lumborum consists of several laminae and is enclosed by the anterior and middle layers of the thoracolumbar fascia (Bogduk 1997, Williams et al 1989) (Fig. 4.5d). The medial portion of the muscle runs from the ilium to the anterior surface of the transverse processes of the lumbar vertebrae, and other fibres travel from the transverse processes to anchor onto the twelfth rib. The lateral portion of the muscle, which belongs to the global system, spans the lumbar area, attaching on the lateral ilium to insert into the twelfth rib without attachment to any vertebrae. The lateral fibres produce primarily a lateral bending moment. The medial portion, while unlikely to make a substantial contribution to lateral flexion (Bogduk 1997), is capable of providing segmental stability via its segmental attachments (McGill et al 1996). Studies investigating the pattern of activation of the quadratus lumborum in functional tasks have been limited because the depth of this muscle means that invasive EMG techniques are required (Andersson et al 1996, McGill et al 1996). In addition, needle insertion for fine-wire EMG is both unpleasant and painful because of the thickness of the fascia surrounding the muscle (P. W. Hodges, M. Comerford, C. A. Richardson, unpublished observations 1995). In two recent studies, which did use fine-wire EMG, recordings were made from a mid portion of the muscle, but there was no clear indication of whether activity was recorded from the lateral or medial portion of the muscle. McGill et al (1996) provided evidence that the quadratus lumborum plays a significant role in the stability of the spine. Muscle activity was measured during a symmetrical bucket-holding task. Activity increased with increasing spinal compression provided through progressive axial loading. Further evidence for the general stabilizing role of the quadratus lumborum was provided by Andersson et al (1996), who found that, unlike the erector spinae (Kipper and Parker 1984), there was no electrical silence of the muscle in full-forward flexion.

While the results of these two studies support the thesis for a stabilizing role for the quadratus lumborum, we regard this muscle as a global stabilizing muscle, capable of controlling the external loads placed on the spine. Interestingly, in patients with back pain, overactivity, tightness and trigger points are often reported by clinicians (Janda 1996, Travell and Simons 1983). Treatment is focused on decreasing activity in the quadratus lumborum rather than increasing it with exercise. The medial portion of the quadratus lumborum may in the future be shown to be functionally separate to the lateral part of the muscle and contribute directly to the segmental support of the spine.

PARASPINAL MECHANISM AND SUPPORT OF THE LUMBAR SPINE: CLINICAL RELEVANCE

The key morphological features of the multifidus that can be related to a role in lumbar stability are the segmental arrangement of the multifidus fascicles (Macintosh et al 1986), the large size of the multifidus at the lumbosacral junction and the close relationship between the multifidus and the zygapophyseal joints. The segmental morphology of the multifidus has implications for rehabilitation. As it is a muscle with segmental innervation and control, rehabilitation can be aimed at specific segments.

The relationship between the multifidus and the thoracolumbar fascia is also important for rehabilitation, as it has been proposed that contraction of the multifidus and the lumbar erector spinae tensions the fascia. It is our contention that the muscles of the abdominal corset that tension the fascias fulfil a vital role in protection of the lumbopelvic region. This mechanism is described and illustrated in Chapter 5.

The multifidus has a high proportion of type I muscle fibres and is well perfused, meaning that it is well suited to a tonic, holding function. EMG analysis has provided further evidence of a tonic or almost continuous activation of the multifidus, particularly the deep fibres. Exercise therapy should be aimed at restoring this function, and an emphasis on activation of the deep fibres for stability is justified. Re-education of the multifidus to promote segmental stabilization is extremely subtle. It is an important principle for therapeutic exercise that isometric contraction of the deep multifidus occurs without spinal or pelvic movement. Patients should be able to contract the muscle slowly.

It has been proved that the multifidus controls the neutral zone and increases segmental stiffness. It has been proposed that contractions of only a very small percentage of the maximum voluntary contraction are required to increase segmental stiffness (Cholewicki and McGill 1996). Furthermore, the deep fibres of multifidus are placed close to the centres of rotation of spinal movement. This means that the length of the muscle fibres remains unchanged in any physiological posture.

The implication for rehabilitation is that isometric contractions of a very small percentage of the maximum voluntary contraction are appropriate, as only small amounts of muscle contraction will be required to protect the vertebral segment. Peripheral feedback from the joint and ligament afferents affects the gamma spindle system (Johansson et al 1991a), and the gamma system biases the spindle towards an increased sensitivity. For this reason, sensory techniques that affect the joint and muscle receptors are important in rehabilitation of the multifidus. Furthermore, the role of the multifidus in maintenance of the normal lordosis provides another important goal of rehabilitation, as it is important that the spine can be adjusted precisely to match the applied loading. Maintenance of the lumbar lordosis requires integration of local, one joint (antigravity) and multijoint/multifunction muscles. Activation of global muscles alone provides insufficient control of the lordosis. As activation of the local muscles (80% of the contribution from the multifidus) decreases forces in the global system, provides stiffness, increases stability and increases compression (Keifer et al 1997, 1998), the multifidus must be re-educated in this role for successful rehabilitation. Integration of local, one joint (antigravity) and multijoint/multifunction muscles must be undertaken for optimal results.

PART 3

The antigravity muscle support system

PART CONTENTS

Chapter 5

Stiffness of the lumbopelvic region for load transfer

Carolyn Richardson and Julie Hides

INTRODUCTION

This chapter initiates the expanded antigravity model of joint protection, which links (via the neural system) the muscles of the trunk, pelvis and limbs for safe load transfer through the body to protect all the weightbearing joints from injury against the high forces of gravity. It explains, as a basis for effective load transfer through the region, how the local muscle system can specifically improve joint stiffness of the lumbar spine and pelvis and enhance the sensory detection of load. Chapter 6 provides the evidence for an antigravity muscle system that links the local and global muscles of the trunk, pelvis and limbs for safe load transfer.

LINKS BETWEEN JOINT STABILIZATION, MUSCLE STIFFNESS AND KINAESTHETIC SENSE

Control of the continuous muscle recruitment for joint stability depends not only on the preprogrammed motor patterns from the cortex but also on the state of the feedback system emanating from the kinaesthetic input. The feedback system is complex and relates to the receptors within the muscle, which provide continuous information to the central nervous system (CNS) on the length and tension being generated in the muscle (for a review see McCloskey 1978). A highly sensitive and accurate information system is required to ensure the control needed to achieve joint support during functional joint movement.

Muscles behave in a similar way to a spring. They resist deformation resulting from internal or external joint loading and tend to return to their original position following lengthening. 'Muscle stiffness', which is a quality reflecting the ratio of force change to length change in the muscle (Johansson et al 1991a,b), is a term used to describe the spring-like qualities of the muscle. Therefore, when a muscle has high stiffness, increased force is required to cause lengthening of the muscle.

Johansson et al (1991a,b) have undertaken much of the neurophysiological research linking muscle stiffness to joint stability. They have described muscle stiffness as having two components: intrinsic and reflex-mediated stiffness. Intrinsic stiffness refers to the viscoelastic properties in the muscle and the existing bonds between the actin and myosin. Reflex-mediated stiffness depends on the excitability of the motor neuron pool, which, in turn, is dependent on the primary spindle afferents set by the degree of stretch of the muscle and the activity of the fusimotor neurons. Muscle stiffness is very closely related to the sensitivity of the proprioceptive sensory organs contained within the muscle itself.

High levels of muscle stiffness in muscles surrounding a joint have been considered a very desirable feature to ensure good stabilization. Recently, descriptions of muscle stiffness have appeared in the biomechanical (Cholewicki and McGill 1996) and the neurophysiological (Johansson et al 1991a,b) literature, with suggestions that muscle stiffness is one of the most critical variables in joint stabilization, with low muscle stiffness generally linked to poor joint stabilization. Muscle stiffness is considered the function of muscle that is most closely related to joint protection and support, rather than the property of muscle strength or endurance. In the development of an in vivo biomechanical model of lumbar stability, Cholewicki and McGill (1996) added muscle stiffness coefficients to their lumbar stability biomechanical model in order to gain more insight into muscle function associated with lumbar stabilization.

Several features of muscle stiffness can be used as the basis for understanding how muscles contribute to joint stabilization. The generation of stiffness in a muscle is linked to the activation of the tonic (postural and slow twitch) motor units (for a review see Burke and Edgerton 1975). The primary muscle afferents potently influence the small gamma motoneurons projecting to the slow-twitch fibres (Johansson and Sojka 1991). Antigravity muscles have a large proportion of gamma motoneuron (fusimotor) representation at the cortex level (Guyton 1981), suggesting that fusimotor activity is a particular feature of muscles controlling the bony skeleton when under the influence of gravitational forces.

The role of muscle stiffness and feedback systems for stabilization, especially under high, unexpected loading of the joint, has always been a matter of debate. Protective reflexes have been shown to be too slow to prevent joint injury (Pope et al 1979). Nevertheless, Johansson et al (1991a,b) viewed the contribution of the spindle system and its fusimotor support more positively. They considered that there is a state of changeable, continuously regulated muscle stiffness at the time of the displacement or trauma that can contribute to joint protection in unexpected loading of the joint. In the knee joint, a link has been established between receptors found in the ligaments of the joint and muscle stiffness (Johansson et al 1991b) (Fig. 5.1).

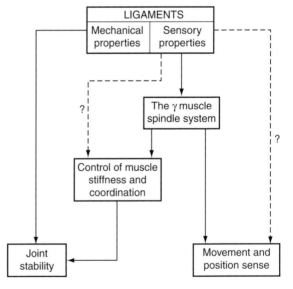

Figure 5.1 Mechanisms by which ligaments may contribute to the regulation of joint stability and proprioception. (Reproduced with permission from Johansson et al 1991a, p. 174.)

The sensory properties of the ligament have been shown to be related to the gamma (fusimotor) spindle system, which, in turn, can determine both muscle stiffness and coordination as well as movement and position sense. In the lumbar spine, stimulation of mechanoreceptors located in the supraspinous ligament, zygapophyseal joints and disc led to reflex recruitment of the multifidus muscle to stabilize the spine (Solomonou et al 1998). The gamma system appears to be the key feature of muscle stiffness. Decreased gamma motoneuron support to a muscle may, therefore, be closely linked to poor joint stabilization.

It is possible that the sensory properties of structures within the joints could be modified by the contraction of the local stability muscles. Besides providing mechanical stability to the joint, local stability muscles could also contribute to the sensory feedback mechanisms associated with the joint structures themselves (i.e. the joint capsules and ligaments). Contraction of these muscles can be associated with a tightening of these passive joint structures and thus indirectly influence their ability to detect movement. In a study involving shoulder movement, tightening of the joint structures with active muscle contraction was found to increase the proprioceptive acuity of the joint (Blasier et al 1994). This may occur in the lumbar spine, where there exists an intimate relationship between the multifidus and the joint capsule of the zygapophyseal joints (see Ch. 4).

This knowledge of the feedback motor control mechanisms and their link to joint stabilization provides the evidence base to address muscle stiffness and proprioception when investigating muscle function associated with joint stabilization. As the tonic motor units of a muscle are linked to these factors, their contribution to the function of a muscle likewise needs to be considered. Tonic motor units are involved in tonic continuous low-load activation of the muscle (Burke and Edgerton 1975). This is in contrast to the strength (high-load) capabilities of muscle function, which are linked to the phasic (fast-twitch) motor units. This emphasis on low-load continuous muscle activation to enhance the ability of a muscle to stabilize joints is strengthened by recent evidence that maximum stiffness can occur at relatively low levels of maximum voluntary contraction because of the multiple factors contributing to muscle stiffness (i.e. intrinsic factors) (Hoffer and Andreassen 1981). In addition, it could be argued that it is the muscle contraction in its shortened range of muscle length that is most critical in establishing the sensitivity and optimal functional capacity of the sensory feedback system of the muscle (Richardson and Sims 1991). A shortened muscle requires increased sensitivity of its spindle system, via gamma motoneuron or fusimotor support, to maintain the shortened length (Guyton 1981).

STIFFNESS OF THE LUMBOPELVIC REGION FOR HIGH-LOAD WEIGHTBEARING

It is our contention that the contraction of a deep musculo-fascial corset, initiated with the maintenance of a neutral spinal posture and firmly pulling in the lower abdominal wall, provides the basic support of the lumbopelvic region for weightbearing, especially under high loading.

The deep musculo-fascial corset

One of the most important functional aspects of the local muscle function (and dysfunction) is the relationship between co-contraction of the transversus abdominis and multifidus muscles and the deep fascial system which surrounds the lumbopelvic region. Our current research is demonstrating that each muscle belly of transversus abdominis, with insertions into the thoracolumbar fascia posteriorly and the abdominal fascia anteriorly, is capable of exerting an effect on lumbopelvic stability through the fascial system.

The realization of the importance of the deep muscle corset concept for the support of the lumbopelvic region has come through the clinical use of real-time ultrasound (Hides et al 1998) (see Appendix, p. 89) and our current research, involving the use of magnetic resonance imaging (MRI). These imaging techniques have allowed the deep musculo-fascial system to be viewed in its normal and dysfunctional state. One important feature of using imaging modalities to examine the corset is that these techniques allow observation of tension and sliding of fascias. As tensioning of the musculo-fascial unit is thought to be a crucial mechanism of

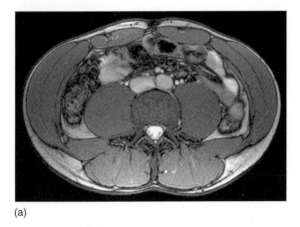
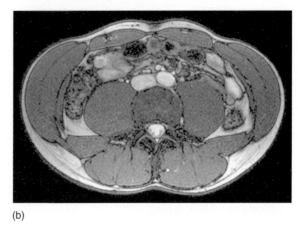

(a)   (b)

Figure 5.2 Magnetic resonance images of a transection through the abdomen at the L4 level to view the 'muscle corset' with (a) a relaxed abdominal wall and (b) during a drawing in of the abdominal wall. Note the shortening contraction of each belly of transversus abdominis.

joint protection and stabilization, this method of investigation has inherent advantages not offered by electromyography (EMG). For example, while fine-wire EMG of the transversus abdominis can detect activity of the muscle, it is impossible to judge whether a concentric or eccentric contraction has occurred and it is impossible to ascertain if tensioning of the fascial system has occurred.

In selected pain-free individuals, a muscular corset is formed automatically in response to a simple instruction to pull in the lower abdomen (without spinal movement occurring). Figure 5.2 shows MRI data demonstrating the relaxed (a) then contracted (b) deep musculo-fascial corset. Importantly, pulling in the abdomen involves symmetrical muscle shortening of each side of transversus abdominis (Fig. 5.2b).

This is visualized using real-time ultrasound imaging in the clinical situation. Real-time ultrasound imaging has a much smaller field of view than MRI. However, its advantages are that it is readily available, is relatively inexpensive and is a safe mode of imaging. Images of the anterolateral abdominal wall can be seen in Figure 5.3. On ultrasound imaging, the fascias are clearly visible, and the three muscles of the anterolateral abdominal wall (obliquus externus abdominis, obliquus internus abdominis and transversus abdominis) are clearly differentiated. There are definite features that can be observed during the drawing in of the

abdominal wall. The features of an optimal pattern of activation include:

1. Transversus abdominis shortens and tensions the anterior abdominal fascia
2. Transversus abdominis thickens in diameter slightly, indicating that it has contracted
3. Transversus abdominis wraps around the waistline (corset action)
4. The dimensions of the obliquus externus abdominis and obliquus internus abdominis remain relatively unchanged
5. The pattern is symmetrical for both sides.

If the abdominal wall is viewed anteriorly, the rectus abdominis on both sides and the anterior fascia can be viewed. If the patient performs a correct activation pattern for the transversus abdominis, the anterior abdominal wall should be seen to move in a posterior direction (Fig. 5.4).

The features of a global pattern of activation include:

1. Transversus abdominis, obliquus externus abdominis, obliquus internus abdominis all thicken and increase their diameters simultaneously, often rapidly
2. Despite contraction of the transversus abdominis, it is evident that the transversus abdominis does not shorten and tension the anterior fascia

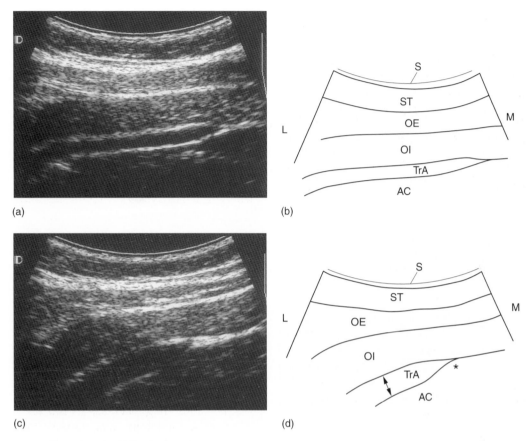

(a) (b)

(c) (d)

Figure 5.3 Sonographic appearance of the anterolateral abdominal wall in transverse section, showing correct pattern of activation for the transversus abdominis. (a) Relaxed abdominal wall. (b) The tissues visible in (a). (c) Correct pattern of activation of the transversus abdominis. Note that transversus abdominis shortens and tensions the anterior abdominal fascia and thickens in diameter slightly, indicating that it has contracted; transversus abdominis wraps around the waistline (corset action) and the dimensions of the obliquus externus abdominis, obliquus internus abdominis remain relatively unchanged. (d) The tissues visible in (c). S, skin; ST, subcutaneous tissue; OE, obliquus externus abdominis; OI, obliquus abdominis internus; TrA, transversus abdominis; AC, abdominal contents; L, lateral; M, medial; *denotes tensioning of the anterior abdominal fascia; ↔, thickening of the transversus abdominis.

3. The transversus abdominis does not wrap around the waistline, and the waistline may in fact, widen rather than narrow
4. The pattern may be asymmetrical between sides.

The sonographic appearance of a global contraction of the abdominal wall is shown in Figure 5.5.

Similarly, the multifidus and lumbar erector spinae are also capable of contributing to the changing tension in the thoracolumbar fascia. The influence of the multifidus and the lumbar erector spinae on the thoracolumbar fascia was investigated by Gracovetsky et al (1977) using a mathematical model. It was proposed in the hydraulic amplifier mechanism that contraction of the muscles exerts a pushing force on the fascia, thus tensioning it and increasing the stiffness of the spine. The insertion of abdominal muscles into the thoracolumbar fascia posteriorly can be seen in Figure 5.6.

Isometric contraction of the multifidus can also be observed using ultrasound imaging (Fig. 5.7). This is best observed in parasagittal section. If the distance from the top of the zygapophyseal joint to the thoracolumbar fascia is measured, this distance is seen to increase on contraction as the myofibrils overlap. It is an important feature to

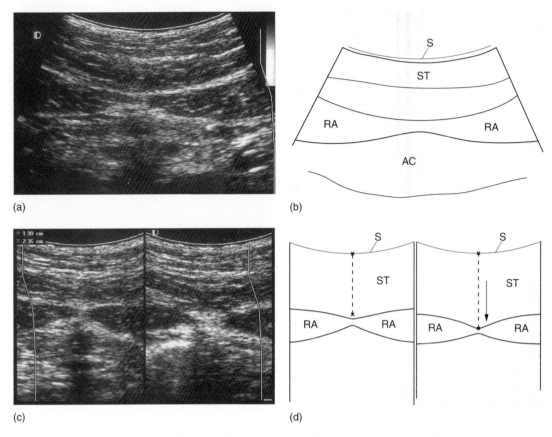

(a)   (b)

(c)   (d)

Figure 5.4 Sonographic appearance of the anterior abdominal wall on correct activation of transversus abdominis. (a) Relaxed abdominal wall. (b) The tissues visible in (a). (c) Split screen view showing displacement of the anterior abdominal wall posteriorly resulting from the correct activation pattern of the transversus abdominis. The image on the left-hand side shows the relaxed abdominal wall. The distance from the skin to the fascia is 1.98 cm. The image on the right-hand side shows evidence of displacement of the anterior abdominal wall, and the distance from the skin to the fascia is 2.36 cm. Imaging anteriorly will also show if there is asymmetry of activation of the transversus abdominis between sides. (d) The tissues visible in (c). S, skin; ST, subcutaneous tissue; RA, rectus abdominis; AC, abdominal contents.

observe that the spine does not move. As the transducer is in contact with the skin, it appears on imaging that the zygapophyseal joints move inferiorly rather than the skin and thoracolumbar fascia move superiorly. In subjects who are unable to perform this isometric contraction, it may be observed that the muscle simply does not contract, or that aberrant patterns are used. These may include a domination of the superficial multifidus fasicles in the pattern, which will generate spinal movement. It is difficult to observe multifidus contraction by the MRI, as the subjects are positioned in supine lying, which compresses the muscle.

In summary, contractions of transversus abdominis as well as the lumbar musculature are capable of changing tension in the fascia. This is demonstrated diagrammatically in Figure 5.8.

The deep corset model of stability would also include the pelvic floor muscles, as explained in Chapter 3 which overviews the abdominal mechanism. It will be argued later in this chapter that the deep corset contraction is also closely linked to other deep muscles of the pelvis and hip.

In order to develop and explain the role of the deep, dynamic muscle corset in relation to weight-bearing, it is important to review the biomechanical models that have been devised in relation to

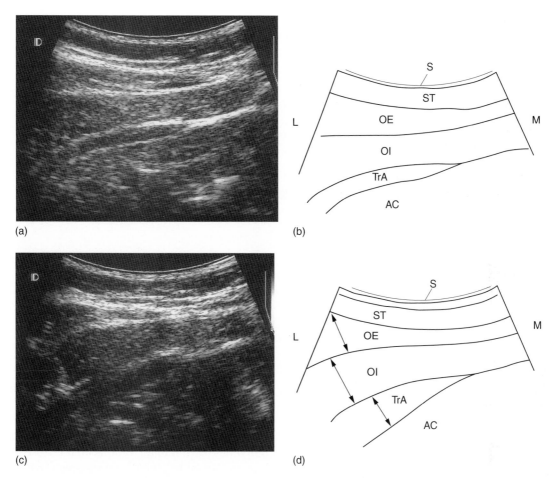

Figure 5.5 Sonographic appearance of the anterolateral abdominal wall in transverse section, showing global activation pattern. (a) Relaxed abdominal wall. (b) The tissues visible in (a). (c) Global pattern of activation. Note that all three muscles of the anterolateral abdominal wall thicken, indicating contraction. However, the contraction of the transversus abdominis does not tension the anterior fascia in this global contraction and does not wrap around the waistline (corset action). (d) The tissues visible in (c). S, skin; ST, subcutaneous tissue; OE, obliquus externus abdominis; OI, obliquus abdominis internus; TrA, transversus abdominis; AC, abdominal contents; L, lateral; M, medial.

weightbearing through the spine as well as weightbearing through the pelvis.

The function of transversus abdominis and multifidus in providing joint stiffness

The importance of neutral spine position for optimal weightbearing and load transfer through the lumbar spine has been emphasized in Chapter 4 in the studies of Keifer et al (1997, 1998). These studies addressed the issue of integration between local and global muscles and highlighted the role of multifidus in maintaining the lumbar lordosis.

The importance of a neutral spinal posture has also been highlighted in other biomechanical perspectives. For example, in a recent text on low back pain, McGill (2002b) detailed the harmful effects of spinal flexion and the 'destabilizing consequences of full flexion' of the spine. This is especially in relation to creep in the passive support structures, which occurs in the dorsal (extensor) aspects of the lumbar spine after prolonged flexion, and which takes some time to re-establish its joint-protective qualities. Therefore, to prevent tissue creep and

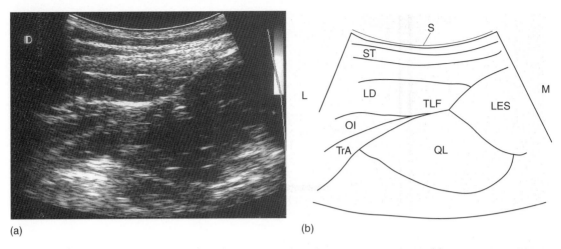

(a)   (b)

Figure 5.6   Sonographic appearance of the posterolateral aspect of the abdominal corset. (a) This image is taken at the level of the third lumbar vertebra and shows the insertion of the transverses abdominis and obliquus externus abdominis into the thoracolumbar fascia. (b) The tissues visible in (a). S, skin; ST, subcutaneous tissue; LD, latissimus dorsi; TLF, thoracolumbar fascia; QL, quadratus lumborum; OI, obliquus internus abdominis; TrA, transversus abdominis; LES, lumbar erector spinae muscles; L, lateral; M, medial.

hence prevent the vunerability of the spine for injury in flexed postures, McGill (2002b) recommended the neutral spinal posture for safety and protection of the lumbar spine for all functional upright tasks as well as for formal strengthening exercises. These models of spinal loading have resulted in increased emphasis on the importance of the neutral spine position for weightbearing, as well as its importance as an optimal position for the integration of the local and global muscle function (expanded in Ch. 6).

The biomechanical aspects of weightbearing in the lumbopelvic region have also been extensively researched by Snijders and colleagues (1995). This team of researchers from Erasmus University in the Netherlands have developed models to explain how the pelvic joints, most importantly the sacro-iliac joints, can resist shear from the force of gravity, as well as resist the extremely high forces developed by the skeletal muscles that have large attachments to the pelvis. Figure 5.9 provides a diagrammatic representation of these concepts (Snijders et al 1995).

The biomechanical model predicts that the action of the transverse fibres of pelvic muscles, such as transversus abdominis, ishiococcygeas and piriformis, can stiffen the sacro-iliac joints (i.e. force closure) and stabilize and support the pelvis for weightbearing, in a similar way to the effects of a belt around the pelvis (Snijders et al 1998). Thus a key function of these transverse muscles for the pelvis is likely to be the control of weightbearing through the lumbopelvic region. Figure 5.10 (from Snijders et al 1995) explains the way a transverse muscle force can be magnified approximately five times (owing to the unique architecture of the human pelvis) to give a compressive force to the sacro-iliac joint. Such an angled force in a more horizontal direction is designed to produce joint stiffness in the coronal plane in order to form a firm platform of pelvic support. Such stiffness is required for efficient and safe, loaded antigravity function in the sagittal plane.

Our recent study completed in collaboration with Snijders and colleagues has studied the biomechanical effect of an independent contraction of transversus abdominis and lumbar multifidus (elicited through instructing the subjects to pull in their abdomen without moving their spine) on the laxity of the sacro-iliac joints (Richardson et al 2002).

Subjects were recruited for the study if they had no low back pain and, on testing with real-time ultrasound, could perform a shortening contraction of transverses abdominis with a drawing in of the abdominal wall. This shortening contraction of transverses abdominis was recorded during the experiment as a real-time ultrasound image in hard

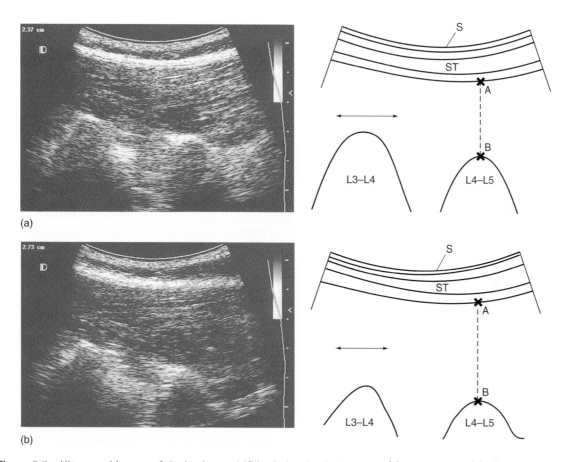

Figure 5.7 Ultrasound images of the lumbar multifidus in longitudinal section: (a) relaxed state; (b) after isometric contraction. The line AB represents the depth of the muscle from its superior aspect to the superior aspect of the L4–L5 zygapophyseal joint. In the relaxed state (a), this is 2.37 cm; on contraction (b), this depth increases to 2.73 cm. S, skin; ST, subcutaneous tissue; ↔, the direction of the fibres in the multifidus.

copy (Fig. 5.11a,b). At this point, it is relevant to emphasize, as explained earlier in this chapter, that the concept of a shortening contraction of transversus abdominis during the draw in manoeuvre is currently being validated in our functional MRI studies.

The subjects were also required to do a 'bracing' contraction, involving all of the abdominal muscles, so that the effect of two different muscle recruitment patterns on pelvic support could be compared. This second abdominal muscle pattern was also assessed visually then recorded using real-time ultrasound (Fig. 5.11a,c). In addition, surface EMG on the abdominal muscles allowed the global response of these muscles, as a result of manoeuvres, to be quantified.

Sacro-iliac joint laxity was measured using Doppler imaging of vibrations. This is a new measurement technique from Erasmus University in which laxity is assessed in the prone, non-weightbearing position. By adding a known vibration to the pelvis from below (via the region of the anterior superior iliac spine), the difference in the resultant frequency of vibration between the sacrum and ilium is measured using Doppler imaging. As these two bones are connected via the sacro-iliac joint, the larger the difference in resultant frequency as it passes through each bone, the greater the laxity in the joint.

The results demonstrated that a specific contraction of the transversus abdominis and multifidus (confirmed using real-time ultrasound) with

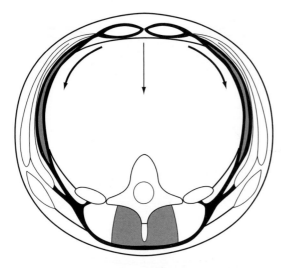

Figure 5.8 The muscle contraction of 'drawing in' of the abdominal wall with an isometric contraction of the lumbar multifidus. The interrelationship and the interaction between these two muscles and the fascial system can be appreciated, and the diagram illustrates how they can work together to give spinal support.

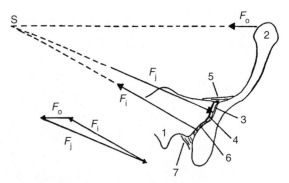

Figure 5.10 Cross-section of the pelvis at the level of the sacro-iliac joints. The application of force by the transversus abdominis and oblique abdominal muscles (F_o), in combination with stiff dorsal sacro-iliac ligaments (F_i), compresses the sacro-iliac joints (F_j). Because the lever arms of the muscle and ligament force are different, the joint reaction force is much greater than the muscle force. 1, Sacrum; 2, iliac bone; 3, joint cartilage; 4, joint space; 5, ventral sacroiliac ligament; 6, interosseous sacro-iliac ligaments; 7, dorsal sacro-iliac ligaments. (Reproduced with permission from Snijders et al 1995, p. 423.)

contraction involving all the muscles of the abdominal wall (Fig. 5.12).

These findings confirm the biomechanical model of the mechanics of the sacro-iliac joint proposed by Snijders et al (1995) in which the transversely oriented muscles such as transversus abdominis are well able to increase the stiffness of the sacro-iliac joints for weightbearing whereas the superficial abdominals are not as efficient. This study has provided some initial evidence of how the transversus abdominis can directly help to stabilize and control the pelvis for weightbearing, and also explains how specific activation of the deep local muscles could exert an effect on pain and pathology of the sacro-iliac joints.

The arguments presented in this chapter have led to two recommended manoeuvres that are essential for loaded function of the lumbopelvic region.

Stiffening manoeuvres to protect and support the lumbopelvic region for weightbearing

The arguments presented in this chapter have led to two recommended manoeuvres that are essential for loaded function of the lumbopelvic region.

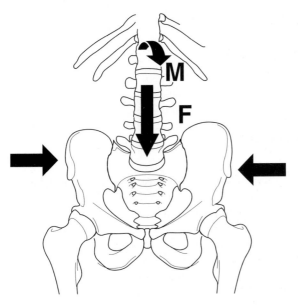

Figure 5.9 Concept that compression of joint surfaces by muscle force helps to prevent shearing. (Reproduced with permission from Snijders et al 1995, p. 420.)

minimal contraction of the superficial abdominal muscles (confirmed with EMG) increased stiffness (or decreased laxity) of the sacro-iliac joints to a greater degree than a higher level 'bracing'

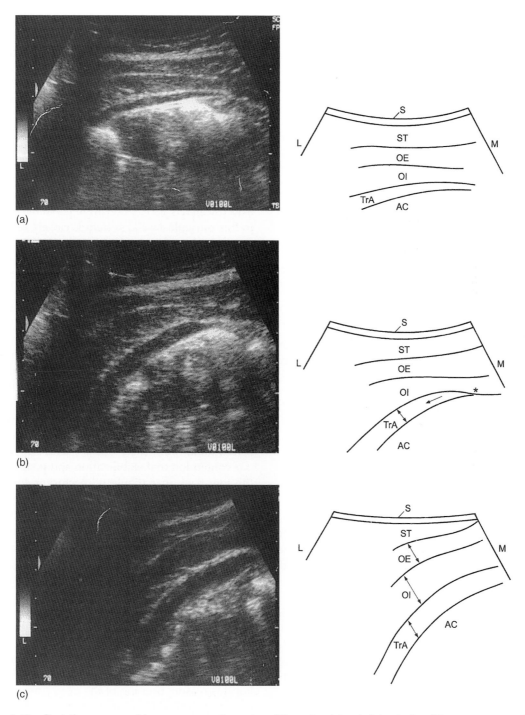

Figure 5.11   Real-time sonographic appearance of muscles of the anterolateral abdominal wall in transverse section during (a) relaxed prone lying; (b) 'draw in' test; (c) 'brace' test. S, skin; ST, subcutaneous tissue; OE, obliquus externus abdominis; OI, obliquus abdominis internus; TrA, transversus abdominis; AC, abdominal contents; L, lateral; M, medial. (Reproduced with permission of Richardson et al 2002, p. 402.)

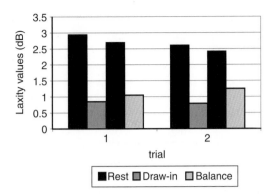

Figure 5.12 Sacro-iliac joint laxity recorded during rest, draw-in exercise and brace exercise. A lower threshold unit represents a stiffer sacro-iliac joint. The draw-in and the brace result in a reduction of joint laxity, but the draw-in test with independent transversus abdominis contraction is more effective. Average values of all subjects measured in two repeated trials. (Reproduced with permission of Richardson et al 2002, p. 404.)

These two conditions apply to activate the local muscles and support the lumbopelvic region for weightbearing.

1. Maintain a neutral lumbar spine (maintain all spinal curves)
2. Draw in the lower abdominal wall, without spinal movement. Check that the corset is activated, i.e. transversus abdominis is forming a shortening (corset) contraction with the manoeuvre, and the lumbar erector spinae are co-contracting isometrically.

Chapters 12 and 15 will explain how the ability to hold neutral spinal curves can be assessed and will discuss research findings that patients with low back pain cannot hold neutral spinal curves in upright working postures. In addition, Chapter 15 explains how to check if transverses abdominis is forming a shortening (corset) contraction automatically in response to the instruction 'draw in the lower abdominal wall' and in this way also assess when the corset cannot be formed, for example, in patients with low back pain.

CLINICAL EVIDENCE OF EFFECTIVENESS OF RETRAINING THE CORSET ACTION

The deep musculo-fascial corset has been implicated in providing the stiffness of the joints of the lumbopelvic region for both movement and weight-bearing function. However, the most significant evidence for importance of the corset in relation to lumbopelvic stability has been in clinical trials where training of this action has resulted in the relief of low back pain symptoms and prevention of recurrence (Hides et al 1996b, 2001, O'Sullivan et al 1997, Golby et al 2001). In these studies, the exercise that is effective in the management of low back pain involves teaching patients to form a dynamic muscle 'corset' involving contraction of transverses abdominis and multifidus. Our current MRI research is also demonstrating that dysfunction in this musculo-fascial system is closely related to the presence of low back pain (Ch. 12).

However, clinical evidence of the effectiveness of retraining the corset action in chronic low back pain has demonstrated that strength training (with the addition of load) is also required to obtain significant improvement in muscle function of multifidus, as assessed by its cross-sectional area (Danneels et al 2000). This can also be inferred from a study where specific stabilizing exercises (teaching the deep corset action) given for 4 weeks did not change the cross-sectional area of multifidus in subjects with chronic low back pain who had undergone surgery (S. Kelley et al 2003, unpublished data). Both these studies lend support for our contention that stabilization and protection of the low back in patients with chronic low back pain also involves higher level strengthening exercise. Our research would seem to suggest that this strengthening exercise should focus on the anti-gravity system, which controls high-load weight-bearing function (Chs 6 and 13).

However, although high-load weightbearing function is important, the initial stage of rehabilitation and prevention (i.e. activation of the deep muscle corset) is recognized as the essential component of developing the joint-protection mechanisms of the lumbopelvic region and forming the 'motor control' building blocks for weightbearing. For this reason, training of the deep corset should remain the initial focus of prevention and rehabilitation programmes (Ch. 14). Once the automatic corset action has been trained, progress to the functional integration of the deep corset with the global muscle system for loaded, antigravity weightbearing can be begun.

APPENDIX: THE USE OF REAL-TIME ULTRASOUND IMAGING IN PHYSIOTHERAPY

Real-time ultrasound imaging has been extensively used in medicine since the 1960s. It allows rapid evaluation of the morphology and pathomorphology of numerous organs and tissues. Its most common application has been in the field of obstetrics, where it has been of special benefit because it does not involve exposure of the fetus to ionizing radiation. Other areas of use in medicine include gynaecology, internal medicine, surgery, orthopaedics, sports medicine, neurology and paediatrics. Ultrasound has proven to be very useful in sports medicine, allowing imaging of muscles, tendons, joints, ligaments and bursae. Real-time ultrasound has proven to be of specific benefit in research and rehabilitation of patients with lumbopelvic pain.

Basic principles and instrumentation

Ultrasound technology is not new and dates back to World War I, where ultrasound was used to detect submarines. It involves sending short pulses of ultrasound into the body and using reflections received from tissue interfaces to produce images of internal structures. Pulsed ultrasound is described by frequency, propagation speed, intensity, attenuation and pulse length (Kremkau 1983). For musculoskeletal imaging, frequencies from 3.5 to 10 MHz are usually used. Similar to the principles taught for therapeutic ultrasound, higher frequencies provide less penetration into the tissues, and lower frequencies are used for penetration into deeper tissues. For imaging, higher frequencies provide less penetration but better image resolution. Lower frequencies provide images of deeper structures, but the trade-off is decreased image resolution. The velocity, or speed, of sound waves in soft tissue is an average of 1540 m/s, and in bone is about 4000 m/s. The sound waves attenuate as they progress through the tissues as a result of reflection, refraction, scattering, absorption and divergence of the beam. At diagnostic frequencies, ultrasound obeys the laws of light in that it is reflected at interfaces, refracts at interfaces and can be focused.

Imaging systems consist of a pulser, transducer, receiver, memory and display. An example of ultrasound equipment is shown in Figure 5.13. Similar to therapeutic ultrasound, diagnostic ultrasound is generated by the piezo-electric effect. This involves conversion of electrical voltages into ultrasound, which is sent into the body, reflected back and reconverted into electrical voltages. For ultrasound imaging, the same transducer is used to send pulses and receive echoes reflected back to it. Various types of transducer are available: multielement transducers of both straight linear and curvilinear arrays. For imaging the multifidus, we have used a 5 MHz curvilinear transducer (Fig. 5.14). It produces a well-defined image of the complex fascial planes of this muscle. This transducer can also be used for the transverses abdominis and generally would be the most useful transducer for this area. For larger patients, a 3.5 MHz transducer may be required. The distance from the transducer to the tissues is determined by travel time. This form of

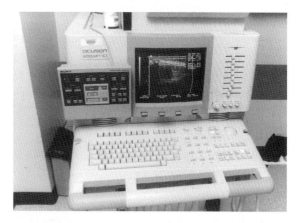

Figure 5.13   Example of real-time ultrasound imaging equipment.

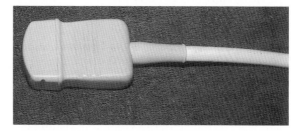

Figure 5.14   A 5 MHz curvilinear transducer used to image the multifidus muscle.

imaging is known as B-mode (brightness mode). Grey scale imaging is a B-mode scanning technique that permits the brightness of the B-mode dots to be displayed in various shades of grey to represent different echo amplitudes (Van Holsbeeck and Introcaso 1992). On an ultrasound image, fluid appears black, whereas reflection from a bone has increased echogenicity and appears white. Muscle often appears black on ultrasound imaging as it is full of fluid (blood).

The advantages of ultrasound imaging are that it is relatively inexpensive and does not involve exposure to ionizing radiation. Its disadvantages are that it is operator dependent, has a limited field of view and its resolution is inferior to MRI and computed tomography scanning.

Use of ultrasound imaging in rehabilitation

The two main uses of real-time ultrasound imaging in rehabilitation are for research and for feedback of muscle activation patterns.

Research

Real-time ultrasound imaging has been used to guide fine-wire electrode placement into the transversus abdominis, internal oblique and external oblique muscles (Cresswell et al 1992a, Hodges and Richardson 1997c). Ultrasound imaging allows visualization of the muscle tissue and the fascias while the needle is being inserted, ensuring accurate placement of the electrodes.

Another research application of real-time ultrasound imaging is measurement of muscle size. This is possible as ultrasound imaging allows measurements in cross-section, thus directly assessing muscle atrophy and hypertrophy. Various muscles have been measured in this way, including quadriceps, anterior tibial muscles and the lumbar multifidus (Stokes and Young 1986, Loo and Stokes 1990, Martinson and Stokes 1991, Hides et al 1992, 1994, 1995, 1996b, Sipila and Suominen 1993, S. Kelley et al 2003, unpublished data, T. Wallwork et al unpublished data). For the multifidus, initial trials were conducted to ascertain if measurement by ultrasound imaging was repeatable (Hides et al 1992). Forty-eight subjects without a history of low

back pain were studied, and multifidus cross-sectional area measurements were performed bilaterally. Results showed good duplication of the measurements and that the multifidus is symmetrical in subjects who have never suffered low back pain. The shape of the muscle varied between male and female subjects. Validity of the measure has also been examined by comparison with MRI (Hides et al 1995). Ten subjects without a history of low back pain were measured using both ultrasound imaging and MRI by blinded assessors. Despite the difference in position of the subjects (prone for ultrasound and supine for MRI), every attempt was made to standardize subject position, as joint position and muscle length may influence cross-sectional area. Figure 5.15 shows a subject in the study undergoing assessment. Multifidus was measured bilaterally at five vertebral levels. Results showed a significant difference in multifidus cross-sectional area between vertebral levels, but no significant difference between the two modalities used. This measure was then used in a longitudinal randomized

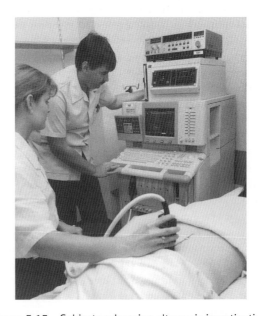

Figure 5.15 Subject undergoing ultrasonic investigation of multifidus cross-sectional area. To replicate the position of the hips in the magnetic resonance scanner, which were flexed, the hips were flexed to the same angle in the prone position by tilting the bottom half of the bed for ultrasound examination.

clinical trial involving subjects with acute low back pain. One group underwent specific multifidus rehabilitation and there was a control group (Hides et al 1996b, 2001). It had been essential to establish repeatability, reliability and validity of the measure prior to its adoption as the study depended upon repeated measures. If measurement error was large, it would have masked the effects of the intervention. Examination of the multifidus in parasagittal section revealed its unusual morphology. Because of depth differences over the course of one vertebral level, landmarks had to be used to ensure that measurements were accurate. The vertebra lamina provided such a landmark. The measurement of multifidus is a difficult parameter and should only be adopted after repeatability and reliability studies have been established.

Ultrasound imaging has also been used to assess the stiffness of the sacro-iliac joint (Damen et al 2002, Richardson et al 2002). Subjects were positioned in prone lying, and vibrations from a mechanical vibrator were applied unilaterally to the anterior superior iliac spine. The vertical vibrations propagated from the ilium to the sacrum, depending on the laxity of the intervening sacro-iliac joint. The vibrations of the ilium and the sacrum were detected by a colour Doppler imaging transducer (Doppler imaging of vibrations). The measure has been validated on measurements made on a model pelvis and on embalmed human pelvises (Damen et al 2002). Reliability has also been demonstrated (Damen et al 2002).

Feedback of muscle activation

One of the main advantages of real-time ultrasound imaging is that muscle contraction can be imaged as it actually occurs. This is very useful in rehabilitation as it can provide direct feedback to the subject and enhances learning.

The use of ultrasound imaging to provide feedback of multifidus muscle activation was reported by Hides et al (1996b). The multifidus was imaged in longitudinal (parasagittal section) and patients were asked to 'swell' the multifidus gently, which was a gentle isometric contraction. On the ultrasound image, the muscle was seen to increase in depth as the muscle contracted, providing immediate visual feedback of muscle activation to the subjects as they

contracted the muscle. The effect of ultrasound as a form of feedback on motor learning of the multifidus isometric contraction has been investigated (K. Van et al 2003, unpublished data; Fig. 5.16). Two groups of subjects without a history of low back pain were taught how to contract the multifidus isometrically but only one group received visual feedback of the contraction. The group who received the feedback of multifidus activation via the ultrasound maintained the skill significantly better than the subjects of the control group. This measurement of the increase in muscle depth of the multifidus on isometric contraction has been shown to be repeatable and reliable (K. Van et al 2003, unpublished data, T. Wallwork et al, unpublished data).

The transversus abdominis, internal oblique and external oblique muscles can be imaged quite easily using ultrasound imaging. The transducer is placed lateral to the umbilicus, on the anterolateral aspect of the abdominal wall. The intimate relationship between abdominal muscles and their fascial attachments can be clearly witnessed using ultrasound imaging. The corset action of the transversus abdominis is easily observed. When the muscle contracts and shortens, it is seen to pull its anterior fascial attachments in a lateral direction. This should occur evenly bilaterally, and if it does, it will pull the anterior abdominal wall in a posterior direction. The features we look for in a good activation pattern are (a) that transversus abdominis tensions its fascial attachment and pulls it laterally; (b) that transversus abdominis wraps around the waistline (corset action); (c) that transverses abdominis thickens slightly; and (d) that internal oblique and external oblique remain relatively inactive. We are currently validating the ultrasound assessment of abdominal activation patterns by comparison with MRI in subjects with and without a history of low back pain. The advantage of the MRI is that the whole corset can be imaged at once, as it has a much wider field of view than the ultrasound imaging. We believe that a symmetrical concentric contraction of the transversus abdominis is the ideal pattern of activation. This study is providing fascinating insights into the corset mechanism and should help to generate simple measurements of corset efficiency.

The relationship between the increase in muscle thickness observed during contraction on ultrasound imaging and EMG activity has been

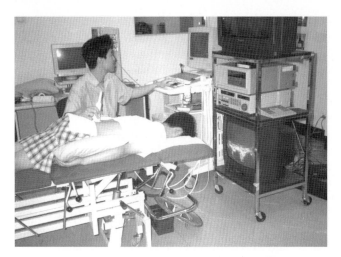

Figure 5.16 Subject performing isometric contraction of the multifidus with visual feedback provided by ultrasound imaging. The subject is viewing the contraction through a hole in the bed, and the ultrasound image is being displayed on a TV monitor and reflected by a mirror, to allow the subject to view the screen with the head placed in the midline.

examined for the transversus abdominis (Hodges et al 2003d). Results showed that the relationship was good for the transversus abdominis and the internal oblique muscle at low levels of maximum voluntary contraction. The relationship was not as close for the external oblique, probably related to the architecture of the muscle and orientation of its fibres. Surface EMG should, therefore, be used in addition to ultrasound imaging of the internal oblique and transversus abdominis to give an adequate indication of activation of the three muscles of the anterolateral abdominal wall. We used this combination of measures to verify the patterns of abdominal activation in our recent study of the effects of muscle activation on the stiffness of the sacro-iliac joint (Richardson et al 2002).

Chapter **6**

The role of weightbearing and non-weightbearing muscles

Carolyn Richardson

INTRODUCTION

The development of exercise principles for the integration of local and global muscles for stability of the lumbopelvic region has been based on an increased understanding of the antigravity joint protection mechanisms. This awareness was also important in order to appreciate how to expand and integrate local muscle function into high-load joint support. In this way, load can be safely and effectively added to the joint support systems during a progressive exercise programme for the treatment and prevention of low back pain.

The antigravity joint protection mechanisms depend not only on the stiffness developed in the lumbopelvic region for weightbearing (Ch. 5) but also on the close links with the antigravity muscle support system of the trunk and limbs. It will be argued in this chapter that effective antigravity joint protection mechanisms rely on the balanced integrated function of weightbearing and non-weightbearing muscles. In order to explain this concept, it is first important to explain how the muscle function involved in protecting joints from injury sits within the framework of upright functional postures.

ANTIGRAVITY MUSCLE SYSTEMS AND THE CONTROL OF POSTURE

Massion (1998) in a review of postural control systems has explained that the function of posture can be divided into two main functions:

- antigravity function, where the opposing force of gravity is considered; and
- providing an interface with the external environment or a reference frame for organizing movement (grasping, reaching).

It is considered that posture develops initially from providing a way to interact with the external environment and that antigravity organization is the last phase of development. This is logical when one considers that the adaption to a weightbearing erect posture is an important task for the sensory motor system in early childhood development. Massion (1998) also proposed that the antigravity organization function of posture can, in turn, be divided into two aspects of function:

- providing the mechanical support necessary to perform movements, including providing joint stiffness and muscle recruitment in the antigravity extensors; such stiffness needs to be adjusted to provide joint support for movement;
- controlling balance and body sway.

Most research into the antigravity organization function of posture has considered the second aspect, that is, controlling balance and body sway in an erect standing posture (Fig. 6.1a), while little research has focused on investigating joint stiffness and muscle recruitment of the antigravity extensors in a flexed, working or loaded posture (Fig. 6.1b).

This chapter deals with the integrated function of weightbearing and non-weightbearing muscles, to produce antigravity joint stiffness and joint protection. The functional patterns of use for the weightbearing and non-weightbearing muscles required for joint protection are not necessarily the same as for the muscles recruited to control balance and body sway.

MODELS TO DEFINE SKELETAL MUSCLE FUNCTION IN ANTIGRAVITY JOINT PROTECTION

An anatomical model

To understand the function of the antigravity joint protection mechanisms and the integration of the

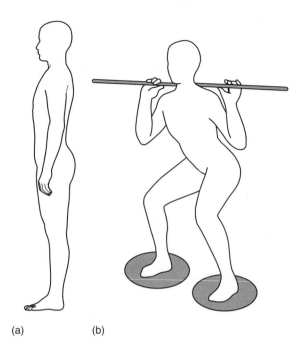

(a)   (b)

Figure 6.1   Comparison between (a) an upright posture and (b) an erect, working or loaded posture.

local and global systems for joint protection, it is first important to differentiate the global muscle synergists into two different anatomical based categories: one-joint (or uniarticular) and multijoint (multiarticular, two or more joints) muscles.

To this point, the focus of the joint protection mechanisms has been on the local and the global (torque-producing) muscles. From a mechanical viewpoint, one-joint muscles are closely related to a single joint position and movement direction, which can be controlled through the muscle contracting isometrically, concentrically or eccentrically. In comparison, multijoint muscles are mechanically multifunctional, affecting many joint movements and are often involved in the control of a single joint in many different directions (van Ingen Schenau et al 1992). Theoretically, these two types of muscle synergist pass over a single reference joint under load and will both contribute to force production in one movement direction (e.g. knee extension).

This chapter focuses on the evidence for the different roles of the two categories of global muscles for antigravity protective function. Joint protection, when opposing the force of gravity, is required for

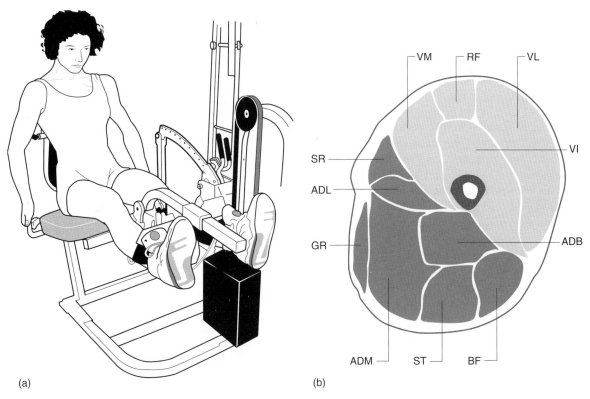

(a)

(b)

Figure 6.2   (a) Resisted knee extension in sitting. (b) Magnetic resonance images depicting quadriceps pattern of use during (a). AD B, adductus brevis; AD L, adductus longus; AD M, adductus magnus; BF, biceps femoris; GR, gracilis; RF, rectus femoris; SR, sartorius; ST, semitendinosus; VM, vastus medialis; VL, vastus lateralis; VI, vastus intermedius. (Reproduced with permission of Tesch 1993, p. 47.)

safe loaded weightbearing. Such joint protection is determined by the muscle recruitment patterns at each joint of the limb opposing gravitational force. As far as the global muscles are concerned, it will be argued that it is predominantly the one-joint (or one area of the spine) extensors of the trunk and limbs that are the weightbearing muscles, providing the mechanical support and joint protection for functional loaded postures (see Fig. 6.1b) and that these muscles are closely linked to the function of the local muscle system. The multijoint muscles, which have multiple functions in relation to joint movement, do not, in normal erect working postures, have a weightbearing role (i.e. they are non-weightbearing muscles).

This concept will be developed using the muscles and joints of the lower limb as the model. The role of the muscles of the upper quadrant in antigravity weightbearing function, and their links to weight

transfer through the trunk, is a topic for our on-going research into weightbearing mechanisms and joint protection.

Recruitment patterns of synergists in open chain exercise loading

Before describing a differential function for one-joint and multijoint muscles, it is first important to recognize that in most loaded exercise situations, both one-joint and multijoint synergists are recruited together to provide the force to oppose the external resistance. For example, resisted knee extension in sitting (Fig. 6.2a) requires the recruitment of all of the quadriceps muscles, including the one-joint vasti and the multijoint vastus medialis oblique. This is illustrated schematically in the functional magnetic resonance images (MRI) by Tesch (1993) depicting high muscle use (white), medium muscle use (grey) and lack of use (black). These MRI images, which are taken before and after a loaded knee extension exercise, demonstrate the pattern of use of the muscles. Figure 6.2b demonstrates the high use (white) of all quadriceps synergists during the exercise. Also important to note is the lack of use (black) of the mutijoint hamstring muscles (antagonists) as well as lack of use of all the adductors muscles of the hip. Consequently, exercise to increasing strength, power and endurance of muscles around a single joint by traditional means involves the use of all muscles in the movement direction of the force, with relaxation of the main antagonist set of muscles. It is likely that such exercise in this example does not include the adductor muscles (Fig. 6.2b). Therefore, it could be argued that reduced function of the adductor magnus, which functions as an extensor of the hip in weight-bearing (reviewed by Hodges and Richardson 1993) could, over a period of time, result in reduced pelvic stabilization for weightbearing.

Recruitment patterns of synergists in closed chain exercise loading

Completely different recruitment patterns of the one-joint and multijoint muscle synergists of the quadriceps occur in closed chain loading. Closed chain loading involves joint compression, with proximal and distal segments moving together to load longitudinally through the body including through the feet.

Compared with open chain loading, closed chain exercise loading highlights the differential function of the one- and multijoint muscles, with the one-joint muscles recruited optimally to oppose external resistance. For example, resisted knee extension in lying (closed chain) (Fig. 6.3a) requires the recruitment of all of the one-joint vasti muscles but does not use the multijoint rectus femoris. This is illustrated schematically in the functional MRI illustrations by Tesch (1993) depicting quadriceps level of use after a loaded, closed chain knee extension exercise in the form of the leg press. Figure 6.3b demonstrates the high use (white) of the vasti synergists during the exercise. Most importantly, there is lack of use (black) of the multijoint hamstring muscles as well as the multijoint hip muscles (e.g. sartorius). This type of

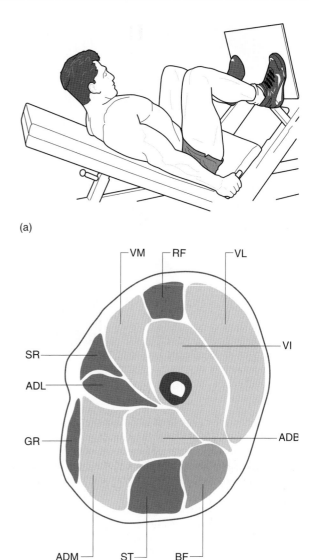

(a)

(b)

Figure 6.3   (a) Closed chain resisted knee extension. (b) MRI depicting quadriceps pattern of use during (a). AD B, adductus brevis; AD L, adductus longus; AD M, adductus magnus; BF, biceps femoris; GR, gracilis; RF, rectus femoris; SR, sartorius; ST, semitendinosus; VM, vastus medialis; VL, vastus lateralis; VI, vastus intermedius. (Reproduced with permission of Tesch 1993, p. 59.)

exercise is also well suited to recruitment of the large one-joint adductor muscles of the hip (e.g. adductor magnus and brevis).

A more functional closed chain exercise would be a 'squat' or 'lunge' exercise. Importantly, the

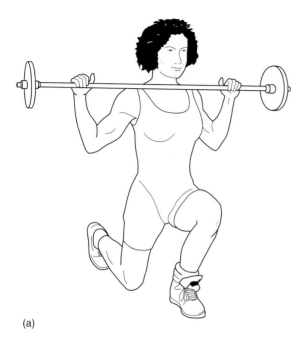

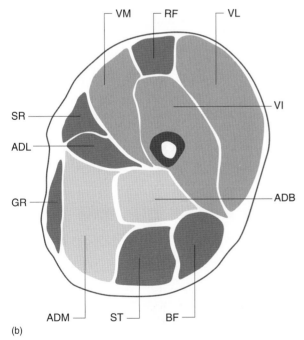

(a)

(b)

Figure 6.4 (a) Lunge exercise. (b) MRI depicting quadriceps pattern of use during (a). AD B, adductus brevis; AD L, adductus longus; AD M, adductus magnus; BF, biceps femoris; GR, gracilis; RF, rectus femoris; SR, sartorius; ST, semitendinosus; VM, vastus medialis; VL, vastus lateralis; VI, vastus intermedius. (Reproduced with permission of Tesch 1993, p. 46.)

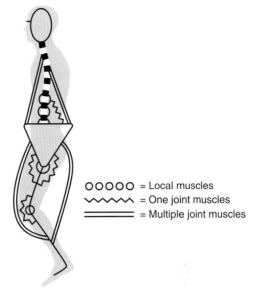

○○○○○ = Local muscles
〰〰〰 = One joint muscles
═══ = Multiple joint muscles

Figure 6.5 The one joint muscles are stretched under the force of gravity in weightbearing, while the multijoint muscles are more likely to be in a more shortened (relaxed) position.

lunge exercise with shoulder load (Fig. 6.4a) has the same muscle recruitment patterns (Fig. 6.4b) as the leg press (Fig. 6.3b; Tesch 1993).

However, although squat and lunge exercise performed in the erect posture are more functional than the leg press, it should be recognized that these exercises also include the balance and sway aspects of antigravity, upright posture function, and it may be more difficult to control the joint loading and levels of individual antigravity muscle recruitment for treatments. This aspect of progressive exercise will be discussed in detail in Chapter 15.

Increasing strength, power and endurance of muscles involving several joints in the kinetic chain in closed chain exercise involves a different set of muscle synergists. From a biomechanical point of view, some muscles (i.e. the one-joint muscles) are stretched under the force of gravity in weightbearing (i.e. closed chain) activities (Fig. 6.5), while the non-weightbearing, multijoint muscles are more likely to be placed in a more shortened relaxed position, as while they are stretched over one joint, they are relaxed over another (Fig. 6.5).

Consequently, it can be argued that the antigravity (one-joint) muscles, which are under stretch (tend to lengthen) with gravity load, are providing joint protection and support in the erect working or loaded posture. These muscles would also be important for the transfer of load in this position.

There is some initial evidence that the local muscles and one-joint muscles are closely linked together in antigravity function. An EMG study of Hodges and Richardson (1993) demonstrated that co-activation of adductor magnus (one-joint hip muscle) and vastus medialis oblique (a local muscle of the knee) was significantly higher in weight-bearing than in non-weightbearing situations. This study also suggested that a strong link may exist between weightbearing function of the muscles of the hip and the knee joints.

Closed chain exercise involving the trunk and upper limbs is likely to present the same pattern of activation that is observed for the trunk and lower limbs (i.e. recruitment of the one-joint antigravity muscles with relaxation of the multijoint muscles). In an MRI assessment of the three heads of the triceps brachii during overhead (antigravity) upper limb extension with heavy weights, Tesch (1993) reported that there was maximal recruitment of the one-joint heads of the muscle, with relaxation of the multijoint head of the muscle (Fig. 6.6). Future research into the possible relaxation of the latissimus dorsi and pectoralis muscle during this type of closed chain exercise for the trunk and upper limbs may prove useful in establishing the

joint protective mechanisms of the lumbopelvic region as well as being useful in the prevention (and treatment) of many shoulder pathologies.

Although the antigravity (one-joint) muscles are recruited in closed chain activity, there is evidence that these muscles providing joint protection and support are not used in some non-weightbearing conditions, for example where body weight is minimized and increasing speed is used to increase the level of muscle contraction for training.

Recruitment patterns of synergists in fast ballistic, open chain exercise

Interaction of the one-joint and multijoint synergists with open chain, ballistic movement (speed loading) results in recruitment patterns that are the direct antithesis to the patterns seen in closed chain loading conditions. That is, this pattern of exercise favours the multijoint muscles, with the antigravity one-joint muscles not responding.

Some of the first evidence for this differential function of one-joint and multijoint muscles came from research involving fast ballistic flexion/extension movements of the knee, involving the quadricep and hamstring muscle groups. Richardson and Bullock (1986) studied subjects performing knee flexion/extension movements in a prone position at progressive increases in speed and with individual muscle recruitment measured with surface EMG. A spring was attached to the ankle at a set angle (Fig. 6.7) to deload the lower

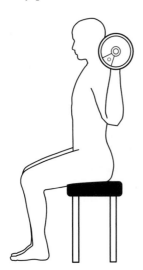

Figure 6.6 Antigravity upper limb extension with heavy weights.

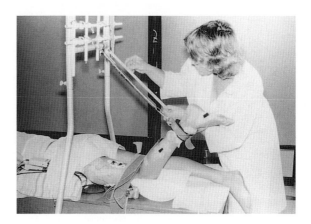

Figure 6.7 The exercise model with a spring attachment to reduce the load of the lower leg to zero during the high-speed ballistic task.

leg and minimize the effect of gravity during the movement. Biomechanical analysis showed how the spring negated the leg load. The movement model, which involved ballistic movement with no time for sensory feedback, was considered to be a largely preprogrammed action (Desmedt and Godaux 1978) and, therefore, operated under 'open loop' motor control conditions. In ballistic movement conditions where the gravitational load cues had been eliminated, recruitment of the multijoint rectus femoris and hamstrings increased significantly with increasing speeds while the recruitment of the one-joint vastus lateralis and the local muscle vastus medialis oblique was not affected (Fig. 6.8). This is demonstrated schematically in Figure 6.9.

Most importantly, the local muscle vastus medialis oblique was recruited tonically in 90% of subjects during the high-speed phasic movement, indicating that it was not involved in lower leg movement when gravitational load cues were eliminated. Interestingly, vastus lateralis was also recruited tonically in 40% of subjects. These results provide some evidence that both the local muscle vastus medialis oblique and the one-joint muscle vastus lateralis do not respond to movement cues given through fast ballistic knee movement. This may indicate that these synergists are recruited together, as proposed earlier in this chapter, for the antithesis of this exercise movement: the antigravity, weightbearing function.

Following this knee muscle research, Ng and Richardson (1990) studied the effect on the function of the lower leg muscles of a 6-week exercise programme involving rapid (ballistic) ankle plantar flexion. While jumping height improved, the isometric strength of the soleus was significantly

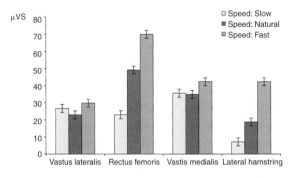

Figure 6.8 Electromyographic activity measured over three movement cycles with the ballistic exercise. Note the relative increase in activity of the rectus femoris and hamstrings (multijoint muscles). (Reproduced with permission from Richardson and Bullock 1986, p. 55.)

AD B = Adductor brevis
AD L = Adductor longus
AD M = Adductor magnus
BF = Biceps femoris
GR = Gracilis
RF = Rectus femoris
SR = Sartorius
ST = Semitendinosis
VM = Vastus medialis
VL = Vastus lateralis
VI = Vastus intermedius

Stand, look down at your right leg, and imagine looking into a slice (cross-section) of your right thigh.

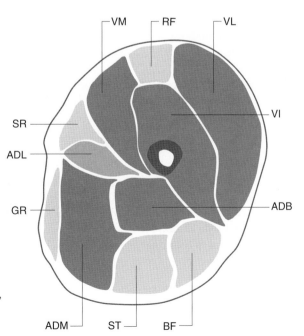

Figure 6.9 The high use of the multijoint muscles and low use of the one joint muscles during non-weightbearing ballistic exercise, adapted from the model used by Tesch.

Table 6.1   Summary of Rood's approach to the differentiation of muscle

	Muscles active in patterns of functional mobility (mobilizers)	Muscles active in patterns of functional stability (stabilizers)
Example muscles	Multiarthrodal muscles, flexors, adductors (vasti)	One-joint extensors and abductors
Fibre type	Fusiform, fibres parallel to the long axis	Bipennate (fan shaped or irregular), fibres run obliquely
Location	More superficial (and more lateral)	Located deeply and more medial
Relationship to joint	Muscle fibres further from the joint on which they act	Fibres cross one major joint
Activity	More active when distal lever is free and non-weightbearing	Function in heavy work, associated with joint compression as in weightbearing
Leverage	More active in light work of smaller lever acting on the larger one, in skill activities	More active in movement of heavier larger object while lighter lever is fixed
Active period	Work to initiate movement and perform bursts of activity (phasic)	Capable of prolonged holding especially in a stretched position (tonic, continuous activity)
Threshold of stimulation	Low	High
Motor units affected	Mainly quick acting	Mainly slow acting

From Stockmeyer 1967.

reduced. Therefore, rapid movement favoured recruitment of the multijoint gastrocnemius, with decreased use of the one-joint muscle soleus. This research is in line with the argument that repetitive rapid movement is more likely to recruit predominately the multijoint muscles.

Of interest, this type of speed loading, especially in non-weightbearing, results in high muscle activation levels, which are accompanied by joint distraction rather than joint compression. With less joint loading involved, this type of exercise is usually more comfortable for the patients with joint injury and pain. However, it is important to consider that this type of exercise loading heavily favours the multijoint muscles and reduces the contribution of the one-joint muscles.

A neurophysiological model

Neurophysiologists Desmedt and Godaux (1978) contributed significantly to knowledge in this area of muscle control. They described two types of voluntary movement. 'Ramp' movements (which can be fast or slow) are those that are continuously controlled by sensory input from the periphery, with motor commands guided by the feedback system. This type of movement is similar to closed kinetic chain function, which demonstrates a dominance of the one-joint, weightbearing muscles. The antithesis of ramp movement is 'ballistic' movement, involving largely a preprogrammed action with minimal possibility of modification (sensory feedback) because of its rapid nature. This is demonstrated in the rapid knee flexion/extension model, which demonstrates a dominance of multijoint, non-weightbearing muscles. Desmedt and Godaux (1978) acknowledged that these represent the extremes of motor function, with most functional activities consisting of a combination of both types of movement.

The differing recruitment patterns of human weightbearing and non-weightbearing muscles at the two extremes of function are very similar to the functional categorization of muscles in animals. Since the last part of the 19th century, physiologists have recognized that 'fast' and 'slow' muscles exist in animals. Denny-Brown (1929) completed histological studies on various animal muscles and came to the conclusion that, as a general rule, the red slow muscles (which exhibit longer twitch contraction duration) form the deeper layers of skeletal muscle, have shorter tendons and consist

Table 6.2   Muscle recruitment with extremes of exercise conditions

Weightbearing muscles	Non–weightbearing muscles
One-joint muscles (and local muscles) Separation in extreme closed loop motor function	*Multijoint/multifunction muscles* Separation in extreme open loop motor function
Exercise: closed chain exercise Static weightbearing Antigravity working postures Joint compression	*Exercise: open chain exercise* Rapid, ballistic movement Eliminate gravity Joint distraction

of units with low threshold for postural reflexes. The extensors at each joint, as an undifferentiated group, belong to this type of muscle, except for the double joint, more superficial extensors, which, together with all flexor groups, develop as more rapidly contracting muscles (i.e. the pale, fast muscles).

Interestingly, it was with these types of study in mind that Rood (1962) developed her theories on muscle types as a basis for rehabilitation. She suggested that fast 'mobilizers' (multijoint muscles) were made up of fast contracting motor units and were involved in rapid skilled movements, while the slow 'stabilizers' (one-joint muscles) consisting of slow-contracting motor units were involved in weightbearing stabilizing function. In 1967, Stockmeyer wrote a clinical interpretation of the Rood approach, which has implications for treatment and prevention of musculo-skeletal injuries such as low back pain. This approach is summarized in Table 6.1.

It could be argued from information provided earlier in this chapter that the ideas of Denny-Brown (1929) and Rood (1962) may be, in many ways, acceptable today. However, as more recent studies of muscle fibre types in humans have established that, unlike animals, skeletal muscles consist of a variable 50:50 mixture of fast and slow twitch muscle fibres, the differences in function of muscle synergists can only be explained in terms of differences in motor control rather than fibre type predominance. This would be an important area for neurophysiological research on which to base exercise models.

In summary, the global muscle synergists (weightbearing and non-weightbearing muscles) demonstrate differential muscle recruitment patterns at the extremes of the ramp (closed chain) and ballistic exercise conditions. Table 6.2 summarizes the extreme conditions of exercise and the muscle synergists involved.

THE CONTROL AND CO-ORDINATION OF ONE-JOINT AND MULTIJOINT MUSCLES

The co-ordination of one-joint and multijoint musles in the dynamic interaction of body segments remains an issue of intense debate in the current motor control literature. Prilutsky (2000) highlighted the 'spring like' behaviour of multijoint muscles, and their efficiency in multijoint movements in facilitating energy transfer between joints; he also provided arguments, from an evolutionary viewpoint, that having only one-joint muscles would produce inefficient movements.

Bobbert and van Soerst (2000), in a commentary on Prilutsky's paper, provided more evidence for the multijoint muscles being considered the solution to the problems of evolution and increasing efficiency of movement. They presented arguments to explain how multijoint muscles are coordinated to favour their force–velocity relationships to give an efficient, skilled performance. The problem from a health science perspective is how the nervous system deals with the resultant unfavourable length-tension relationships in the one-joint muscles, which must offer 'directional restraint' to the joints through all ranges of functional movement. This would be the most challenging to one-joint muscle control when they are in their shortened position, with resultant unfavourable length–tension relationships (see Ch. 7).

Interestingly, Bobbert and van Soerst (2000) reflected on the hypothesis of van Ingen Schenau et al (1994) who suggested that one-joint muscles are recruited in high-energy tasks based on spindle information in order that these muscles can be activated in their shortened range. They suggested that other sensory information relating to movement information, including the line of action of the forces, would be more important for the multijoint muscles. Chapter 7 lends support to these theories that one-joint and multijoint muscles can be separated in terms of reliance on different types of sensory information, and it goes on to argue that the one-joint system primarily has a weightbearing (antigravity) role while the multijoint system has a non-weightbearing role.

Therefore, although a better movement performance would be expected if all muscles were multijoint, we propose that, for the health field, the one-joint muscles should be considered the solution to the problems of evolution, where their roles in the adjustment of the body segments to an erect posture (against the forces of gravity) and in supporting and protecting the weightbearing joints during functional movement become the most important issues of motor control, in relation to the co-ordination of the one- and multijoint muscles.

BASIS FOR AN ANTIGRAVITY EXERCISE MODEL

The separation of function of non-weightbearing and weightbearing muscles at the extremes of the motor control continuum has important implications for rehabilitative and preventative exercise. Non-weightbearing muscles are facilitated in ballistic motor tasks at one extreme of the control model while weightbearing muscles are facilitated at the other extreme (i.e. in ramped (closed chain) motor tasks). This could be how impairments develop through lack of use of the weightbearing muscles,

and overuse of the non-weightbearing muscles, when the ballistic motor function is dominant. This model could also form the basis of treatment of overactive non-weightbearing muscles, and underactive weightbearing muscles, as the closed chain exercise models are likely to facilitate weightbearing muscle function and 'turn off' the more active non-weightbearing muscle system.

It was argued in Chapter 5 that providing joint stiffness (and muscle stiffness) to the lumbopelvic region for high-load antigravity function of muscles requires very specialized motor control strategies for that region. The second part of the integration phase, with the local muscles integrating with the global muscles, is gained through focusing on the close links between the local and the weightbearing muscles and, therefore, the muscle corset (Ch. 5) combined with closed chain exercise for the weightbearing muscles (and which differentiates weightbearing from non-weightbearing muscles) would be the rehabilitative and preventative exercise of choice.

Training and improving the joint protection mechanisms is based on normal function of the muscle system for joint protection (Chs 2–6) as well as on changes that occur in the muscle system with dysfunction associated with prolonged deloading (Ch. 7), injury (Ch. 8) and pain (Ch. 9). This chapter has focused on the functional categorization of synergistic muscles, and the various patterns of muscle function related to the addition of load to the joints in exercise. Chapter 7 will deal with deloading and loss of antigravity function and how it differentially affects the weightbearing muscles (including local muscles) in a different way to the non-weightbearing muscles; this leads to impairments in the joint protection mechanisms and to the development of joint injury.

SECTION 3

Impairment in the joint protection mechanisms: concepts

Chapter 7

The deload model of injury

Carolyn Richardson

INTRODUCTION

Numerous research studies have been undertaken by many health-related professions in an effort to find the aetiology of mechanical low back pain and generate effective preventative strategies. The development of mechanical low back pain is considered by many clinicians and researchers to be a consequence of tissue loading, which results (often over long periods of time) in tissue failure in structures associated with the vertebral discs as well as other joint structures of the spine (e.g. zygopophyseal joints) and pelvis (e.g. sacro-iliac joints). McGill (2002b), an internationally respected researcher in low back pain disorders and their prevention, explained that the prediction of risk of tissue damage occurs when the applied load is greater than tissue strength. Tissue damage is most commonly considered to result from the application of high forces to the body (e.g. high impact or compressive loading to the spine or through incorrect lifting and working techniques). Such tissue failure can result in the development of painful symptoms from a variety of potential pain sources in the region. This process could occur in one single incident or through accumulated trauma over longer periods of time.

In line with these concepts of increased tissue loading leading to tissue failure and subsequent pain, most strategies for prevention address the issue of high tissue loading and concentrate on methods of reducing the forces and loads on the spine. Biomechanical and anatomical research studies have led to an evidence base for the many methods of lowering spinal loads (review by McGill 2002b). These include the very important strategies of posture training, focusing on neutral spine, and instructing on safe ways of lifting and moving heavy objects and reducing asymmetry during lifting and other functional tasks.

It is important to realize that tissue failure results in joint injury and pain, with subsequent changes in muscle function, including muscle size (inhibition) as well as motor control changes. These issues need to be considered for management of low back pain and are detailed in Chapter 8 (injury) and Chapter 9 (pain).

This chapter deals with the aetiology of low back pain from a different, new perspective to that of the high-load model of injury. Prediction of tissue damage to the joints increases owing to the neuromuscular plasticity of muscle in response to a reduction in weightbearing (deloading). While this concept is not, in itself, new, the argument presented in this chapter is that weightbearing muscles and non-weightbearing muscles are differentially affected in deloaded situations. The former, which are primarily involved in joint protection, tend to atrophy, become more fatiguable and exhibit specific sensory motor changes. The latter, by comparison, tends to hypertrophy, become less fatiguable and display the antithesis of the sensory motor changes depicted in the weightbearing muscles. It is these selective impairments in weightbearing and non-weightbearing synergists that we propose may affect joint stress and eventually lead to injury of the joint structures and pain.

MUSCULO-SKELETAL CHANGES WITH DELOADING THE WEIGHTBEARING KINETIC CHAIN

In this context, 'deloading' refers to a reduction in weightbearing load, or a decrease in the sensory information available to the central nervous system about gravity and loads. It is important to emphasize that deloading refers to an absence of weightbearing rather than a reduction in overall activity.

The muscle dysfunction occurring with deloading may take several decades to reach the point where joint injury and pain develop. Therefore, research requires specialized methodology that

can quicken the process. These approaches include animal studies involving immobilization, tenotomy or suspension of lower limbs; bedrest studies involving subjects (with no pathology) lying in bed for 2–3 months; and humans and animals living for short periods in microgravity.

The opportunity to study this area of motor control has been provided through our current involvement in space (microgravity) research, where skeletal muscle function, owing to the reduction in gravitational sensory load cues, can be deduced from the impairments that develop when gravity is minimized.

Neuromuscular plasticity in response to deloading

Neuromuscular plasticity represents the ability of the nervous system to adapt and change the control as well as the properties of skeletal muscle (including the properties of the slow and fast twitch fibres) in response to both therapeutic input (i.e. treatment modalities) and environmental stimuli (Kidd et al 1992). An environmental stimuli that could cause changes in the muscle system and its control is deloading the skeleton through minimizing the effect of gravity on the body. Many physiological research studies have investigated the effect of minimization of gravity on the body and the neuromuscular system.

The new model of injury proposes that musculo-skeletal injury can occur as a result of deloading the skeleton in a situation where there is a decrease of sensory information available to the nervous system about gravity and loads. This causes loss of function and weakness in the 'antigravity' muscle system: the local and one-joint muscles, which have a major role of protecting the joints from injury (see Chs 2, 3, 4, 5 and 6).

In addition, it will be argued that the antigravity muscle system will become less active and begin to be recruited more phasically during movement. Importantly, this change in function, which affects the muscles responsible for the control and protection of the underlying joint, is likely to change significantly the weightbearing loading patterns of the joint and thus increase the likelihood of joint injuries developing over extended periods of time.

Muscle changes

One of the most obvious impairments with deloading is muscle atrophy. Atrophy and decreased cross-sectional area (White and Davies 1984, Appell 1990 (review), McComas 1996) are the most obvious effects of deloading, with power more affected than expected from the degree of muscle atrophy (Antonutto et al 1999). The significance of these 'atrophy' impairments in relation to function lies not only in the fact that they are mainly present in the one-joint antigravity extensors but also that they are closely related to motor control problems that develop in the recruitment patterns of these extensors.

General muscle atrophy is combined with preferential type 1 atrophy (Appell 1990 (review), La Dora 2002) and increased contractile velocities (Fitts and Brimmer 1985). There is a loss of tonic function in antigravity one-joint muscles as deloading triggers fast fibre function with fast myosin expression (Fitts et al 1998). Microgravity and other deloaded conditions result in a change in fibre type in the one-joint extensors with a loss in type I (slow-twitch) fibres to the more fatiguable type II (fast twitch) fibres (Edgerton et al 1995, Fitts et al 2000). Increased fatiguability as a result of deloading has been found in rats (Grichko et al 2000). Zetterberg et al (1983), in a study of idiopathic scoliosis, reported that muscles on the deloaded side of the spinal curve demonstrated an increase in fatiguability, with less tonic (type I) fibres and increased IIb/IIa ratios. The muscles on the weightbearing convex side of the spine had reduced fatiguability, with an increase in type I fibres and increased IIa/IIb ratios.

There is some evidence that local muscles of the joint may be more affected in deloading. Studies on the vastus medialis (a muscle related to joint protection) have demonstrated that this muscle changes the most of all the quadriceps in microgravity conditions (Musacchia et al 1992). Muscles such as vastus medialis, deep fibres of soleus and intrinsic lumbar muscles appear to show the greatest loss of mass in microgravity (reviews: Fitts et al 2000, LeBlanc et al 2000). This may indicate the sensitivity of deep local muscles to deloading.

There is evidence that the multijoint muscles are unaffected in microgravity conditions. It has been reported by Hather et al (1992) that the cross-sectional area of the quadriceps is decreased by double that of the hamstrings. Most importantly, the rectus femoris showed no change in cross-sectional area. LeBlanc et al (2000) reported that hamstrings were unaffected by microgravity after 17 days in space. In addition, while knee extension strength was reduced by 19% with head-down bedrest, there was no change in knee flexion strength (i.e. hamstrings, Dudley et al 1989).

Few studies have been performed on the muscles of the lumbopelvic region in relation to the effects of deloading. In a microgravity study involving rats in a non-restricted environment, the external obliques were found to hypertrophy because of their frequent use as trunk rotators (Fijtek and Wassersug 1999). This finding was reversed in experiments where the rats movement was restricted (Fijtek and Wassersug 2001).

Thus research is beginning to produce evidence that changes in weightbearing and non-weightbearing muscle synergists occur as a result of deloading, and that local muscles may be the most affected of the weightbearing group. This mechanism-based hypothesis has been described previously in Richardson (2002).

There is also evidence that the changes in muscle could result from the effects of deloading on the sensory system. Sensory receptors affect recruitment patterns to the muscle, which then, via neuromuscular plasticity, may lead to changes in the muscle fibres themselves.

Changes in the sensory–motor system

By far the most compelling evidence for an independent antigravity system that is controlled independently to movement has come from microgravity research on both human and animal subjects, where pain and injury are not present. Roy et al (1991) suggested that 'Space flight to include recovery appears to be an excellent model to study the rapid remodeling of the neuro-muscular unit in the absence of disease and direct neural trauma'.

A loss of proprioception (load cues) has been linked with the muscle changes observed in deloading. Recktenwald et al (1999), in a study on monkeys, reported that microgravity induces changes in the 'gravitational or load related cues', which results in a 'biased recruitment away from the antigravity muscles'. For example, the antigravity (monoarticular) extensors of the lower limb are more affected in microgravity conditions than the flexors (Dudley et al 1989, Oganov et al 1991, Recktenwald et al 1999). In addition, rats exposed to 120 days of hypokinesia, demonstrated a lower excitability of the motoneuron pool of the extensors, with no change in the flexor pool (Jiang et al 1992). This research suggests that the lack of gravitational load cues affects the one-joint extensors but has no effect on the flexors.

Further, animal studies have indicated that, rather than the receptors (e.g. spindles) being affected directly, it may be the gamma (fusimotor) system which is the most affected in environments where minimal gravitational force is present. Through studying the effect of microgravity on the lower leg muscles of rats, Kawano et al (2002) deduced that muscular adaptation in gravity is closely related to how afferent input is modulated. According to Kanemura et al (2002), minimizing gravity reduces the gamma motoneuron activity and, therefore, implicates gamma efferent input to the muscle spindles as an important feature causing the impairments in muscles that occur with deloading of the skeleton. In line with these arguments, physiologists have reported that the antigravity muscles have more gamma representation in the cortex (Guyton 1981).

These findings have important implications for the development of injury when one considers the close relationship already shown to exist between joint protection mechanisms and the gamma muscle system. In relation to sensory motor changes, Johansson et al (1991a,b) (Johansson and Sojka 1991) have demonstrated that an essential element in the protection of joints by the muscles comes through the gamma support of the muscle spindle system, a proprioceptive receptor mechanism used to enhance the muscles' ability to detect load (see Ch. 5). Through their research on the ligaments of the knee, these researchers have linked the sensory properties of ligaments (i.e. the mechanoreceptors present in the ligaments), with increasing the activation of the gamma motoneuron pool.

This picture becomes even more intriguing when joint mechanoreceptors, which are closely linked to the gamma fusimotor system, were found to be reduced in number as a result of deloading in animal studies (Kanemura et al 2002). This argument that mechanoreceptors are directly affected by deloading has important implications for low back pain, as mechanoreceptors could not be found in the thoracolumbar fascia of patients' chronic low back pain, where usually they are present (Yahia et al 1992, Bednar et al 1995).

The role of the proprioceptive system in deloading has been further developed by Roll et al (1998). These researchers studied the sensory–motor loops involving proprioceptive afferents and found an adaptation with a reduction in gain in the loops especially in the antigravity muscles. This could explain the changes from tonic to more phasic motor unit activity in these muscles. Interestingly, it is reported that a reversal of flexor and extensor muscle activity occurs, with the tonic vibratory reflexes increased significantly in the flexor muscles, which demonstrate increased tonic activity, and significantly reduced in the antigravity extensors, which demonstrate reduced tonic activity (Roll et al 1993).

The link between deloading and the motor control of posture has also been studied. Baroni et al (2001) studied postural mechanisms in two astronauts exposed to long-term weightlessness. The subjects could still control their centre of mass in dynamic posture but had major problems with static postural control, namely orientation of the body segments. The authors argued that this may indicate that static and dynamic postural regulations are controlled separately in humans. These issues have also been addressed in Chapter 6.

It is important that the point is made that the changes reviewed in this chapter refer to the antigravity weightbearing mechanisms. Deloading (immobilization) seems to have the opposite sensory–motor effect on the hand muscles, which are mainly used for skilled function (Duchateau and Hainaut 1990).

RELEVANCE OF MICROGRAVITY RESEARCH TO PREVENTION OF MUSCULO–SKELETAL INJURY

Microgravity (deloading) research has many implications for the prevention of musculo-skeletal injury. It has verified the differentiation of muscles into weightbearing and non-weightbearing categories and has assisted in developing the methods which we use clinically to reload the weightbearing muscles and reduce activity in the non-weightbearing muscles.

Differentiation of muscles into two functionally different synergistic groups

It has been argued that, because of the neuroplasticity of the nervous system, deloading gradually causes muscle changes as well as motor control changes in both the antigravity muscles and the multijoint muscle system. These are summarized in Table 7.1. Based on the muscle changes that occur in microgravity, weightbearing can be used to distinguish muscle function with reference to the joint protection mechanisms. Weightbearing

against the force of gravity in flexed working postures is closely linked to antigravity muscle function, closed chain exercise (Ch. 6) and closed loop motor control, relying heavily on sensory feedback. This is the domain of the antigravity (one-joint and local) muscles. At the other extreme, open chain movement with the absence of weightbearing and gravitational load cues (sensory feedback) is the domain of the multijoint muscles. Table 7.2 gives a summary of the two functional muscle groups.

Methods of reloading the weightbearing muscles

In essence it is the antigravity weightbearing system that is under the stretch of gravity which may lose the ability to detect load in the deloading process. For this reason, it will be the synergist

Table 7.1 Muscle changes in 'deload' conditions

Characteristics	Antigravity weightbearing muscles	Non-weightbearing muscles
Muscle type	One joint muscles (and local muscles) of the kinetic chain	Multijoint/multifunction muscles
Cross-sectional area	Decreases	No change or an increase
Effect of deloading		
Fibre type change	Slow twitch fibres to fast twitch	No change
Motor unit change	Tonic to phasic shift	Phasic to tonic shift
Gamma motoneuron support	Less	No change
Tonic vibratory reflexes	Decreased	Increased
Fatiguable	More	Less

Table 7.2 Muscle recruitment with extremes of motor control conditions

	Antigravity weightbearing muscles	Non-weightbearing muscles
Muscle type	One joint muscles (and local muscles)	Multijoint/multifunction muscles
From Chapter 6	Closed chain exercise	Open chain exercise
	Static weightbearing	Rapid, ballistic movement
	Antigravity working postures	Eliminate gravity
	Joint compression	Joint distraction
	Fast and slow 'ramp' contractions	Phasic on/off contractions
From Chapter 7	Closed loop conditions	Open loop conditions
	Maximize sensory feedback	Minimal sensory feedback
	Maximize proprioceptive load cues	Minimal proprioceptive load cues
	Focus = antigravity function	Focus = non-weightbearing movement
Injury/pain	Prevention/treatment	Cause

group most affected by deloading. Importantly, Kanemura et al (2002) suggested that exercise under gravitation loads (weightbearing) is important for rehabilitation after deloading (especially in relation to the knee).

One of the most important observations from microgravity research in relation to training is the critical nature of the gamma (fusimotor) system. This system, which is closely associated with the joint protection mechanisms, appears to be targeted in deloaded situations, and this could lead to the muscle impairments developing in the antigravity musculature. This lack of gamma support to the load detectors (muscle spindles) of antigravity muscles would be more crucial in weightbearing activities in erect postures, where the one-joint (antigravity) extensors would be in their shortened position. Muscles that need to detect load in their shortened positions (i.e. one-joint antigravity muscles) require efferent input (fusimotor activity) to the spindles to ensure that these receptors are sensitive to stretch, even though the muscle is shortened. This would especially relate to joint protection in upright, walking activities on uneven ground, where load cues must be detected even when the weightbearing muscles are not in a stretched position. This would be even more difficult when the one-joint muscles have been lengthened by poor postural position and the length–tension relationship has changed to favour a lengthened position (Sahrmann 2002). This likely poor joint protection by the muscle system in upright weightbearing activities may be one reason why patients with low back pain report difficulties and pain when walking in soft sand or on very soft surfaces (S. Roll, personal communication).

The local muscle system may be even more sensitive to the deloading process because of its likely close relationship to the joint proprioceptors and the large percentage of muscle spindles found in these muscles (Peck et al 1984). The development of a muscle corset, through drawing in the abdominal wall (Ch. 5), requires a shortening contraction. The level of fusimotor support to achieve and hold this shortening contraction cognitively in order to develop lumbo-pelvic stiffness (Ch. 5) may be important in the local muscles, which are not directly stretched by gravity. If the effect of deloading was to reduce fusimotor support and

influence the sensitivity of the proprioceptive system (to detect and respond to load), then patients with low back dysfunction would lose the ability to perform a corset action (Ch. 12). It is very interesting that patients with low back pain also have a loss of mechanoreceptors in the thoracolumbar fascia (Bednar et al 1995). As the mechanoreceptors are closely associated with the activation of the gamma motoneurons, impairment of the proprioceptive system of the lumbopelvic region in patients with low back pain could be explained by these changes.

Methods of reducing overactivity in non–weightbearing muscles

Problems in the gamma support system with deloading may also influence the non-weightbearing system, where increased reflex muscle activity may result. Importantly for rehabilitation, reloading of the weightbearing muscles may reduce this activity in the non-weightbearing muscles. Future research studies may show that exercise specifically for the weightbearing muscles is an effective method of lengthening tight, overactive non-weightbearing muscles.

As deloading causes problems in the joint protection mechanism and considerably increases the risk of musculo-skeletal injury, it is relevant to review the many situations that can lead to deloading, in an effort to optimize injury prevention.

LIFESTYLE FACTORS RESULTING IN DELOADING

There are many human lifestyle factors that may lead, over time, to significant deloading of the skeleton and the development of common musculoskeletal problems, such as low back pain. Lifestyle factors that can cause deloading of the skeleton can be grouped as factors associated with (a) deloaded upright and sitting postures, (b) non-weightbearing exercise/environments, and (c) decreased gravitational load cues

Deloaded upright and sitting postures

Maintenance of flexed postures

One way in which high forces of gravity can cause injury and pain to the joint structures is when there are changes to more flexed static and working postures, both in sitting and standing. This would occur if individuals 'gave in' to the high force of gravity and the body gradually progressed into a flexed 'relaxed' posture, resting on the passive joint structures, with the trunk and hip extensor muscles 'turning off' and with the possible domination of the trunk and hip flexor muscles over time (Fig. 7.1).

These events are best understood by considering the evolutionary development of the human musculo-skeletal system, which has required that muscles and bones slowly adapt their function to the high gravitational forces acting on the body during upright functional tasks (Fig. 7.2).

If humans succumb to the force of gravity during daily activities, for example having poor (flexed) sitting postures in comfortable chairs while watching television or when working at

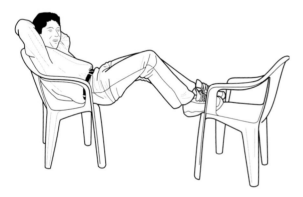

Figure 7.1   Relaxed lifestyle in the sitting position.

computers, or when lifting with a flexed or bent spine, the dangers of injury and the development of low back pain are known but the exact aetiology has remained elusive. It is usually considered in terms of changes in tissue creep with lumbar flexion and the resulting reduced passive joint protection mechanisms (Chs 5 and 6). However, considering the muscle system, it is the trunk and hip extensor support system of muscles that keep the body lifted and erect in extension and prevents its collapse into flexion (Fig. 7.2). Therefore, with gradual increase in flexed postures, the resulting deloading of the weightbearing extensor muscles, with reliance on passive structures, would lead to the development of motor control impairments, as previously described.

There are also several other physiological changes that may occur in the weightbearing muscles with changing postures which could be important in the development of pathology. These factors would also need to be reflected in clinical assessment and exercise treatment techniques. The main problem would be the change in the length–tension relationships in muscles lengthened under gravity loading (e.g. gluteus maximus). It is considered that the extensor, one-joint muscle system would gradually become weak and lengthened, with the addition of sarcomeres and changes in the length–tension curves (reviewed by Sahrmann 2002). This would affect the ability of these muscles to contract and support the lumbopelvic region in their shortened range.

These impairments in the weightbearing muscles would lead to a cycle of increasing deterioration in

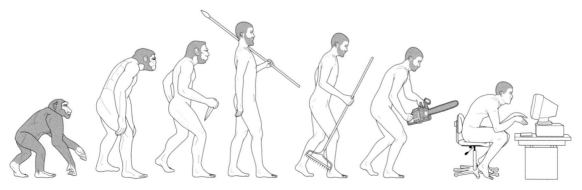

Figure 7.2   The evolutionary development of an antigravity erect posture and the gradual lifestyle changes that are reversing these postures.

(a)   (b)

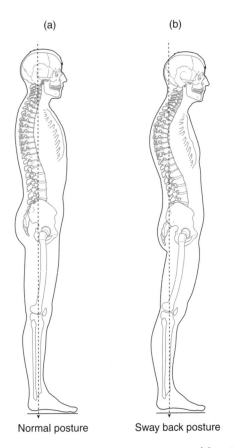

Normal posture   Sway back posture

Figure 7.3 Normal and sway back posture: (a) upright normal posture; (b) sway back. (Adapted from Kendall and McCreary 1983.)

their antigravity function. The right side of Figure 7.2 shows how starting to bend from the full upright position during daily tasks would give rise to deterioration in antigravity function of the extensor muscle system, which would gradually weaken and lengthen; further bending with gravity would follow.

There is also evidence that the local multifidus muscle is 'turning off' when the lumbar spine is in a flexed position for an extended period. In an electromyographic (EMG) study on cats, Williams et al (2000) showed that holding the lumbar spine in flexion led to changes in the firing patterns of the multifidus. Within minutes, the multifidus began firing in phasic erratic bursts and lost its joint protective role. This has been described in Chapter 11.

Maintenance of other deloaded postures

It is not just the flexed postures that will result in deloading of muscles which normally protect the joints of the body from gravity. Many variations of upright postures, for example the sway back posture (Fig. 7.3) would lead to a reliance on the passive structures of the spine and result in increased activity of the less-fatiguable, multifunction external obliques and hamstring muscles to hold the weight-bearing postures. O'Sullivan et al (2002) studied levels of muscle activity in slumped and sway back postures and found that internal oblique, superficial lumbar multifidus and thoracic erector spinae were less active in passive postures.

Non-weightbearing exercise

Repetitive sports or occupational skills that involve fast repetitive ballistic activities, especially if open chain, would also gradually result in decreased use of the antigravity weightbearing muscles (Fig. 7.4). This was explained in Chapter 6. There is some evidence that increased training involving rapid (ballistic) repetitive sports can lead to the development of musculo-skeletal injury. An example of changing patterns of motor control, similar to that seen in deloading, has been detected in a common musculo-skeletal injury, patellofemoral pain syndrome. This pain syndrome is very common in sports such as running and cycling, involving rapid repetitive muscle work with reduced static weightbearing components.

Rehabilitation of chronic patellofemoral pain syndrome involves retraining the vastus medialis oblique, the quadriceps muscle that is responsible for the control of the patella. It is an imbalance between a 'weak and inefficient' local muscle, vastus medialis, compared with the rest of the quadriceps muscles, especially vastus lateralis, that has been considered to be an important factor in the aetiology of the condition (Pevsner et al 1979, Paulos et al 1980).

A non-weightbearing test that assessed the activation patterns of muscles in relation to a fast repetitive movement of the knee appears to be very sensitive in detecting the changes in the motor control patterns in the quadriceps muscles

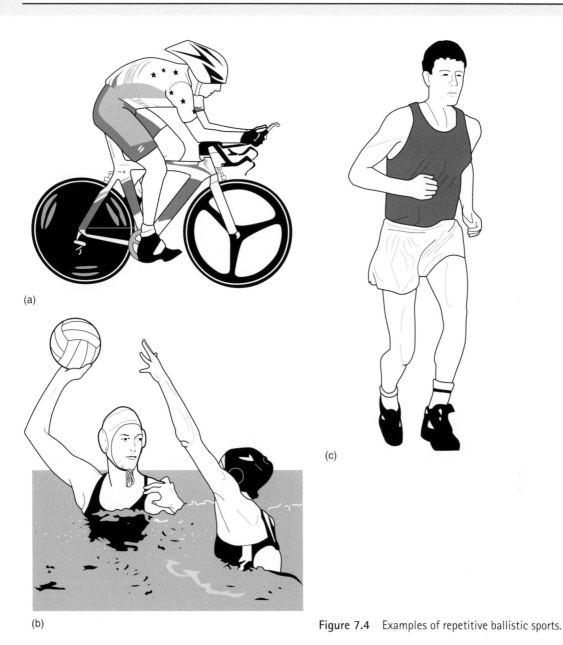

(a)

(b)

(c)

Figure 7.4   Examples of repetitive ballistic sports.

(Richardson and Bullock 1986, also described in Ch. 6). Richardson (1987a,b) reported that changes in the pattern of recruitment of vastus medialis oblique occurred in patients with chronic patellofemoral pain syndrome compared with that in healthy matched controls. The latter had a predominantly tonic activity in vastus medialis (Fig. 7.5a), whereas the muscle in the former displayed phasic patterns of recruitment (Fig. 7.5b). This would concur with the predicted changes resulting from deloading of the weightbearing muscles. Perhaps lack of gravitational load cues over long periods of time could be the cause of patellofemoral pain syndrome in some athletes.

Other changes in the control of vastus medialis in patellofemoral pain syndrome are also of interest. In healthy control subjects, the vastus medialis was shown not only to work tonically in response to rapid movement cues but also to display the same levels of muscle activity over three increasing

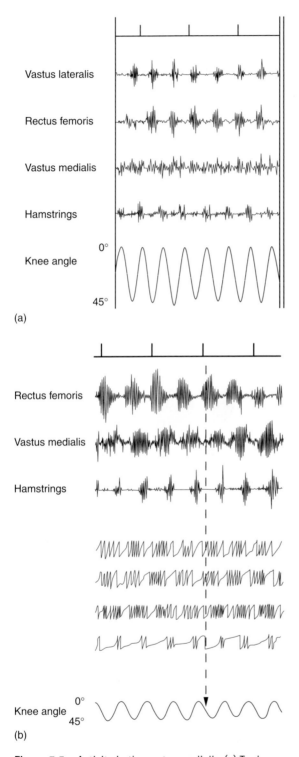

(a)

(b)

Figure 7.5 Activity in the vastus medialis. (a) Tonic activity in normal subjects. (b) The phasic patterns present in patello-femoral pain syndrome.

speeds of the movement cycle. This was in contrast to the rectus femoris and hamstrings (non-weightbearing muscles), which contracted in a phasic way in line with the biomechanical analysis of the movement and increased their activity in response to increases in speed of the non-weightbearing knee flexion–extension movements (see Ch. 6). In contrast, patients with patellofemoral pain syndrome demonstrated highly significant increases in the magnitude of integrated EMG in vastus medialis, with increasing speeds of the test movement, in a similar pattern of recruitment to that detected in rectus femoris and hamstrings. That is, the local (weightbearing) muscle, vastus medialis, in a dysfunctional state began to respond to movement cues in a similar way to the multijoint (non-weightbearing) muscles. This is indicative of motor control changes occurring in the muscle. Deloading may have played a large role in these changes, developing over periods of time. Similar changes occurring in the transversus abdominis muscle (Ch. 10) and in the deep multifidus (Ch. 11) have been detected in patients with low back pain. Deloading could contribute to the changes reported in these muscles.

This non-weightbearing knee flexion–extension test is being used by our group as an outcome measure for the Berlin bedrest study currently being undertaken in Europe. Initial results on four subjects have indicated that a tonic-to-phasic shift in recruitment patterns does occur in vastus medialis oblique after removal of weightbearing for an 8-week period.

Interestingly, a study by Richardson and Sims (1991) demonstrated that, compared with non-cyclists, competitive cyclists were unable to maintain an inner range holding contraction of gluteus maximus. This would appear to reflect an impairment that could develop in the gluteus maximus of cyclists owing to the ballistic, non-weightbearing nature of their sport and the reduced use of the weightbearing muscles. Water sports and repetitive running activities may also reduce the use of the weightbearing muscles and gradually lead to impairments developing in the weightbearing muscles.

A 6-week training programme, involving ankle plantarflexion in standing, was undertaken by Ng and Richardson in 1990. Instead of increasing weightbearing load (e.g. as may be used to strengthen the ankle plantarflexors (gastrocnemius and soleus)), the exercise progression involved increasing the speed at which the exercise was undertaken, at weekly intervals. Results indicated that jump height had increased after the 6-week training period but that the isometric contraction of the soleus muscle had significantly decreased during training. Therefore, speed loading had improved the skill of the activity but had resulted in decreased function of the one-joint extensor at the ankle. The impairment in soleus may affect ankle protection and support and may, in time, result in injury to the ankle.

Non–weightbearing environments

Several types of environment lead to a decrease in gravitational load and loss of weightbearing, for example immobilization, bedrest, prolonged sitting, less loading of the antigravity extensors in sedentary lifestyles (e.g. age or occupation related) and microgravity (space) (Fig. 7.6). In addition, some occupational groups working in environments with less gravitational load would be at risk of loss of their joint protective mechanisms over time because of the effect of deloading on the control of the muscle system. Changes in the joint protective mechanisms can be expected, not only in astronauts but also in occupational groups such as deep water divers and pilots of high-performance aircraft, where normal gravitational loading conditions are not present (Fig. 7.7). Interestingly, James (2001) commented that these occupations are subject to 'skeletal degeneration', although the reasons for the changes have not been fully explored.

Decreased gravitational load cues

Other situations that effectively deload the musculo-skeletal system occur in lifestyles that lack input from gravitational load cues related to uneven or changing surfaces of support. Muscle recruitment from direct vertical loading (i.e. in squatting activities where the body weight is lifted against gravity) may be regularly performed by most individuals. However, it has been argued earlier in this chapter that maintaining muscle recruitment for joint support in erect postures

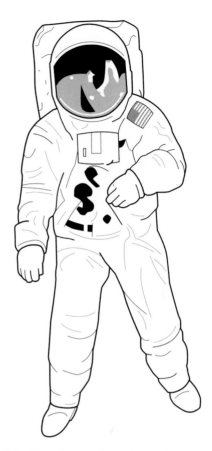

Figure 7.6   The microgravity environment.

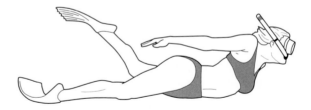

Figure 7.7   Deep sea divers.

during activities such as walking on uneven, soft, moving surfaces or slopes requires a highly sensitive proprioceptive system to react to the gravitational load cues. Individuals may not be regularly subjected to this type of loading, that is, when the antigravity muscles are in a shortened position but must still detect changes in load. Therefore, walking in solid shoes on even, firm surfaces (Fig. 7.8) may lead, over time, to lack of use of the antigravity muscle system, and muscle impairments could develop.

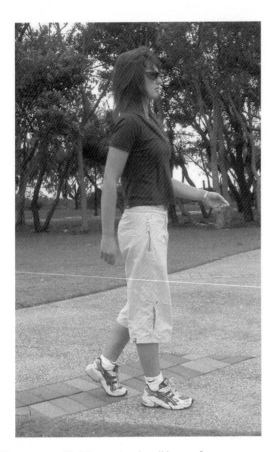

Figure 7.8   Walking on hard walking surfaces.

IMPLICATIONS FOR PREVENTION OR TREATMENT EXERCISE PROGRAMMES

Neuromuscular plasticity in response to specific exercise training

Skeletal muscle tissue is very mutable and neuromuscular plasticity can also occur in response to therapeutic input (i.e. treatment modalities). Therefore, specifically directed exercise can prevent or reverse the effects of deloading and the subsequent breakdown of tissue.

The specific exercise prevention and treatment strategies for the expanded 'segmental stabilization training' model of exercise are directed to changing the pattern of joint loading so that the joint can safely cope with the high forces of gravity and other types of loading. This specific type of exercise involves slowly increasing gravitational load cues in weightbearing or simulated weightbearing, including the process of reloading the antigravity

(one-joint) muscles, while unloading and minimizing the activity of the multijoint muscles (Ch. 6).

From a neurophysiological viewpoint, the one-joint and local muscles operate independently at the opposite extreme of motor control continuum (i.e. ramp or 'closed loop' conditions). Therefore, a suitable countermeasure exercise technique would be closed chain exercise with gradually increasing gravity-related load cues while ensuring that the local muscle system of the lumbopelvic region is activated during the exercise (Ch. 5).

It would be important to recognize in prevention/rehabilitation programmes that adding too much load or allowing fatigue to develop would lead to compensation patterns, with dominance of the multijoint muscles and decreased activation of the antigravity muscles.

The key to the activation of the antigravity muscles lies in the sensory mechanisms providing information of the body weight via the weightbearing joints and muscles. Antigravity muscles need continuous sensory information for the maintenence of continuous muscle tone or state of 'preparedness' to allow their optimal functional integration with the multijoint non-weightbearing muscle system.

Sensory information from all the weightbearing joints and muscles would contribute to maintaining or developing the tonic background activity in the antigravity weightbearing musculature, which gradually would change its morphology through neuromuscular plasticity. This process is the antithesis of the neuromuscular plasticity occurring with deloading. Table 7.2 summarizes the type of exercise suitable for not only reloading the antigravity weightbearing muscles but also unloading the multijoint non-weightbearing muscles. Maximizing proprioceptive load cues (Table 7.2), which includes the use of uneven surfaces (Fig. 7.9), balance boards, mini trampolines, as well as whole body vibration given in combination with antigravity closed chain exercise (Fig. 7.10), will be described in more detail in Chapter 15.

Assessments of muscle/motor control problems

The consideration of muscle control as divided into two groups related to gravity and weightbearing has allowed muscle dysfunctions to be predicted

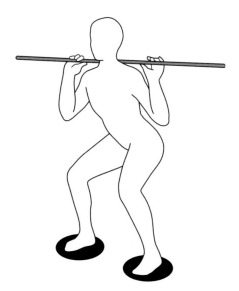

Figure 7.9   Closed chain exercise with uneven surfaces.

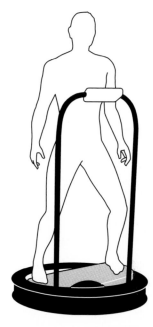

Figure 7.10   Closed chain exercise with whole body vibration.

and measured. Clinical assessments of muscle/motor control problems have been devised to enable predictions on the relative contribution to joint support and protection by individual muscle synergists. These clinical assessments will be explained in Chapters 12 and 15. In addition, laboratory assessments of the recruitment patterns allows patterns that optimize functional and safe weightbearing to be studied and analysed.

Microgravity creates an environment in which the development of injury and pathological processes caused by minimizing the effects of gravity can be studied within a short time frame. Consequently, our research team is using space research to study the effects of deloading on the lumbopelvic region and to examine the aetiology of gravity-related skeletal health problems such as mechanical low back pain and arthritis of the weightbearing (hip) joints. Currently we are involved in the European Space Agency's Berlin Bedrest Study, where our new laboratory measures of the weightbearing function of muscles of the lumbopelvic region are being tested.

Chapter 12 will discuss the problems in the weightbearing and non-weightbearing system that have been detected in patients with low back pain on Earth.

Chapter **8**

Joint injury

Julie Hides

INTRODUCTION

Injury to a joint or associated passive structures will have direct effects upon muscle function and control and needs to be understood if rehabilitation programmes are to be efficient and effective. Most importantly, it appears that the effects of joint injury on muscles are different for the three categories of muscle (local, one-joint and multijoint/multifunction). It will be argued in this chapter that inhibition of muscles appears to occur most frequently in local and one-joint muscles, and that the dysfunction occurring is related to a loss of tonic function in these muscles. Multijoint/multifunction muscles are rarely inhibited. In fact, their activation may increase as a compensation strategy (see Ch. 12). Investigations of muscle inhibition have been conducted on both human and animal subjects. Most human studies have used the knee as the joint of choice for investigation of the effects of injury, as this is one of the few joints of the body with ready access to the individual muscles which control the joint, allowing direct measures of reflex inhibition to be performed. In comparison, studies of inhibition of the spinal muscles that have used indirect measures as direct measures are too difficult to perform in this region. Pain has devastating effects upon muscle control, and pain models will be discussed in Chapter 9. The focus of this chapter will be reflex inhibition, which can occur in the absence of pain and can persist well after pain has completely subsided. It is important to study the effects of joint injury on the muscles and the possible neurophysiological mechanisms involved to guide and develop principles for optimal rehabilitation.

REFLEX INHIBITION

Definition

Reflex inhibition of a muscle has been defined as the situation that occurs when sensory stimuli impede the voluntary activation of a muscle. These afferent stimuli usually arise from injury to a joint at which the muscle functions (Morrissey 1989). Hurley and Newham (1993) similarly defined reflex inhibition as being elicited by abnormal afferent information from a damaged joint, resulting in decreased motor drive to muscle groups acting across the joint. Reflex inhibition causes weakness directly and may also contribute to muscle atrophy. Weakness then predisposes the joint to further damage (Stokes and Young 1984a). This atrophy may occur rapidly (Stener 1969). It is not clear what causes reflex inhibition or which specific receptors are stimulated (Stokes and Young 1984b). Reflex inhibition is reported to hamper alpha motorneuron activity in the anterior horn of the spinal cord (Stokes and Cooper 1993), but animal research has implicated the gamma motorneuron system (He et al 1988).

To understand the phenomenon of reflex inhibition and how it could influence therapeutic exercise design, it is necessary to review briefly the possible neurophysiological pathways involved.

Neurophysiological pathways

The specific sensory pathway involved in reflex inhibition is not known. It involves joint afferents and articular nerves, terminating in the spinal cord. Interestingly, the main sensation attributed to the joint is pain (Schiable and Grubb 1993). Joints are supplied by articular branches descending from main nerve trunks or their muscular, cutaneous and periosteal branches (for review of joint innervation, morphology, types and location of joint receptors, see Freeman and Wyke 1967, Schiable and Grubb 1993). Studies performed on inflamed joints have shown that inflammation increases the mechanosensitivity of articular afferents and that sensory units are sensitized during inflammation (Schiable and Grubb 1993). Mechanosensitivity is altered by both physical changes that occur during inflammation (e.g. synovial effusion) and chemical changes. The pathways from joint afferents have extensive projections in the spinal cord (Craig et al 1988). Animal research has shown that the sensory input from the knee joint is conveyed to interneurons, motoneurons and supraspinal structures, including the cerebral cortex and the cerebellum. Information from the afferents ascend in the dorsal columns and in the spinothalamic, spinoreticular and spinocerebellar pathways (Johansson et al 1991b). Electrical stimulation of the posterior articular nerve of the cat knee joint has been shown to excite interneurons (Gardner et al 1949), motoneurons (Eccles and Lundberg 1959a,b) and neurons of the spinocerebellar (Haddad 1953) and spinocervical (Harrison and Jankowska 1984) tracts in the lumbar spinal cord. A number of transmitters, neuromodulators and receptors are involved in spinal cord activity when nociceptive input from joints is processed (Schiable and Grubb 1993). Variables such as joint inflammation affect the levels of transmitters and neuromodulators present in the dorsal root ganglion and the spinal cord.

The sensory pathways involved in reflex inhibition are complex. Animal research has been conducted to investigate motor reflexes, where reflexes in limb muscles and reflex discharges in motoneurons have been elicited by either electrical stimulation of articular nerves or activation of receptors in the joint capsule or the joint ligaments. Electrical stimulation of articular nerves provided the first evidence that reflex motor pathways actually exist (Gardner 1950, Eccles and Lundberg 1959a,b, Hongo et al 1969, Lundberg et al 1978). Activation of receptors in the joint capsule (either directly or by pressure applied by inflation of the joint) and the joint ligaments confirmed this motor response (Ekholm et al 1960, Grigg et al 1978, Baxendale et al 1987). Motor reflexes may be considered as a feedback mechanism from the joint back to the joint since sensory information arising in the joint may influence the motor output to the muscles that move and stabilize the joint (Schiable and Grubb 1993). It is interesting to examine the pattern of muscle wasting found in studies of reflex inhibition, as this information may help to guide specific rehabilitation approaches.

Patterns of muscle wasting

Most research concerning patterns of muscle wasting in reflex inhibition has been conducted at the knee joint. Evidence of patterns of motor responses has been provided by the classic study of Ekholm et al (1960), which involved stimulation of joint receptors by pinching the joint capsule. This led to inhibition of knee extensors and facilitation of knee flexors. These results have been used to explain the common finding of isolated wasting of the quadriceps with hamstring sparing in knee joint injuries. Furthermore, several studies have shown that the pattern of reflex responses in the spinal cord can be changed by the induction of joint inflammation using chemical stimulants that activate fine afferent fibres (Woolf and Wall 1986, Ferrell et al 1988, He et al 1988). The response to inflammation was a pronounced and prolonged increase in alpha motoneuron excitability in the flexor muscles. The prolonged facilitation of the flexor reflex did not require any ongoing input (i.e. peripheral activation) of the afferent fibres (C fibres) to modify the functional response of the spinal cord. This shows that sensory and motor alterations are found after peripheral tissue injury. These findings may describe a possible mechanism for the development of flexion contractures as seen in arthritic patients (Ferrell et al 1988) and also may relate directly to joint resting positions in acute joints.

In summary, these studies have demonstrated that sensory stimuli can exert potent effects on motorneuron excitability. Preferential inhibition of extensor motoneurons and facilitation of flexor motoneurons has been demonstrated when receptors in the joint capsule have been activated (Ekholm et al 1960). Evidence of flexor motoneuron facilitation has been provided by joint inflammation studies.

Reflex inhibition and selective muscle atrophy

While classic studies have provided evidence of inhibition of extensors and facilitation of flexor muscles at the knee joint, further investigations have provided evidence that the inhibition response may be specific to parts of muscles. Studies have used the H reflex to assess the effects of experimental effusion on the different parts of the quadriceps in human subjects (Kennedy et al 1982, Spencer et al 1984). The H reflex was elicited by selective recruitment of Ia spindle afferents in the femoral nerve by a consistent low-voltage stimulus. This generated a reproducible quadriceps contraction. Within the spinal cord, this transmission comes under the influence of modulating sensory inputs, acting through the internuncial pool. The inputs arriving from the articular receptors can facilitate or inhibit the H reflex. By maintaining a constant stimulus, Kennedy et al (1982) and Spencer et al (1984) were provided with an indirect assessment of the activity of articular afferents by measuring the degree of the quadriceps contraction using elctromyography (EMG) as they increased the volume of the intra-articular fluid in the subjects' knees. Experimentally induced effusions used to stimulate joint receptors in human knee joints led to preferential inhibition of the vastus medialis muscle. Similar findings of selective vastus medialis muscle inhibition measured using EMG have been reported by Wise et al (1984) in patients with patellofemoral pain syndromes. It has been reported that the rectus femoris muscle is the component of the quadriceps muscle group least affected by inhibition following injury (Stener 1969, Wolf et al 1971). Imaging techniques have similarly been employed to provide information on selective atrophy of parts of muscle groups; however, results are conflicting. Gerber et al (1985) reported selective atrophy of the vastus medialis muscle, while others suggested a more uniform atrophy (Halkjaer-Kristensen et al 1980, Young et al 1982, Richardson 1987b). Although some of the findings in this area are contradictory, the weight of the evidence provided would suggest that parts of muscles can be selectively inhibited.

Evidence of dysfunction of the multifidus in patients with acute low back pain has been provided in the form of a segmental decrease in multifidus cross-sectional area (Hides et al 1994, see Ch. 11). Subjects with acute/subacute, unilateral, first-episode low back pain were investigated. The decrease in multifidus cross-sectional area occurred rapidly (within days) and was found to be significantly greater in subjects with a duration of symptoms of less than 2 weeks than in those with a longer duration of symptoms. The decreased multifidus size was localized to the side of painful symptoms in patients with unilateral low back pain. Possible causes of decreased multifidus size include reflex inhibition, pain inhibition and disuse atrophy. The rapidity of onset and localized distribution of the decrease in muscle size suggest that disuse atrophy was not the cause and that a selective mechanism (most likely reflex inhibition) was in operation (Hides et al 1994).

Examination of the possible mechanism of selective inhibition of part of a muscle group is intriguing. In the case of the knee joint, there is no neurophysiological explanation as yet for the common clinical finding of isolated wasting of the quadriceps with hamstring sparing in knee joint injuries. It is the sensory innervation of the injured joint or structure that is the crucial element in reflex inhibition. From definitions of reflex inhibition, sensory stimuli impede the voluntary activation of a muscle. The afferent stimuli arise from injury to a joint at which the muscle functions. However, in the case of the knee joint, the nerves that supply the joint are derived from the obturator, femoral, tibial and common peroneal nerves (Kennedy et al 1982). The segmental supply of the knee joint and capsule is, therefore, widespread (from L2 to S3). On the basis of the sensory innervation of the knee joint, almost any muscle in the lower limb could potentially be inhibited. Yet, the actual response is isolated to the quadriceps group, which is innervated by the femoral nerve (L2–L4), and an even more specific effect has been observed in part of the quadriceps (the vastus medialis). This finding implies that input from the joint is processed and modulated in the spinal cord to produce a specific effect in specific muscles and even parts of muscle. This has led to clinical definitions of reflex inhibition, such as that by Hurley and Newham (1993), who defined reflex inhibition as resulting in decreased motor drive to muscle groups acting across the joint, as the specific nature of the actual response seen clinically is not yet clear.

A similar argument applies in the case of localized segmental inhibition of the lumbar multifidus in patients with acute low back pain. The innervation of the zygapophyseal joints is derived from branches of the dorsal rami (Bradley 1974). The capsule receives a number of branches from either two nerves (the medial branch of the dorsal ramus

at that level and the level above (Bradley 1974, Bogduk and Twomey 1987) or three nerves (one spinal nerve higher, one lower and the spinal nerve of the level in question (Wyke 1981, Paris 1983). Lumbar discs are supplied by the sinuvertebral nerves, which are recurrent branches of the ventral rami that re-enter the intervertebral foramen to be distributed within the intervertebral canal (Bogduk and Twomey 1987). Each lumbar sinuvertebral nerve supplies the disc at its level of entry into the vertebral canal and the disc above; that is the L3–L4 disc is supplied by the L3 and L4 sinuvertebral nerves. There are countless other vertebral structures that are innervated and could be injured in acute low back pain. Yet the response to injury in the case of the multifidus, as with the knee joint, is specific and localized to the part of the multifidus muscle that crosses the affected vertebral segment (Hides et al 1994). As the effects of reflex inhibition are localized and specific to the injured joint or segment, this information will influence the approach to rehabilitation, which will need to be equally specific to be effective.

Reflex inhibition and joint position

Studies have been conducted on joint position to determine if position affects reflex inhibition. Investigators have used experimentally and non-experimentally induced joint inflammation, nerve stimulation and joint effusion to investigate this relationship.

Models of experimentally induced joint inflammation have been used to investigate the position in which animals hold their injured limbs. This position has been described as a semiflexed or 'resting position'. Induction of joint inflammation by chemical stimulants that activate joint afferents is known to alter the pattern of reflex responses in the spinal cord (Woolf and Wall 1986, Ferrell et al 1988, He et al 1988). He et al (1988) showed that inflammation of the cat knee produced significant and often large increases in the response of flexor motoneurons to local pressure and movement of the leg. However, some flexor motoneurons were inhibited by the inflammation. The inhibitory reflex response modified the stereotype flexion response to allow the joint to be kept at a midrange, or 'resting', position. This position is one where the nociceptive joint afferents are least activated (Schaible and Grubb 1993).

Acute experimental joint inflammation at the ankle showed that the resting activity and reflex excitability of the majority of fusimotoneurons supplying specifically the ankle extensors was inhibited (Berberich et al 1987). Investigations using electrical stimulation of afferent nerves have also shown effects on specific muscle groups. Flexor gamma motoneurons were particularly excited, where mixed effects were demonstrated in the extensor gamma motoneurons (Johansson et al 1986). This evidence of facilitation of the flexor neurons and inhibition of extensor neurons in inflamed joints indicates that joint position may be relevant when selecting the position of the joint for facilitation of muscle activation.

In human subjects, knee joint effusion is known to produce quadriceps inhibition (DeAndre et al 1965, Jayson and Dixon 1970, Stratford 1981, Kennedy et al 1982, Spencer et al 1984). It has been proposed that joint distension stimulates the type I corpuscles and produces afferent impulses leading to quadriceps inhibition (Jayson and Dixon 1970). In one classic study that investigated this phenomena, the effects of human knee joint effusion and increased articular pressure were investigated in normal patients and patients with rheumatoid arthritis (Jayson and Dixon 1970). Intra-articular pressure and quadriceps inhibition was least in 30 degrees of knee flexion. Similar findings with respect to joint position were found when EMG was used to assess the electrical activity of the quadriceps in a group of patients with painless acute knee effusions (Stratford 1981). The findings were also confirmed in animal studies, where changes in discharge patterns were observed in inflated cat knees. Lowest discharge rates were observed when the joint was in mid position. Synovial pressure was normally lowest when joints were positioned in a resting position but rose and often became positive during knee flexion (Ferrell et al 1986).

In summary, evidence of the importance of a neutral or mid-range position has been provided through investigations of inflamed and effused joints. To minimize the effects of inhibition, the joint should be positioned in a neutral position (Krebs et al 1983). This is especially relevant in the acute situation, where both inflammation and effusion may be present. Evidence of the importance of a neutral position, particularly for the extensor muscles, has been provided from inflammation studies.

Magnitude and duration of reflex inhibition

The effects of reflex inhibition are known to be extremely rapid, with inhibition reported to occur within hours (Stokes and Young 1984b). The magnitude and duration of reflex inhibition following injury is also unexpectedly high. In a study of patients undergoing menisectomy, quadriceps inhibition became more pronounced over the first 24 hours (80%) and was still very severe at 3–4 days after the operation (70–80%) (Stokes and Young 1984). Even 10–15 days postoperatively, there was still 35–40% inhibition. This occurred despite the fact that patients were discharged from hospital, were experiencing minimal or no pain and were fully weightbearing. Other EMG studies of quadriceps muscle have supported these findings with regard to the persistence of reflex inhibition. Krebs et al (1983) found decreased quadriceps activity 3 or more weeks postmeniscectomy, and Santavirta (1979) found EMG changes up to at least 12 weeks after surgery.

A similar persistent effect of injury was seen in the multifidus muscle in patients with acute low back pain. Subjects were monitored weekly for 4 weeks, and then at 10 weeks after injury. In 90%, pain was completely diminished at 4 weeks. Subjects then resumed full premorbid activity levels for work, sport and leisure for 6 weeks. Despite full resumption of activity over this period, multifidus muscle size was not restored at 10 weeks in subjects who did not receive specific intervention to reactivate the multifidus (Hides et al 1996). This provides further support for the argument that the most likely cause of decreased multifidus cross-sectional area in patients with acute low back pain is reflex inhibition.

Further evidence regarding the rapidity and duration of reflex inhibition comes from biopsy studies. Biopsy analysis has been used in an attempt to determine the relative effects of reflex inhibition on different muscle fibre types. Häggmark et al (1981) showed that type I atrophy occurred very rapidly (within the first week) following knee joint injury. In a cross-country skier who was treated operatively, there was a fall of 81% to 57% in slow-twitch fibres of the quadriceps. Despite the fact that the patient received very early active rehabilitation, it took some months for the quadriceps to return to its pre-injury fibre distribution.

POSSIBLE EXPLANATIONS FOR RAPID MUSCLE RESPONSE TO REFLEX INHIBITION

Muscle atrophy is known to occur very rapidly in the case of reflex inhibition (Stener 1969). In the clinical situation, rapid atrophy of muscle is also a commonly observed phenomenon. Yet, the actual mechanism of rapid muscle atrophy in reflex inhibition is as yet not fully understood.

The size of muscle fibres is determined multifactorily, with influence exerted by various factors including activity and innervation, hormones, growth, stretch and nutrition (Jennekens 1982). Muscle atrophy is one of the most common responses of a muscle fibre to a loss of neural influences, to processes that prevent normal contractile activity and to various pathological stimuli (Cullen and Mastaglia 1982). It involves a phase of negative growth and a regression in volume. The mechanisms underlying myofibre atrophy are not fully understood. Shrinkage of a cell or tissue may be brought about by an increase in the normal rate of protein degradation, by a reduction in protein synthesis or by both processes together (Goldberg 1975). The actual enzymes involved in the degradation of muscle protein have not been identified. Proteinases that are present in muscle and capable of breaking down myofibrillar proteins have been examined in animal studies. In rats, myofibrillar protein breakdown can be rapid during myofibre atrophy, with a potential for total myosin degradation within 6–9 days (Schwartz and Bird 1977). However, the intracellular control mechanisms of protein degradation are not understood (Cullen and Mastaglia 1982).

In order to understand the mechanism of rapid muscle atrophy in reflex inhibition, it is useful to review explanations of decrease in muscle size in conditions such as denervation atrophy and disuse atrophy. Reports of the time taken for a decrease in muscle fibre size as a result of denervation vary. It is common to find reports of atrophy of human muscles taking a few weeks to become evident following denervation (Jennekens 1982). Animal research models have commonly been adopted for atrophy studies because of ethical restrictions. Muscle fibres of the Australian opossum atrophy rapidly in the initial weeks following denervation. Atrophy becomes evident in cats after a month, and rats show evidence of decreases of approximately 20% within 3 weeks (Jennekens 1982). A more rapid rate of muscle atrophy in humans has been documented in immobilization studies. Muscle weight, fibre size and muscle strength decrease most dramatically during the first week of immobilization (Appell 1990). In the rat gastrocnemius muscle, a weight loss of 30% had occurred within the first 3 days of immobilization (Max et al 1971). Similar findings have been reported for muscle fibre size, with little further reduction in fibre diameter after 1 week (Appell 1986). Consequently, the rapid atrophy described in immobilization studies provides a basis for examining possible mechanisms at a muscular level involved in reflex inhibition.

Rapid muscle atrophy is a commonly observed clinical phenomenon in various conditions. Following spinal cord injury, a decrease in quadriceps depth of 16% within days of injury has been reported using ultrasound imaging (Taylor et al 1993). Up to 50% of quadriceps depth was lost in the first 3 weeks following injury. Clinical observations would suggest that rapid atrophy is more evident in certain muscles following injury, for example the quadriceps and especially the vastus medialis muscle in knee joint injuries. This may reflect varying susceptibility of different fibre types. It has been suggested that extensor (i.e. antigravity) muscles undergo more severe atrophy than flexors in reflex inhibition. This has also been demonstrated in immobilization studies and has been explained in terms of the greater amount of type I fibres in vastus medialis than in other components of the quadriceps, making the former the most vulnerable to immobilization-induced atrophy (Appell 1990). Furthermore, Appell (1990) suggested that muscles that function as antigravity muscles, cross a single joint and contain a relatively large proportion of slow fibres that are most vulnerable to atrophy owing to immobilization. This may well also be the case in reflex inhibition and may explain the finding of rapid atrophy of the multifidus, which has similar muscular characteristics. Dysfunction of the multifidus has also been found in the deep ventromedial corner of the muscle. The known anatomical distribution of type I and type II fibres may provide an explanation for this finding. The numerical proportions of the fibre types are not constant throughout the cross-sectional area of the muscle, with type I fibres tending to predominate in a deeper plane, nearer to the trunk or limb axis than type II fibres (Jennekens et al 1971, Johnson et al 1973, Pullen 1977). If these deep type I fibres are more susceptible to atrophy, this could explain the location of the changes found in the multifidus. Furthermore, type I muscle fibres are innervated by beta motoneurons (Landon 1982), which are frequently activated and receive a more continuous impulse flow from the motoneurons in the spinal cord than the type II fibres, which receive stimulation in the form of bursts of impulses (Burke and Edgerton 1975, Burke 1980). The greater susceptibility of slow fibres may relate to their dependence on tonic and ongoing neural input, and it may also depend on their more rapid rates of turnover and thus a higher rate constant for protein degradation (Goldberg 1967).

At a biochemical level, rapid muscle atrophy may be explained in terms of increased protein degradation, the autophagic response and decreased succinate dehydrogenase (Appell 1990). Increased protein degradation results in a net loss of muscle protein during atrophy. Evidence of autophagic activity has been demonstrated in atrophic muscle. Lysosomal enzymes may be important in the initiation of muscle atrophy. Succinate dehydrogenase activity decreases as a consequence of muscular disuse in animals (Booth 1978) and humans (Häggmark et al 1981). These changes further highlight the susceptibility of type I fibres, as they are dependent on oxidative metabolism.

In conclusion, rapid muscle atrophy is known to occur in reflex inhibition. The mechanisms involved at a muscular level may be similar to those described for disuse atrophy, which also leads to rapid muscle atrophy. Disuse atrophy presents a similar pattern of muscle dysfunction as demonstrated in the multifidus, with type I muscle fibres being predominantly affected, parts of muscles more affected than others and deep portions of the muscle specifically affected. This pattern is also seen in conditions of deloading (Ch. 7).

Summary

Injury to joints and joint structures has devastating effects on muscles surrounding the joints. The effects are rapid, localized, potent and long lasting. The muscles surrounding and intimately linked to the joints are the most affected when joint injury occurs. Antigravity muscles are more affected than flexor muscles. Multijoint/multifunction muscles are rarely affected by reflex inhibition. Muscle inhibition may persist well after painful symptoms have subsided. The link between reflex inhibition and the gamma motoneuron system may help to answer some of the intriguing unresolved questions surrounding the reflex inhibition mechanisms. There are distinct similarities between the patterns of muscles that are affected by reflex inhibition and by deloading. It is important to understand the susceptibility of the muscles that protect the joints in conditions of joint injury and deloading, as this information is vital for developing principles of therapeutic exercise. These are discussed in Chapter 14.

CLINICAL RELEVANCE

In the patient with lumbopelvic pain, there could be many mechanisms at play that could disturb muscle function. Consideration of neurophysiological mechanisms provides many basic principles for rehabilitation. Principles of therapeutic exercise that can be derived from the research on reflex inhibition include:

- excite the motoneuron pool;
- commence rehabilitation early;
- perform rehabilitation regularly;
- decrease stress on joint structures;
- exercise under painless conditions;
- use low-load exercise.

Excite the motoneuron pool

Reflex inhibition involves inhibition of the spinal motoneurons. Retraining must, therefore, focus on exciting the inhibited motoneuronal pool. Stener and Petersen (1962) stated that retraining was very important after injury, as the muscles that are inhibited will not be retrained automatically. Various strategies exist to enhance muscle retraining. The two possibilities are actively to decrease inhibition and/or facilitate the inhibited muscles. Decreasing muscle inhibition involves decreasing stress on joints and avoidance of pain. Facilitation will be more successful if factors actively causing or perpetuating reflex inhibition can be minimized. Facilitation may actually work in two ways in inhibition. It is known that sensory stimuli can block other afferent sensory stimuli in the spinal cord (Wolf 1978). Cutaneous sensory nerve stimulation can increase motoneuron excitability in humans. Facilitation techniques may reduce inhibition either by preventing activation of inhibitory synapses (disinhibition) or by increasing the excitability of anterior horn cells (Stokes and Young 1984a) or the gamma spindle system.

Techniques of facilitation have been described in the proprioceptive neuromuscular facilitation literature (Knott and Voss 1968). Techniques include manual contact, verbal commands, stretch facilitation, traction and approximation, and resistance. Manual contacts use pressure as a facilitating mechanism. Communication with the patient may include manual contact and the use of visual and verbal cues. Preparatory commands can be made more meaningful by demonstration of the desired movement and by providing a visual cue. Patient motivation may be positively influenced by verbal cues. Muscle stretch may be used to facilitate muscle contraction because of the physiology of the stretch reflex. The stretch reflex can be used to initiate voluntary motion as well as increase strength and enhance a response in weak motions. Vibration may also be used to stimulate muscle via the stretch reflex. Traction (or separation of joint surfaces) and approximation (compressing the joint surfaces) affect the joint receptors, which are receptive to alterations in joint position. Traction and approximation are used to stimulate the proprioceptive centres supplying the joint structures themselves. Remembering that peripheral feedback from the joint and ligament afferents affects the gamma spindle system (Johansson et al 1991b) and biases the spindle towards an increased sensitivity, provides a good basis for the inclusion of sensory techniques in the 'segmental stabilization retraining' approach, when the aim is to promote tonic contractions of the appropriate muscles.

EMG biofeedback has been successfully used to retrain inhibited quadriceps muscles (LeVeau and Rogers 1980, Krebs 1981, Wise et al 1984). Biofeedback techniques provide auditory and visual feedback, which are important for re-education of muscle function especially in the motor learning phase (Martenuik 1979). In isometric strengthening programmes, the addition of EMG biofeedback has been shown to lead to greater strength gains than with isometric exercise alone (Lucca and Recchuiti 1983). Increases in strength associated with biofeedback could result from both motor unit firing rate and recruitment patterns (Asfour et al 1990). Real-time ultrasound has also been used to provide feedback of muscle activation.

Commence rehabilitation early

It is important to commence rehabilitation of inhibited muscles early following injury, as the effects of reflex inhibition are known to occur as rapidly as within hours (Stokes and Young 1984a). This is an important principle to consider if reversal of the inhibition is the goal of the intervention. The frequency, intensity and duration of the exercise regimen should be tailored to the individual (Morrissey 1989) and should be of an intensity, frequency and duration that results in a training effect but does not result in increased inflammation (and increased muscle inhibition) of the injured joint. The fact that reflex inhibition lasts for such a long period of time following injury supports the concept that facilitation of the motoneuronal pool should be commenced as early as possible in an attempt to curtail these prolonged effects.

Perform rehabilitation regularly

As the goal of treatment is to increase the excitability of anterior horn cells and to stimulate the gamma spindle system, it can be argued that bombardment of the inhibited motoneuronal pool, through regular performance of exercises, would be necessary to promote overriding of the inhibitory sensory stimuli. The greater sensitivity of type I muscle fibres to disuse, pain and reflex inhibition than type II fibres also has implications for the frequency of rehabilitation required. It has been demonstrated that the type I fibres (which are connected to low-threshold motoneurons) receive a more continuous impulse flow from the motoneurons in the spinal cord than the type II fibres, which receive stimulation in the form of bursts of impulses (Burke and Edgerton 1975). Häggmark and Eriksson (1979) proposed that occasional exercise sessions would maintain type II fibres, but that type I fibres would require a more constant nervous activation. More constant nervous activation would require frequent and regular rehabilitation sessions, aimed at restoring the oxidative potential of the type I fibres.

Decrease stress on joint structures

The importance of decreasing stress on joint structures for rehabilitation relates to preventing or minimizing the effects of reflex inhibition. Evidence of the importance of a neutral or midrange position has been provided through investigations of inflamed and effused joints. To minimize the effects of inhibition, the joint should be placed in a neutral position (Krebs et al 1983). This is especially relevant in the acute situation, where both inflammation and effusion may be present. Effused and inflamed joints should be exercised only within a range of motion that does not stimulate afferent inhibitory impulses (DeAndre et al 1965). Evidence of the importance of a neutral position, especially for the extensor muscles, has been provided from inflammation studies.

Exercise under painless conditions

Although reflex inhibition can occur in the absence of pain, pain is capable of causing inhibition in its own right. With respect to pain inhibition and its possible effects on fibre type, Gydikov (1976) demonstrated that painful stimulation of the sural nerve caused selective inhibition of type I muscle fibres, whereas 'tactile' stimulation caused facilitation. If pain directly affects type I fibres, this must also direct the rehabilitation programme towards specific exercises that stimulate these fibres. This relates to the frequency of exercise, the amount of load applied during exercise and the type of contraction. It has been proposed that isometric exercises are more appropriate especially when pain is an inhibitory factor, as isometric exercises involve less joint movement and, therefore, in general, less pain production (Bower 1986).

Use low-load exercise

One of the strongest arguments for implementation of low load initially for patients with lumbopelvic pain relates to the response of inhibited muscles to resistance. Resistance to muscle contraction is generally considered as one of the most effective muscle facilitation techniques, as the number of activated motor units increases approximately in proportion to the magnitude of the resistance (Knott and Voss 1986). However, muscle activity can be inhibited by resistance to contraction in the pathological situation (Janda 1986). Janda (1986) proposed that increased loading in this case will cause a decrease of activity in the muscle being loaded. To continue the exercise against the applied resistance, the inhibited muscle will be eliminated from the movement pattern and replaced by other non-inhibited muscles. Repetition of exercises in this case could further intensify muscle inhibition and, under these circumstances, exercise against resistance may harm the patient.

Further evidence for low-load exercise relates to fibre type. Stimulation of type I fibres, which are affected by reflex inhibition and pain inhibition, requires low-intensity holding contractions suitable for type I oxidative fibres. It has been shown that repeated isometric training increased the oxidative potential of the quadriceps muscle (Grimby et al 1973), suggesting that frequent low-load exercises of this type may be of benefit in rehabilitation of patients with inhibition.

Chapter 9

Pain models

Paul Hodges

INTRODUCTION

In recent years, there has been increasing interest in the neurobiology of pain. This field has grown out of the realisation that the spectrum of chronic back pain disorders cannot be reduced to a simple biomechanical model asserting that stimulation of peripheral nociceptors is responsible for pain (reviewed by Butler 2000). Instead a model must include consideration of the multiple plastic changes in the nervous system that may mediate the perpetuation of pain and the interaction between biological, psychological and social elements of the pain experience. With this paradigm shift, there has been a tendency in some circles to reject the biological in favour of the other two elements. It is not the purpose of this chapter to review the field of pain neurobiology but instead to consider the interaction between the experience of pain and the motor control of spinal stability. Readers interested in reading further in the area of pain neurobiology and the psychosocial aspects of pain are referred to key texts in that area by Butler (2000) and Waddell (1998).

Many authors report changes in the control of the trunk muscles in people with low back pain. Although there is considerable disagreement regarding the nature of these changes, we have consistently found that the effects are different on the deep local muscles than on the superficial global or multisegment muscles of the lumbopelvic region. The specific changes in motor control of the multiple muscles systems will be described in Chapters 10–12. This section will review two key issues: first, whether changes in motor control precede or follow the onset of low back pain and, second, the possible mechanisms for the effect of pain on motor control. Recent data indicate that experimentally induced pain may replicate some of the changes identified in people with low back pain. In Chapter 7, it was argued that 'deloading' induces changes in the muscle system that may lead to changes in control, resulting in irritation of nociceptors and pain. Although this may be true, it is also plausible to consider that pain may lead to changes in motor control and that these changes may be responsible for the recurrence of low back pain. Similarly, the effect of injury on motor control may play a role, as described in Chapter 8. Considering the spectrum of pain disorders, it is plausible to consider that elements of all may be involved in the incidence of low back pain.

WHICH COMES FIRST: PAIN OR MOTOR CONTROL CHANGES

It is not certain whether pain causes changes in motor control or whether motor control changes lead to pain, or both. Farfan (1973) and Panjabi (1992a, b), amongst others, have presented models suggesting that deficits in motor control lead to poor control of joint movement, repeated microtrauma and pain. Consistent with this model, Janda (1978) has argued that people who have mild neurological signs (e.g. minor coordination difficulties) are more likely to have pain as adults. Furthermore, slow reaction times have been linked to increased risk of musculo-skeletal injury (Taimela and Kujala 1992). As described in Chapter 7, deloading may lead to changes in motor control that could lead to pain via similar mechanisms. However, the converse may also be true. Perhaps pain leads to changes in motor control. While neither possibility can be ruled out, numerous studies have replicated the changes in motor control identified in people with low back pain by the experimental induction of pain. For instance, injection of hypertonic saline into the lumbar longissimus muscle to produce transient pain induces changes in the feedforward responses of the local muscle (transversus abdominis) that are similar to those identified as clinical pain (Hodges et al 2003e, see

Ch. 10, Fig. 9.1). Changes in global muscle activity differed between individuals. However, activity of at least one superficial trunk muscle was increased in all subjects. This variability in the response of the superficial muscles to pain is consistent with clinical observations. In separate studies, loss of relaxation of the erector spinae muscles, which is present in low back pain, has been replicated during trunk flexion (Zedka et al 1999a; Fig. 9.2) and gait (Arendt-Nielsen et al 1996) by experimentally induced pain. These are just a few specific examples of replication of clinical changes in motor control. Therefore, if pain occurs, this may provide the initial trigger for changes in motor control. It may be hypothesized that minor injury and pain may result if demand placed on the spine exceeds an individual's ability to maintain spinal stability, for example during lifting or in a motor vehicle accident, this may initiate a vicious cycle. Similarly, if pain is initiated for another cause, for instance from disc swelling from unloading, a similar cycle of events may be initiated. Considering that pain can be responsible for changes in motor control, it is important to consider the possible mechanisms for this effect.

POSSIBLE MECHANISMS FOR THE EFFECT OF PAIN ON MOTOR CONTROL

A number of mechanisms have been proposed to explain the effect of pain on motor control (Fig. 9.3). These include changes in excitability at the spinal or cortical level, changes in proprioception or afferent mediated control, or specific cortical effects imparted by aspects of pain, such as its demand on central nervous system (CNS) resources, stress or fear. The following sections consider each of these possible mechanisms.

Direct effects of pain on motor control

Widespread changes in excitability have been identified at many levels of the motor system during pain. Acute experimental pain has been shown to cause changes in spinal motoneuron activity (Matre et al 1998, Svensson et al 1998, 2000). For instance, increased stretch reflex amplitude of the soleus muscle has been reported after intramuscular injection of hypertonic saline (Matre et al 1998).

(a)

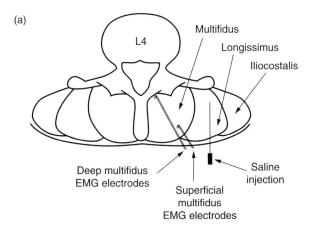

(b)

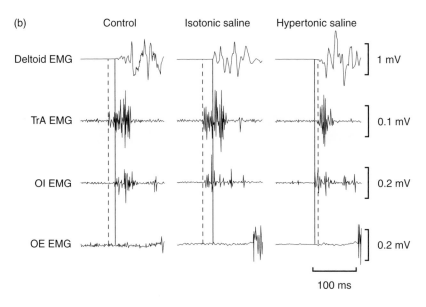

Figure 9.1 Effect of experimentally induced pain on motor control of transversus abdominis (TrA). (a) Pain was induced by injection of hypertonic saline into the paraspinal muscles at the L4 level. (b) When subjects rapidly moved an arm in response to a light, the response of the TrA was initiated before the deltoid in trials without pain and in trials with injection of non-painful isotonic saline. When the arm was moved during pain, the onset of TrA activity was delayed. There was no change in activity of obliquus internus (OI) or externus abdominis (OE) for this subject. (Adapted from Hodges et al 2003e.)

Others have reported reduced amplitude of motor potential evoked by transcranial magnetic stimulation over the motor cortex in response to experimental pain (Valeriani et al 1999). However, these responses may be specific to task or specific to muscle, as other studies have reported no changes in excitability of the motoneuron or motor cortex (Gandevia et al 1996, Zedka et al 1999b). Those authors argued that changes in motor drive may occur 'upstream' of the motor cortex, for instance involving areas associated with motor planning. As mentioned in Chapter 8, reflex inhibition of motoneuron excitability has also been suggested to occur in association with swelling (Spencer et al 1984) and injury to joint structures (Ekholm et al

1960), which has been argued to indicate polysynaptic inhibition at a spinal level (Stokes and Young 1984a). While this may be a factor in clinical populations, it cannot explain the findings of studies of experimental pain that is not associated with oedema and injury, and similar effects cannot be produced by injection of similar volumes of isotonic saline into muscle (Graven-Nielsen et al 1997, Hodges et al 2003e).

Evidence from several groups argues that changes in trunk muscle activity in low back pain may not be mediated by simple changes in excitability. Zedka et al (1999a,b) were unable to identify changes in the short-latency response of the paraspinal muscles to a mechanical tap to the

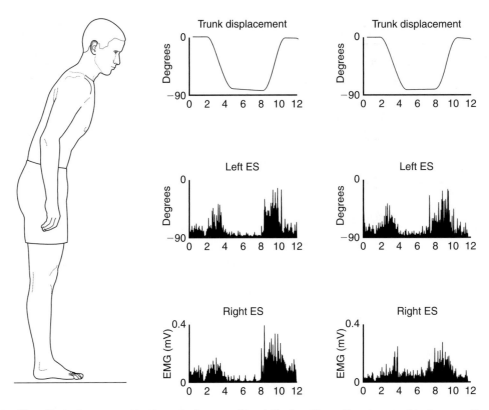

Figure 9.2 The effect of movement to the end of range of trunk flexion. Normally, when a subject moves, the erector spinae (ES) muscles are silent on electromyography (i.e. the flexion-relaxation phenomenon). However, when a person is given experimental pain the period of silence disappears. This also occurs in people with clinical back pain. (Adapted from Zedka et al 1999a.)

muscle following pain induced by injection of hypertonic saline into the muscle (changes in this component would be consistent with changes in motoneuron excitability) (Fig. 9.4). These authors did find changes in later components of the response that can be influenced by input from higher centres. Similarly, we have shown several changes in coordination of the trunk muscles in association with pain that are inconsistent with a change in excitability or delayed transmission of the motor command. For example, when people move an arm rapidly, normally the response of transversus abdominis is independent of the direction of arm movement (Hodges and Richardson 1997b). If the delay in response observed during pain was a result of a change in excitability, it may be predicted that the response would remain consistent between movement directions, although delayed when people have pain. However, this is not the

case (Hodges and Richardson 1996, 1998, Hodges et al 2003e; see Ch. 10).

Consistent with the identification of changes in motor planning, there is compelling evidence that pain has strong effects at the supraspinal level (Venna et al 1994, Derbyshire et al 1997, Lorenz and Bromm 1997, Kuukkanen and Malkia 1998, Luoto et al 1998, 1999, Hodges 2001). Both short- and long-term changes are thought to occur with pain in the activity of the supraspinal structures including the cortex. Many studies have reported changes during experimental pain in the activity of regions of the brain involved in movement planning and performance (see Derbyshire et al 1997). One area that has been consistently found to be affected is the anterior cingulate cortex (Peyron et al 2000). The anterior cingulate cortex has also been reported to be chronically active in people with chronic low back pain (Hsieh et al 1995) and has long been

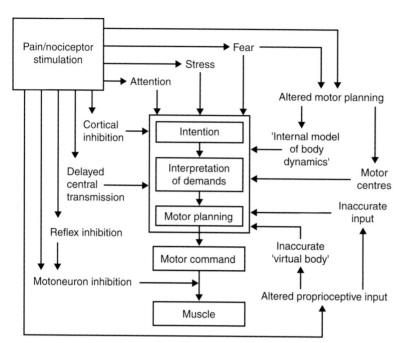

Figure 9.3 Possible mechanisms by which pain can affect motor control. Multiple mechanisms have been proposed. It is unlikely that the simple inhibitory pathways (left) can mediate the complex changes in motor control of the trunk muscles. The most likely candidates are changes in motor planning via a direct influence of pain on the motor centres, fear avoidance or changes in the sensory system. (Adapted from Hodges and Moseley, 2003.)

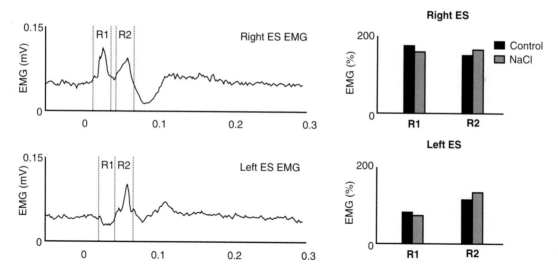

Figure 9.4 When a tap is applied to the right paraspinal muscles, there is a short-latency reflex response. This is not changed during experimental pain (injection of hypertonic saline, NaCl). This indicates that there is no change in excitability of the motoneuron following pain. ES, erector spinae; EMG, electromyography; R, refex response. (Adapted from Zedka et al 1999a.)

thought to be important in motor responses, with its direct projections to motor and supplementary motor areas (Price 2000). Hypothetically, at least, activation of these cortical regions during pain may influence movement control directly and mediate the changes reported above. Other authors have identified increased areas of somatosensory cortex activated by noxious cutaneous stimulation of the finger and back in people with low back pain (Flor et al 1997). Furthermore, the activated area increased as a function of the duration of their pain. These changes may contribute to the perpetuation of pain in the absence of peripheral nociception, but they may also contribute to the motor changes. Further work is required to clarify these findings as they relate to motor control.

Effect of the attention–demanding aspects of pain on motor control

Although nociceptive stimulation and pain may disrupt motor output directly, it is also possible that an effect is caused by aspects of pain, such as its attention-demanding requirements, stress or fear. In terms of attention demand, it is widely considered that pain utilizes attentional resources, probably by virtue of its direct relevance for survival (reviewed by Price 2000). In view of the finite nature of information-processing resources, this may compromise the attention associated with movement performance. Several studies support this hypothesis. For example, increased latencies and/or error rates in the presence of pain have been indicated by recordings of event-related potentials in the cortex (Rosenfeld et al 1992), brain imaging studies (Derbyshire et al 1997), cognitive performance tasks (Crombez et al 1998, 1999; Eccleston and Crombez 1999) and a combination of these methods (Lorenz and Bromm 1997). Therefore, pain may lead to changes in movement coordination as a result of the increased demand placed on information-processing resources. While several authors have identified slower reaction times in people with low back pain, which may be attributable to this mechanism (Luoto et al 1999), we have recently shown that performance of an attention-demanding task does not replicate the changes in trunk muscle activity seen in people with low back pain (Moseley et al 2001). In this study, subjects rapidly moved an arm in response to a visual stimulus while performing an attention-demanding task. Although the reaction time of the arm movement was delayed, the response of the deep local trunk muscles (transversus abdominis and deep multifidus) occurred earlier relative to the deltoid response (i.e. opposite to the changes seen in low back pain). There was no change in the activity of the superficial abdominal or paraspinal muscles. Therefore, although attention demand may influence many elements of movement

performance, it is unlikely to explain the effects seen in the local and global muscles in low back pain.

Effect of stress on motor control

A further possibility is that the stress associated with pain produces the change in control of the trunk muscles. Numerous studies have shown that stress (i.e. perception of threat) may affect motor control (Jones and Cale 1997, Weinberg and Hunt 1976, van Galen and van Huygevoort 2000). Notably, trunk muscle activity during a lifting task was altered when the task was performed in the presence of psychosocial stressors (Marras et al 2000) and shoulder muscle activity during a keyboard task was altered by work-related stress (Ekberg and Eklund 1995). Furthermore, changes in paraspinal muscle activity in patients with chronic pain have been linked to subjective measures of distress and anxiety, rather than just the intensity of pain (Flor and Turk 1989, Flor and Birbaumer 1992, Vlaeyen et al 1999). We have tested the effect of stress on the postural response of the trunk muscles during rapid arm movements by repeating the attention-demanding task described above, but with negative feedback of performance and other negative psychosocial cues (Moseley et al 2001). Although the addition of stress did not replicate the changes observed with experimentally induced pain, there was a delay in the response of the deep local trunk muscles relative to tasks when the attention demand was non-stressful, indicating some effect of stress.

Effect of fear of pain and (re)injury on motor control

An alternative argument is that the changes in control may relate to the fear associated with pain. The notion that fear is important in behavioural and motor output associated with pain is not new, and the fear-avoidance model has gained considerable support in the literature (reviewed by Vlaeyen and Linton 2000). In brief, the fear-avoidance model argues that fear of pain and (re)injury prevents normal return to activity, which leads to deconditioning and disability (Vlaeyen and Linton 2000). Although the primary application of the fear-avoidance model has been in consideration of behavioural response to pain and injury, corresponding findings have been reported in the pattern of motor control (Main and Watson 1996). Several studies have reported differences in trunk muscle activity between fearful and non-fearful patients with back pain. For instance fearful patients have a greater reduction in endurance of the paraspinal muscles (Biedermann et al 1991) and less relaxation of the paraspinal muscles at the end of trunk flexion (Watson and Booker 1997) than non-fearful patients and controls. Furthermore, it has been suggested that patients with chronic low back pain have increased paraspinal muscle activity when they are exposed to personally relevant stressors but not when they are exposed to general stressors (Flor and Birbaumer 1992). Finally, when pain-free subjects rapidly move an arm but are subjected to moderately painful electrical shocks to the back that are unpredictable in time and amplitude, the response of transversus abdominis and deep multifidus is delayed in a manner that is similar to that seen with experimentally induced low back pain (Moseley et al 2001). While the last finding does not confirm that fear or anticipation of pain causes the changes seen in people with low back pain, it does suggest that fear may at least replicate the changes. Moreover, it is possible that both pain and fear of pain act directly on the motor centres through a common mechanism. It is important to consider that fear of pain may explain why people who have a history of pain, but no present pain, have delayed activity of transversus abdominis (Hodges and Richardson 1996). Furthermore, if fear of pain can disrupt the normal control of the trunk muscles, this may provide a link between psychosocial factors and physiological changes that lead to recurrence of pain. It could also be interpreted that these changes in motor control are an adaptation to limit loading and prevent recurrence. However, we propose that these adaptive strategies may provide a short-term solution with long-term sequelae (see below).

Effect of inaccurate sensory input on motor control

An additional factor to consider is that accurate control of movement is dependent on the sensory element of the motor system. Inaccurate afferent input would affect all aspects of motor control from simple reflex responses (e.g. those arising from stimulation of mechanoreceptors in the muscles (Zedka et al 1999a) or other elements of the spine (Indahl et al 1995, Solomonow et al 1998)) to complex movements that are dependent on an accurate 'internal model of body dynamics' (see Gurfinkel 1994), which allows the CNS to predict the interaction between internal and external forces. Several studies have reported decreased acuity to spinal motion in low back pain (Taimela et al 1999) and impaired ability to reposition accurately in those with low back pain (Gill and Callaghan 1998, Brumagne et al 2000). In addition, muscle spindle sensitivity is altered by pain (e.g. Pedersen et al 1997) and muscle activity (Gandevia et al 1992). Consequently, any change in activity may adversely affect perception of movement. Finally, several studies have argued that sensory acuity may be reduced by fatigue (Carpenter et al 1998); thus decreased muscle endurance with injury or pain may lead to impaired sensory acuity via increased fatiguability. In view of these changes, it may be argued that inaccurate sensory input may be responsible for many of the changes in motor control that have been identified. It has been argued that altered proprioceptive input may result from changes in activity of the deep muscles, caused by damage to receptors, or structures in which the receptors are situated, or by changes in the interpretation of proprioceptive input in the presence of pain. For instance, reorganization of the somatosensory cortex has been identified in chronic pain (Flor et al 1997) and proprioceptive input may stimulate central nociceptive pathways and be perceived as pain (reviewed by Hoheisel and Mense 1989). Whatever the mechanism, proprioceptive re-education should form part of intervention for low back pain.

Why are there consistent changes in the local system?

If pain or other supraspinal mechanisms such as fear can disrupt motor control, why does this lead to the relatively consistent finding of reduced activity of deep local spinal muscles and increased activity of the superficial global muscles? The explanation may lie in the pain-adaptation model of Lund and colleagues (1991). This model stipulates that, in the event of pain, the alteration in motor control serves to limit movement. During movement, this involves a decrease in agonist muscle activity and increased antagonist activity to limit the velocity, force and range of movement (Svensson et al 1995). This pattern of response has been observed in clinical and experimental pain studies for many regions of the body including the jaw (Svensson et al 1995) and trunk (Zedka et al 1999a). In terms of control of a segment such as the trunk, the response may also involve general stiffening of the body segment(s) by muscle co-activation. Panjabi (1992a,b) and Cholewicki et al (1997) predicted that such a response would increase vertebral control and is consistent with augmented activity of the large, superficial trunk muscles.

Consistent with this proposal, there is evidence of relative stiffening of the spine in pain. Moe-Nilssen et al (1999) reported reduced trunk movement during gait during experimentally induced pain, and Henry (2001) showed that trunk movement following a support surface translation is reduced during pain. Hypothetically, if the general stiffness of the spine is increased, the CNS may perceive the demand for 'fine-tuning' to be diminished, leading to reduced activity of the deep local spinal muscles despite the potential long-term sequelae of this strategy (see below). This is consistent with data which suggest that postural activity of the trunk muscles is reduced or delayed when the perceived stability of the spine is increased (Hodges et al 1997b, Stokes et al 2000). After resolution of the pain, this adapted strategy may also resolve or, in the presence of ongoing fear of pain or other reinforcement, persist to chronicity. This hypothesis requires investigation.

CLINICAL SIGNIFICANCE

If the experience of pain can cause changes in motor control, this has several key implications for re-education of motor control in people with low back pain. A key issue to consider is that while the changes outlined above may not be responsible for motor control changes in all people with back pain, the effects of pain and its wider elements is likely to impart ongoing effects on the accuracy of motor control and may require specific attention in clinical management.

Consequence of changes in control

As outlined in Chapter 2, the local and global muscles impart specific elements of the control of spinal stability. Any change in the coordination of these systems is likely to lead to reduced accuracy of spinal control. Briefly, a reduction of the fine-tuning of intervertebral control and increased global stiffening of the spine may decrease overall spinal motion, but with reduced accuracy of control of intervertebral motion. Furthermore, excessive activity of the global muscles may increase spinal loading and reduce the contribution of spinal motion to spinal control strategies. These issues will be considered in more detail in Chapter 10.

Implications for exercise intervention

These data have several important implications for exercise for muscle control. First, although pain may not be the key factor in development of motor control changes in all people with back pain, its presence is likely to be associated with perpetuation of ongoing motor control changes, contributing to the ongoing cycle of 'pain–motor control dysfunction–pain'. An important issue from the preceding discussion is that actual pain may not need to be present, as 'fear' or anticipation of pain and (re)injury may have similar effects. This may be a major factor why people who have recovered from an episode of low back pain have motor control changes even when they are in remission.

Second, the demand for accurate motor control is likely to be increased in people with low back pain because of microtrauma to the passive elements of the spine and of peripheral sensitization (see Butler (2000) for review of peripheral sensitization). If passive support for the spine is reduced, this must be compensated by changes in motor control. Numerous studies of experimental trauma have indicated large changes, particularly in the neutral zone (Panjabi 1992a). Therefore, motor control must adapt to compensate for this reduction in stability and control (Panjabi 1992b). The second issue is that numerous changes occur in the nervous system, including plastic changes in the spinal cord and higher centres, as well as changes in the periphery. If peripheral sensitization is present, then the requirement for control of intervertebral motion is likely to be increased to avoid nociceptive stimulation. In either case, this may lead to recurrence if motor control is compromised by pain or potential pain.

Third, the potential for pain to lead to changes in motor control indicates that other strategies which may assist in the resolution of pain, either in the short or long term, are likely to be beneficial. Therefore, the pain-relieving effects of other therapeutic modalities play an important role in management of muscle and control dysfunction. Furthermore, consideration of the psychosocial aspects of pain may require consideration. If an individual has elements of fear of pain or (re)injury in their presentation, these may need to be addressed before motor control changes can be resolved. Many studies indicate that these changes are prevalent in people with low back pain, and methods have been devised to assess and manage these elements. The reader is referred to Butler (2000), Main and Spanswick (2000) and Moseley and Hodges (2003) for further consideration of these issues. A key finding of the studies of pain, fear and stress is that there is interdependence of the biological, psychological and social aspects of the pain experience, and in many cases all elements will require consideration. It is also important to consider that physical intervention may lead to improvements in other non-physical aspects of a patient's presentation. For instance, as motor control education makes a patient responsible for their own recovery, this may lead to positive outcomes in terms of changing the patient's locus of control, which is an important aspect of cognitive behavioural approaches (reviewed by Main and Spanswick 2000). A final consideration is that it would be naive to argue that all back pain can be resolved by motor control re-education, and all dimensions of the neurobiology of pain must be considered.

SECTION 4

Impairments in the joint protection mechanisms in low back pain

Chapter **10**

Abdominal mechanism in low back pain

Paul Hodges

INTRODUCTION

There has been considerable interest in the function of the abdominal muscles in people with low back pain. Early studies of trunk muscle function focused on the strength and endurance of these muscles in patients with chronic low back pain (Thorstensson and Arvidson 1982, Suzuki and Endo 1983). The results of these studies have been variable. For instance, some show reduced strength and endurance (Suzuki et al 1977) while others do not (Thorstensson and Arvidson 1982). It has been suggested that these changes may be more related to inactivity than to pain (Thorstensson and Arvidson 1982). Furthermore, the importance of changes in strength and endurance is unclear, as maximum strength and endurance are infrequently required in function and these parameters indicate little of how the muscles are used. More recently, the increased understanding of the importance of the motor control of lumbopelvic stability has led to the emergence of investigations of the control and coordination of the abdominal muscles. Although considerable variability has been identified in terms of changes in the control of the global muscles, we have found consistent evidence of changes in activity of the transversus abdominis. This section reviews the scope of changes in the abdominal muscles and highlights the relevance of these findings for clinical practice in light of biomechanical models of spinal stability. Changes are described in terms of the specific motor control strategies and then the clinical relevance of these findings in terms of the effect on the control of lumbopelvic stability.

CHANGES IN CONTROL OF THE LOCAL MUSCLES

Changes in feedforward control

As mentioned in Chapter 2, feedforward strategies are preplanned by the nervous system and represent the pattern of muscle activity initiated by the central nervous system in advance of predictable challenges to lumbopelvic stability to prepare for the perturbation. As such, these strategies provide evidence of changes in the manner in which the neural system considers it appropriate to meet the demands of internal and external forces. Several studies have investigated the onset of muscle

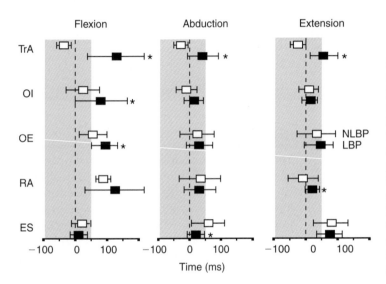

Figure 10.1 Onset of activity of the trunk muscles with movement of the arm in each direction for individuals with and without low back pain. The vertical dashed line indicates the onset of deltoid activity. With movement in each direction, the onset of transversus abdominis (TrA) precedes the onset of deltoid in pain-free individuals but is significantly delayed with each direction of movement. OI, obliquus internus abdominis; OE, obliquus externus abdominis; RA, rectus abdominis; ES, erector spinae; LBP, low back pain; NLBP, no low back pain. (Adapted from Hodges and Richardson, 1996.)

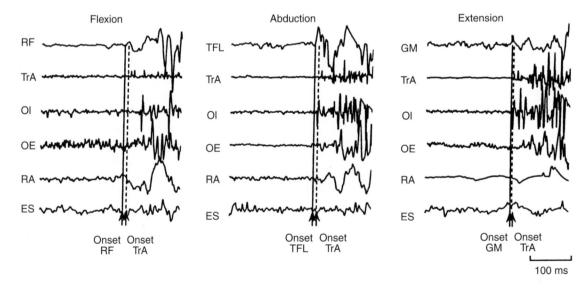

Figure 10.2 Raw electromyographic activity of the abdominal (rectus abdominis (RA), obliquus externus abdominis (OE), obliquus internus abdominis (OI) and transversus abdominis (TrA)), superficial multifidus (MF) muscles and the prime movers of hip flexion (rectus femoris (RF)), abduction (tensor fascia latae (TFL)) and extension (gluteus maximus (GM)) with hip flexion, abduction and extension performed by a patient with low back pain. The onset of activity of the prime mover of the limb is denoted by a line and TrA is denoted by a fine dashed line. There is delayed onset of the TrA, occurring after that of the prime mover. (Reproduced with permission from Hodges and Richardson, 1998, pp. 46–56.)

activity in association with rapid limb movements (Hodges and Richardson 1996, 1998). These studies investigated people with chronic recurrent low back pain when their pain was in remission. The most consistent finding was delayed activity of transversus abdominis with movements of the arm (Fig. 10.1) and leg (Fig. 10.2) in all directions. Activity of transversus abdominis was absent in the period before movement and, therefore, failing to prepare the spine for the perturbation resulting from limb movement. In view of the evidence described in Chapters 2 and 3, this is consistent with a compromise in the control of intervertebral motion. In association with the changes in activity of transversus abdominis, the activity of the superficial abdominal muscles was only delayed with specific movements. A major finding was that the change in transversus abdominis activity could not be explained by 'inhibition' of the response or delayed transmission in the central nervous system. As discussed in Chapter 9, the normal response of transversus abdominis is not dependent on the direction of force acting on the spine, and the muscle provides a non-direction-specific contribution to lumbopelvic stability. The response of transversus abdominis in people with low back pain is earlier with shoulder extension than the other movements, which is similar to the response of the superficial trunk muscles (Hodges and Richardson 1996, Moseley et al 2003). In other words, the normal differential control between the local and global systems is no longer present. As mentioned in Chapter 9, this change in differential control has been replicated in healthy individuals by experimentally induced pain.

Further evidence for a change in motor planning has come from studies in which the preparation for movement is varied. In a healthy population, the reaction time of the arm movement is delayed when the preparation for movement is reduced (Fig. 10.3). This is associated with a slowing of the response of the global abdominal muscles in line with the limb movement, but there is no slowing of the response of transversus abdominis (Hodges and Richardson 1999a). Instead, the response of transversus abdominis maintained a constant reaction time. This finding provides further evidence for differential control of the local and global muscles. Although this finding may be

interpreted to suggest that control of transversus abdominis occurs at a more primitive level of the nervous system, recent data from studies of transcranial magnetic stimulation of the motor cortex confirm that cortical inputs do contribute to the ongoing postural activity of transversus abdominis (Hodges et al 2003f). However, when people with back pain perform that same task with variable preparation for movement, the activity of transversus abdominis is delayed along with the other abdominal muscles (Hodges 2001). Taken together, these findings are likely to represent a change in motor planning.

Recently it has been questioned whether a change in timing of transversus abdominis in the order of milliseconds can have a significant influence on spinal control (McGill 2002b). However, the temporal aspects of transversus abdominis activity are only a small element of the extent of changes in control identified for this muscle and the temporal data simply represent a window of opportunity through which the control of transversus abdominis has been investigated and changes in control have been identified. In reality, widespread changes in control of transversus abdominis exist in people with low back pain. For instance, the threshold for activation of transversus abdominis is increased in people with low back pain (i.e. activity of transversus abdominis is not initiated until arm movements are performed with greater velocity (Hodges and Richardson 1999) than required in control subjects (Hodges and Richardson 1997c; Fig. 10.4), and tonic activity of transversus abdominis is reduced (Hodges et al 2003e). However, tonic activity during sustained and repetitive tasks is likely to have feedback-mediated components as well, and this is discussed in the next section.

Changes in feedback-mediated control

In feedback-mediated control, the neural control system initiates a response of the trunk muscles to afferent input from an unpredicted perturbation (Massion 1992). Changes in a variety of reflex responses have been identified in musculoskeletal pain syndromes, although most commonly investigated for the paraspinal muscles (e.g. Wilder et al 1996, Leinonen et al 2001). Although no studies

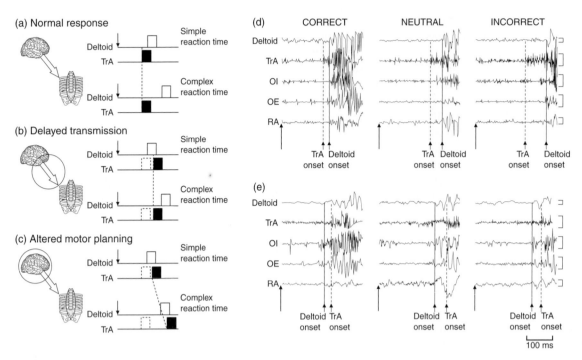

Figure 10.3 Effect of movement preparation on the response of the trunk muscles in association with limb movement. (a) When the reaction time for arm movement is increased in individuals without low back pain by increased task complexity, the reaction time of the muscle responsible for limb movement is increased but that of transversus abdominis (TrA) remains unchanged. The stimulus to move is indicated by the arrow. (b) If the delay in onset of activity of TrA in those with chronic low back pain results from delayed transmission of the descending command in the nervous system, it might be expected that the onset of TrA activity would be delayed but the general strategy would remain unchanged (i.e. the response of TrA would maintain a constant temporal relationship to the movement stimulus between conditions). The dotted boxes indicate the response of TrA in a person without low back pain (i.e. as for (a)). (c) If the response of TrA does not maintain a constant temporal relationship to the movement stimulus in conjunction with an increased reaction time for arm movement, this would suggest a change in strategy rather than a simple delay in transmission of the descending command. (d and e) Representative raw electromyographic (EMG) recordings from a control subject (d) and a subject with chronic recurrent low back pain (e). Responses are shown for all muscles in each of the preparatory conditions for trials of shoulder flexion. The solid and dashed lines denote the onsets of deltoid and TrA EMG, respectively. The large arrow at the bottom left of each panel indicates the time of the movement stimulus. Note that, for the control subjects, the reaction time of TrA did not increase along with that of deltoid, rectus abdominis (RA), obliquus externus abdominis (OE), obliquus internus abdominis (OI) as the preparation for movement decreased. However when people with low back pain performed the same task, the reaction time of TrA was increased with the other muscles. That is, the data are consistent with the altered motor planning option shown in (c). (Adapted from Hodges 2001.)

have yet investigated the activity of the transversus abdominis in response to unexpected perturbations, several studies have indicated changes in tasks that incorporate feedback contributions, such as tonic activity. Notably, tonic activity of transversus abdominis, which is normally observed during repetitive trunk (Cresswell et al 1992a) and limb (Hodges and Gandevia 2000a) movements,

is reduced during experimentally induced pain (Hodges et al 2003e) (Fig. 10.5). In addition, the relative electromyographic (EMG) activity of rectus abdominis and the EMG activity recorded with electrodes over the inferiolateral abdominal wall was altered in people with chronic low back pain during a voluntary task to move the abdominal wall inwards (O'Sullivan et al 1997). Notably,

(a)

(b)

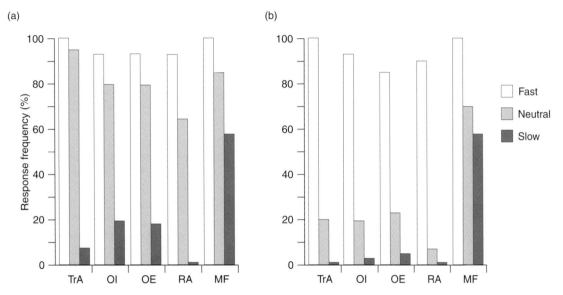

Figure 10.4   Frequency of trials in which a response of each of the abdominal (rectus abdominis (RA), obliquus externus abdominis (OE), obliquus internus abdominis (OI) and transversus abdominis (TrA)) and superficial multifidus (MF) muscles was present with movement of the upper limb at each of three different speeds of limb movement: fast (~300°/s), natural (~150°/s) and slow (~30°/s). (a) Controls; (b) patients with a history of low back pain. The frequency of response of all the abdominal muscles is reduced from the natural speed condition for the subjects with low back pain, thus suggesting that the threshold speed for trunk muscle activation is increased when people have low back pain. (P W Hodges and C A Richardson 1999.)

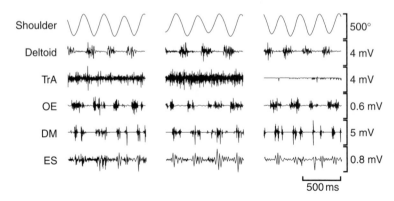

Figure 10.5   Reduction of tonic activity of transversus abdominis following experimentally induced pain. Activity is shown for a representative subject during repetitive arm movement during control trials without pain, following non-painful injection of isotonic saline and during pain following hypertonic saline. TrA, transversus abdominis; OE, obliquus externus abdominis; DM, deep multifidus; ES, erector spinae. (Adapted from Hodges et al 2003e.)

performance of a similar voluntary task of abdominal movement has been associated with timing of transversus abdominis activity in an arm movement paradigm (Hodges et al 1996).

Recent studies have also identified changes in the activity of transversus abdominis using ultrasound imaging. Changes in muscle thickness, fascicle pennation angle and fascicle length can be measured with ultrasound imaging and are related to muscle activity (Herbert and Gandevia 1995, Misuri et al 1997, Maganaris et al 1998, Hodges et al 2003d). When healthy individuals performed gentle isometric leg efforts, automatic recruitment of the abdominal muscles, including transversus abdominis, could be detected, indicated by an increase in thickness (Ferreira et al 2003). Notably, activity of transversus abdominis occurred with movement in opposing directions. This was confirmed with intramuscular EMG recordings. However, when people with low back pain performed the same task, the increase in thickness of transversus abdominis was less, particularly in one direction (Ferreira et al 2003).

CHANGES IN CONTROL OF THE GLOBAL MUSCLES

In contrast to the impaired activity of the local abdominal muscles, activity of the global muscles is often augmented. In studies of experimentally induced pain, activity of at least one of the global muscles was increased when pain was increased (Hodges et al 2003e). However, there was considerable variability in the characteristics of this response between subjects. This finding is consistent with the clinical observation of considerable individual variation in presentation. When arm movement tasks have been investigated in people with clinical low back pain, few changes in global muscle activity have been identified; the changes seen include a combination of delayed and earlier onsets of activity (Hodges and Richardson 1996). The reason for the failure to identify augmented

global activity is likely to be because of the grouping of results, failing to identify individual differences.

Key recent findings have indicated delayed relaxation of the superficial abdominal muscles, particularly obliquus externus abdominis, when a mass was unexpectedly removed from the trunk (i.e. unloading) (Radebold et al 2000), and greater activity of the obliquus externus during rotation efforts (Ng et al 2002a). In the studies of trunk unloading, subjects were positioned in standing with the pelvis supported and a mass attached to a rope connected to either the front or back of the trunk. When the mass is released, activity of muscles on the opposite side of the trunk must reduce for the trunk to maintain an upright position (Radebold et al 2000). When patients with low back pain performed this task, the time to relaxation of the obliquus externus abdominis was increased (i.e. indicative of overactivity) (Fig. 10.6). Two important features are worthy of note. First, the delayed offset of activity was associated with increased antagonist co-activation of anterior and posterior muscles. Second, not all subjects had a modified response and a proportion of subjects had normal activity. As unloading responses are

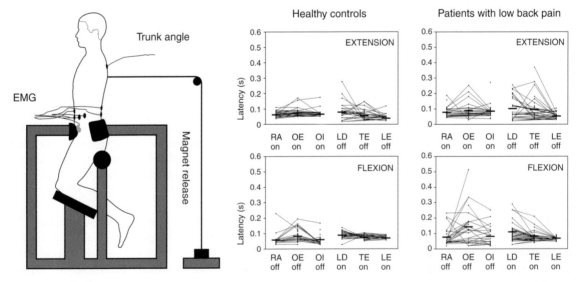

Figure 10.6   When a load is rapidly removed from the trunk, activity of the trunk muscles must reduce for the trunk to maintain an upright posture. When a load is removed from the back (bottom panels) activity of obliquus externus abdominis (OE) must reduce. This reduction in activity is delayed in a subset of people with chronic back pain (right bottom panel). RA, rectus abdominis; OI, obliquus internus abdominis; LD, latisimus dorsi; TE, thoracic erector spinae; LE, lumbar erector spinae; EMG, electromyography.

generally regarded to be a result of reduction of gamma support for contraction (Angel et al 1965), delayed offset may indicate a deficit in the sensory system or a change in descending drive to the motoneuron pool. Notably, in a follow-up study, these authors identified that the change in offset of activity was associated with impaired postural control in sitting (Radebold et al 2001).

The other recent example of overactivity relates to activity of the oblique abdominal muscles during trunk rotation efforts. When subjects with and without low back pain performed isometric rotation at varying levels from 30 to 100% maximal torque, those with low back pain had greater activity of obliquus externus abdominis (and decreased multifidus activity) (Ng et al 2002a) and reduced fatigue rate for the right obliquus externus abdominis (Ng et al 2002b). Consistent with other studies, these data provide additional evidence of augmented global muscle activity.

CHANGES IN OTHER ELEMENTS OF THE ABDOMINAL MECHANISM

Changes in control of the diaphragm and pelvic floor muscles

No studies have directly assessed the postural activity of the diaphragm and pelvic floor muscles in people with low back pain. However, there are several interesting anecdotes from the literature that require consideration. As mentioned in Chapter 3, the changes in trunk control that occur during increased respiratory demand are similar to those seen in people with low back pain. Notably, when respiratory demand is increased and movement inititated, postural activity of transversus abdominis, diaphragm and pelvic floor muscles is reduced in association with rapid limb movement (Hodges 2001) and support surface translation (Hodges et al 2003c) while global muscle activity is increased (Hodges et al 2003c). As this occurs chronically in people with respiratory disease (Hodges et al 2000b), it may be predicted that people with respiratory disease may have increased incidence of low back pain. Interestingly, people with asthma are 50% more likely to have back pain than those without (Hurwitz and Morgenstern 1999) and people who are sick listed for back pain are more likely to take longer to return to work if they have concomitant respiratory disease (Nordin et al 2002). Although these data do not confirm a causal link between biomechanical changes in the efficiency of the spinal control mechanism, they do suggest that it may be possible. Irrespective of the link between respiratory disease and low back pain, the presence of respiratory disease is likely to complicate the rehabilitation of trunk muscle control.

Similar links between pelvic floor muscle function and low back pain have been identified. For instance, men and women with incontinence have almost double the incidence of back pain than people without incontinence (Finkelstein 2002). While further work is required, these data argue that these systems may need to be addressed in people with low back pain.

Changes in control of the posterior abdominal wall muscles

For many years, it has been noted clinically that quadratus lumborum and psoas major have increased activity in people with low back pain (Travell and Simons 1983, Janda 1996). Many therapeutic techniques have been developed based on this, including stretches (Janda 1996), connective tissue and trigger point techniques (Travell and Simons 1983), and even botulinum injections (Lang 2002), although no studies have investigated changes in activity in people with low back pain. One study identified a reduction in the cross-sectional area of psoas on the side of back pain in people with sciatica (Dangaria and Naesh 1998). Several factors require consideration. First, it is plausible that different components of these muscles (medial and lateral quadratus lumborum, and anterior and posterior psoas major) respond differently to pain. For instance, considering the data presented in Chapters 2, 3 and 9, it may be predicted that the long global/multisegmental lateral fibres of quadratus and anterior fibres of psoas may be augmented, and the segmental portions impaired. This has been considered from a clinical context (Gibbons 2001). Second, in view of the data from Euler models of control of buckling forces, strategies have been developed to train the activity of quadratus lumborum in people with low back pain (McGill 2002b). While this may provide a strategy to optimize the control of spinal orientation, further investigation from clinical trials is required to determine whether this leads to improved clinical outcomes.

CLINICAL IMPLICATIONS

The data described above appear to indicate that the deep/local and superficial/global abdominal muscles are commonly affected in an opposite manner by the presence of pain. Hypothetically, this may result in reduced efficiency of fine-tuning of intervertebral control (see Ch. 2). As mentioned above, the superficial muscles are inefficient for controlling intervertebral motion and can only do so at the 'cost' of increased spinal loading and co-activation. Furthermore, this augmented global muscles activity is likely to reduce the normal movement of the spine. As movement is important for dissipation of forces and minimization of energy expenditure, this has detrimental consequences for spinal health. Furthermore, as activity of the global muscles must be 'diverted' to intervertebral control, this is likely to compromise the ability of these muscles to deal with the control of orientation. This follows the hypothesis of Cholewicki et al (1997), who suggested that excessive activity in the superficial muscles might be a measurable compensation for poor passive or active segmental support.

For rehabilitation there are several issues to consider. First, re-education of the activity of the deep local abdominal muscles is essential to restore the normal fine-tuning of intervertebral motion. Second, rehabilitation must consider the normal characteristics of control that are impaired in low back pain, such as tonic activity, early recruitment and differential control of the deep and superficial muscles. Third, a goal in the management of many patients will be the reduction of activity of the global muscles. This requires specific assessment to determine the strategy adopted by an individual patient. It is important to emphasize that the presentation in low back pain is highly variable and individual. As such, no simple model can explain all variations. While a strategy of increased and decreased activity may be common, it is naive to expect this situation to explain all presentations and careful assessment is the key to management of patients.

Finally, co-ordination of the multiple functions of the abdominal muscles requires consideration. For instance, if a patient has incontinence, specific attention may be required to retrain the control of the pelvic floor muscles as co-ordinated activity of the pelvic floor muscles are essential for functioning of the abdominal stability mechanism. Retraining of pelvic floor muscle function may require specialist intervention. Similarly, if a person has respiratory disease, there is likely to be increased difficulty for co-ordination of stability and respiratory functions. However, in all patients, it is critical to ensure that respiratory co-ordination is achieved. Notably, as the superficial abdominal muscles depress the rib cage and are involved in forced expiration (DeTroyer and Estenne 1988), increased activity of these muscles in people with pain may lead to compromised respiratory function, for example restricted movement of the chest wall. Therefore, attention must be paid to restoring normal respiratory movements.

Chapter **11**

Paraspinal mechanism in low back pain

Julie Hides

DYSFUNCTION OF THE MULTIFIDUS

There is evidence of dysfunction in the paraspinal muscles in patients with low back pain; this has been detected through measures of muscle activation, fatiguability, muscle composition and muscle size and consistency. The back extensors as a group can become dysfunctional in patients with low back pain, but particular attention here will be given to the lumbar multifidus muscle.

Muscle activation

Several general investigations of activation of the paraspinal muscles using surface electromyography (EMG) have discriminated patients with low back pain from asymptomatic controls (Cassisi et al 1993, Grabiner et al 1992) by demonstrating differing patterns of activation between the muscle groups with various tasks (Nouwen et al 1987, Soderberg and Barr 1983). Sihvonen et al (1991) studied the lumbar multifidus muscle more specifically and used EMG with surface and fine-wire electrodes to examine activation at the L4 and L5 vertebral levels in 87 patients with low back pain and 25 asymptomatic subjects during forward flexion and the return to the upright position. In addition to EMG, Sihvonen et al (1991) further examined patients with low back pain using plain and mobility radiographs to measure the mobility between lumbar vertebrae during trunk flexion. The activity levels in the segmental multifidus differed between the two groups. General EMG results for the raw intramuscular activity in subjects with low back pain showed that during lumbar extension there was decreased activity in both segments studied compared with controls. In the 28 patients with segmental instability, defined as a greater than 4 mm sliding between lumbar vertebrae during flexion on full-sized radiographs, the EMG results were different at different segments. There was less activity at the unstable level during concentric back activity, suggesting decreased muscular protection at the hypermobile level, the opposite of what is logically required.

Fatiguability

Fatiguability infers potentially inadequate muscular support over extended periods of time. There is evidence that fatigue of paraspinal muscles is more prevalent in patients with low back pain than in control subjects. Fatigue can be defined in mechanical terms as the point at which a contraction can no longer be maintained at a certain level (isometric fatigue) or when repetitive work can no longer be sustained at a certain output (dynamic fatigue) (Andersson et al 1989). Fatigue studies on spinal muscles can be divided into mechanical studies and EMG studies.

Differences between patients with low back pain and asymptomatic controls have been detected using a mechanical method of testing the isometric endurance of the trunk extensors as a group (Nicolaisen and Jorgensen 1985, Jorgensen and Nicolaisen 1987). While no differences were detected in the trunk extensor strength between patients with low back pain and controls, the former were shown to have significantly less endurance than control subjects, indicating greater fatiguability. Such studies have a disadvantage in that they do not permit specific investigations of particular muscles within the back extensor group. The use of power spectral analysis of muscle activity, using EMG with multiple electrode placements, has allowed assessment of individual paraspinal muscles.

In studies where the lumbar multifidus has been specifically examined in patients with low back pain and control subjects, differences between the fatigue rates of this muscle have been detected using power spectral analysis of EMG activity. Biedermann et al (1991) examined the multifidus and iliocostalis lumborum in patients with chronic low back pain and demonstrated that it was the multifidus that demonstrated the greater fatigue rates in the patients compared with normal control subjects. Roy et al (1989) also compared subjects with a history of chronic low back pain with asymptomatic control subjects and again showed that the multifidus muscles of the patients demonstrated significantly higher fatigue rates than did the controls. They extended their studies and investigated high-performance athletes (male rowers). The fatigue rates correctly identified all control subjects and 93% of the subjects with low back pain (Roy et al 1990). As an aside from a rehabilitation perspective, it is pertinent to note that in these elite and highly trained athletes, local muscle dysfunction of the multifidus was present despite rigorous general training regimens. This supports the use of a different exercise approach to address this dysfunction in the multifidus.

Composition

Studies examining changes in type I and type II muscle fibres in patients with low back pain have been conducted in order to provide insight into paraspinal muscle dysfunction. The two main parameters of multifidus muscle composition that have been examined in patients with low back pain are muscle fibre size and muscle fibre internal structure.

Several biopsy studies of the lumbar multifidus muscle have been conducted on patients with low back pain, undergoing lumbar surgery. Selective atrophy of type II muscle fibres has been shown (Fidler et al 1975, Jowett et al 1975, Ford et al 1983, Mattila et al 1986, Zhu et al 1989, Rantanen et al 1993) but the significance of this atrophy to low back pain is unclear as it has also been reported in cadaveric specimens from individuals who in life had no history of lumbar disorders (Mattila et al 1986, Rantanen et al 1993). Changes in the internal structure of type I fibres of the multifidus muscle have been shown in patients with low back pain, although it appears that the size of these fibres remains generally unaffected (Ford et al 1983, Bagnall et al 1984, Mattila et al 1986, Zhu et al 1989, Rantanen et al 1993, Kawaguchi et al 1994). The fibres have been described as core-targetoid and moth-eaten in appearance, and these internal structural changes are considered abnormal for healthy muscle (Mattila et al 1986). Changes in the internal structure of type I fibres occur quickly. They have been demonstrated in biopsy specimens of subjects with a symptom duration of only 3 weeks (range 3 weeks to 1 year) (Ford et al 1983). One recent study has compared multifidus biopsies between sides in patients with lumbar disc herniation (Yoshihara et al 2001). Intraoperative biopsies were taken from L4 and L5 bands of the multifidus on the affected and non-affected sides. Results showed that the mean size of the type I and type II muscle fibres on the affected side and vertebral level were significantly smaller than on the non-affected side. Nerve root impairment led to atrophy of the muscle fibres, with structural changes in the multifidus only at the affected vertebral level. Similar findings were reported by Zhao et al (2000). Animal studies have shown that trauma to the multifidus increases in relation to the length of time of retraction of the muscles during the surgery (Gejo et al 2000). Magnetic resonance imaging (MRI) showed that multifidus muscle regenerated in 21 days after surgery when retraction was 1 hour or less. If retraction was 2 hours or more in length, increased extracellular fluid was seen and muscle regeneration was incomplete.

The long-term sequelae of type II muscle fibre atrophy and type I internal structural changes of the multifidus have been determined in a study of patients undergoing surgery for low back pain (Rantanen et al 1993). Muscle biopsy specimens were obtained from patients at operation for lumbar disc herniation and after a postoperative follow-up period of 5 years. Patients were divided into two groups (positive or negative outcome) on the basis of their functional handicap at the 5-year follow-up. Biopsy specimens collected at operation from all subjects showed evidence of type II muscle fibre atrophy and type I fibre internal structural changes. At follow-up, there were no significant changes in atrophy between the patient groups. In contrast, changes in the internal structure of type I muscle fibres were dramatically different between the groups. Moth-eaten and core-targetoid fibres were seen in the initial multifidus biopsy samples of all patients. In the positive-outcome group, the presence of both these internal structure abnormalities decreased. In contrast, the negative-outcome

group showed a marked increase in the frequency of these abnormalities, the increase being the greatest in moth-eaten fibres (the percentage of moth-eaten fibres increased from 2.7 to 16.7%).

The results of this study indicated for the first time that pathological structural changes in the multifidus muscle found at long-term follow-up correlated well with the long-term clinical outcome. Functional recovery after disc surgery was associated with curtailment of structural abnormalities in the multifidus muscle, especially in the type I muscle fibres. These findings highlight the potential clinical importance of dysfunction in this muscle. It seems that the pathological changes seen originally at initial biopsy could be reversed by adequate surgical and physical therapy management.

Size and consistency

Dysfunction of the lumbar muscles in patients with low back pain has also been demonstrated using imaging modalities that allow assessment of muscle size or cross-sectional area and muscle consist-ency. Atrophy in terms of decreased size of the paraspinal muscles has been demonstrated using imaging techniques, including computed tomography (CT) scanning, MRI and ultrasound imaging. Muscle atrophy has also been visualized by CT and MRI. Decreased muscle density can be caused by fatty infiltration (increased fat/muscle fibre ratio) or actual fatty replacement of fibres (Laasonen 1984, Mayer et al 1989). Some investigators have combined measurements of the multifidus and the lumbar erector spinae muscles (paraspinal muscles), while others have investigated the multifidus specifically.

The paraspinal muscles

Several studies have provided evidence of paraspinal muscle atrophy in patients with chronic low back pain or in patients postoperatively (Mayer et al 1989, Tertti et al 1991, Cooper et al 1992, Alaranta et al 1993, Hultman et al 1993, Parkkola et al 1993). In most instances, this has been ascribed primarily to disuse and deconditioning (Mayer et al 1989, Tertti et al 1991, Cooper et al 1992, Hultman et al 1993, Parkkola et al 1993). Two studies have examined the paraspinal muscles of patients with low back pain in more detail and have shown

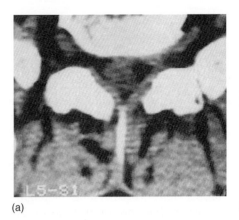
(a)

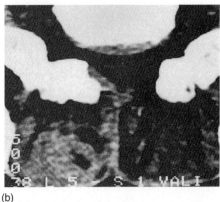
(b)

Figure 11.1 Computed tomography scans taken from the L5 to S1 level. (a) Before surgery, when disc protrusion facet arthrosis and lateral stenosis at this level was noted. (b) After left hemilaminectomy was performed, showing multifidus muscle atrophy at the corresponding vertebral level (L5–S1). (Reproduced with permission from Sihvonen et al 1993, p. 578.)

differences between sides and vertebral levels (Laasonen 1984, Alaranta et al 1993). In an examination of postoperative patients, Laasonen (1984) showed that, when atrophy was partial, it always included atrophy of the medial portion of the multifidus. In unilateral cases, paraspinal muscles were shown to be 10–30% smaller on the affected side than on the unaffected side. Fatty degeneration of the paraspinal muscles was also evident. A positive relationship between the fat content of the paraspinal muscles at the lumbosacral junction and results of a disability index was demonstrated in patients with chronic low back pain and after lumbar surgery (Alaranta et al 1993). This relationship between fat content and disability was not demonstrated at other vertebral levels, thus highlighting the fact that investigation of muscle atrophy in patients with low back pain must be directed to several vertebral levels if the relevant changes are to be discovered.

The multifidus muscle

The effects of low back pain on muscle size have been investigated in postoperative patients (Sihvonen et al 1993, S. Kelley et al 2003 unpublished data), patients with acute/subacute low back pain (Hides et al 1994, 1996b; Hides et al 2001) and patients with chronic low back pain (Danneels et al 2000, 2001; Kader et al 2000; S. Kelley et al 2003 unpublished data; T. Wallwork et al 2003 unpublished data).

The direct effects of lumbar surgery (iatrogenic trauma) on the lumbar multifidus muscle were examined by Sihvonen et al (1993). They demonstrated that, in some cases, lumbar surgery for spinal stenosis and/or disc herniation could lead to severe changes in the multifidus muscle (Fig. 11.1). Two groups of subjects were studied: those with a poor outcome and those with a good outcome from surgery. It was found that patients could have similar outcomes in surgical terms of successful nerve decompression and absence of stenotic regrowth. Nevertheless, they could have different functional recoveries. A variable related to poor outcomes was multifidus muscle atrophy, which was more prevalent in patients with the poorer postoperative outcomes.

Multifidus cross-sectional areas have been measured from L2 to L5 using ultrasound imaging by a trained ultrasonographer in 19 male subjects before and after spinal surgery (S. Kelley et al 2003 unpublished data; Fig. 11.2). There was a segmental decrease in multifidus cross-sectional area in patients with chronic low back pain with disc protrusion and radicular leg pain prior to surgery when compared with control subjects. The greatest difference occurred at the L4 and L5 vertebral levels. Mean values for multifidus cross-sectional area for subjects with chronic low back pain and normal subjects are presented in Table 11.1. Preoperatively, there was significant negative correlation between multifidus cross-sectional area at the L4 and L5 vertebral levels and low back

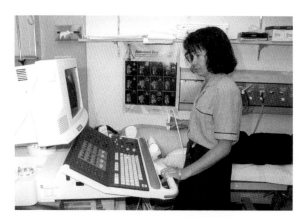

Figure 11.2   Trained sonographer performing measurement of multifidus cross-sectional area on a patient with chronic low back pain prior to spinal surgery.

Table 11.1   Comparison between mean multifidus cross-sectional areas at vertebral levels L2 to L5 for 45 normal subjects and 19 subjects with chronic low back pain measured preoperatively

Vertebral level	Mean multifidus cross-sectional area (cm^2 (SE))	Confidence interval
Normal (control)		
L2	2.33 (0.12)	2.09–2.57
L3	3.5 (0.16)	3.18–3.81
L4	5.03 (0.2)	4.64–5.42
L5	6.34 (0.17)	6.01–6.68
Chronic low back pain		
L2	2.31 (0.21)	1.89–2.72
L3	2.91 (0.27)	2.37–3.45
L4	3.4 (0.33)	2.73–4.07
L5	4.1 (0.29)	3.52–4.68

SE, standard error.
From S. Kelley et al 2003, unpublished data.

pain: those subjects with more low back pain showed greater wasting of the multifidus. Subjects were reimaged postoperatively and followed for 1 year following surgery. Interestingly, there was no further decrease observable in multifidus cross-sectional area following surgery. However, that is not to say that atrophy had not occurred within the muscle itself, as changes in muscle consistency

were not graded on the ultrasound images. It was noted in this study that intramuscular swelling was commonly present, which may have masked atrophy in the cross-sectional area measurements. Other studies have reported muscle atrophy following spinal surgery. Long-term follow-up in this study indicated that multifidus atrophy was long lasting and had not improved at the 1-year assessment. At the 1-year follow-up, there was a significant correlation between leg pain and multifidus atrophy, a finding which has previously been reported (Kader et al 2000).

Multifidus atrophy appears to be a common finding in patients with chronic low back pain. In a recent MRI study of 78 patients with low back pain (with and without leg pain), changes in multifidus muscle consistency were graded as mild (fatty or fibrous tissue replacement less than 10%), moderate (replacement less than 50%) and severe (greater than 50%) (Kader et al 2000). Degeneration of multifidus was present in 80% of the subjects with low back pain and was seen most commonly at L4–L5 and L5–S1 vertebral levels. Of the 78 patients with low back pain, 66 (85%) had degenerated lumbar discs on MRI, most commonly also at L4–L5 and L5–S1. While there was a trend towards a correlation between severity of muscle atrophy and intensity of pain, the most significant correlation demonstrated was between multifidus muscle atrophy and leg pain (radicular and non-radicular) ($p < 0.01$).

Evidence has now been presented that the cross-sectional area of the multifidus is selectively decreased (when compared with other muscles) in those with chronic low back pain compared with controls (Danneels et al 2000). Cross-sectional areas of the multifidus, lumbar erector spinae and psoas were obtained using CT scanning. Only the multifidus was statistically smaller in patients with low back pain than in controls. This atrophy was only significant at the lowest lumbar level, supporting the concept of level-specific changes in the multifidus (a finding also reported by S. Kelley et al 2003, unpublished data). Further evidence for this phenomenon has recently been provided for patients with chronic low back pain using ultrasound imaging (T. Wallwork et al 2003 unpublished data). In this study, three blinded assessors were involved. One measured multifidus cross-sectional

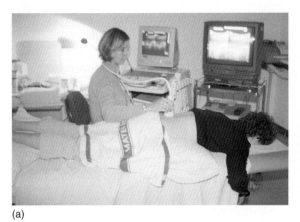 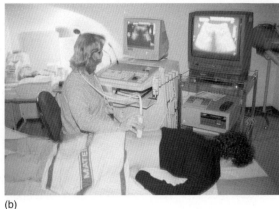

(a)   (b)

Figure 11.3   Assessment of the multifidus using real-time ultrasound imaging. (a) Assessment of multifidus activation (isometric contraction) in a patient with chronic low back pain. The transducer was placed parasagittally to image the multifidus in the plane of the zygapophyseal joints. A split-screen technique was used to ensure that the relaxed and contracted images were taken in the same plane. (b) Measurement of multifidus cross-sectional area of a patient with chronic low back pain using real-time ultrasound imaging by a blinded assessor. Repeatability and reliability of these measurement techniques were established prior to testing.

area. The second assessor asked subjects to contract the multifidus isometrically at each vertebral level and measured the change in multifidus depth as the muscle contracted using ultrasound imaging (see Ch. 5) (Fig. 11.3). The third assessor performed a clinical assessment, including manual examination, palpation for multifidus atrophy and palpation of segmental isometric contraction of the multifidus. Results showed that not only was the cross-sectional area of the multifidus significantly decreased in the patients with low back pain, but activation of the muscle was also significantly decreased compared with the controls. The level-group interaction confirmed that the decreased activation of the multifidus was a segmental response that correlated with the vertebral levels detected by both clinical examination and measurement of cross-sectional area on ultrasound imaging.

We have investigated the lumbar multifidus in patients with acute low back pain using real-time ultrasound imaging. In the first study, the cross-sectional area of the multifidus was measured in 26 patients with first-episode acute unilateral low back pain of a mean duration of approximately 2 weeks, and in 51 normal subjects. In patients with low back pain, the muscle on both sides was measured at all vertebral levels from the second lumbar to the first sacral vertebra (Hides et al

1994). In the 51 normal subjects, the cross-sectional area was measured at L4, and in 10 subjects measurements were made from L2 to L5. Marked side-to-side asymmetry of the cross-sectional area of the multifidus was found in the patients with low back pain but not in the normal subjects (Fig. 11.4). The smaller muscle was found at the symptomatic segment, was on the side ipsilateral to symptoms and was confined predominantly to that one vertebral level. The magnitude of the between-side difference was $31 \pm 8\%$. In normal subjects this was $3 \pm 4\%$. Figure 11.5 shows this difference in asymmetry for patients at the level of symptoms and at L4 for all the normal subjects. Such a comparison between the two groups is considered valid since the degree of asymmetry in normal subjects was similar at all vertebral levels. The changes occurred quickly. One subject was measured within 24 hours of injury and displayed the asymmetry. Therefore, a likely explanation for the mechanism is inhibition of the segmental multifidus (see Ch. 8).

Following on from the findings from the initial study, a randomized clinical trial was conducted. The aim of this research was to monitor if the multifidus muscle recovered spontaneously over time and to evaluate any effect of specific rehabilitation of this segmental dysfunction. Thirty-nine subjects

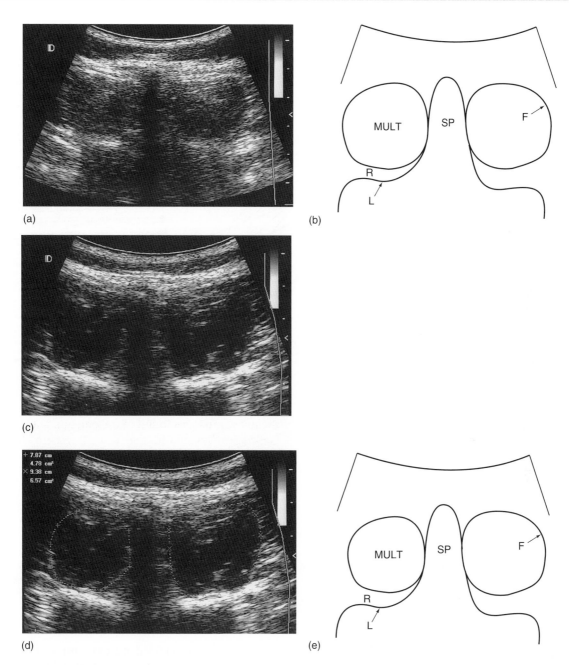

Figure 11.4   Sonographic appearance of the multifidus (axial image) at the level of the fifth vertebra. (a) A normal subject. (b) The multifidus muscle (MULT) in (a) is bordered by the vertebral lamina/zygapophyseal joint (L) inferiorly, the spinous process (SP) medially, fascia, fat and skin superiorly, and the fascia between the multifidus and the lumbar longissimus and iliocostalis (F) laterally. The brightness seen at the interior border of the multifidus is reflection (R) of sound waves from the vertebral lamina and zygapophyseal joints. Acoustic shadowing is seen inferior to this landmark, as the ultrasound waves are unable to penetrate the bone. (c) A patient with unilateral left-sided low back pain. (d) In this image the borders of the multifidus have been traced to demonstrate the asymmetry. (e) The multifidus on the left (symptomatic) side in (d) is 4.78 cm², while the larger multifidus on the right side is 6.57 cm². This represents a decrease on the left side of 27%.

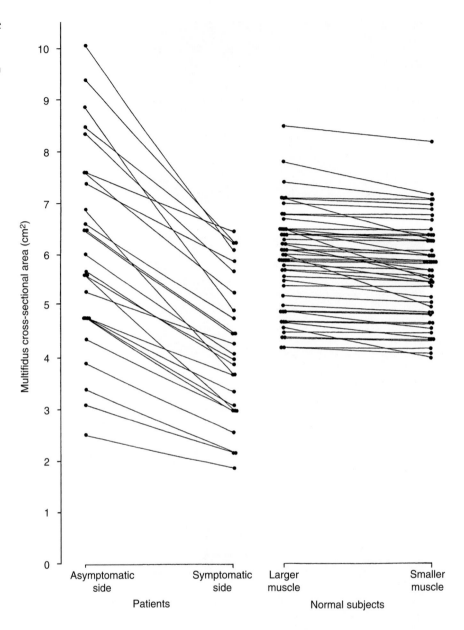

Figure 11.5 Between-side differences in multifidus cross-sectional area in patients with low back pain ($n = 26$). These patients showed greater asymmetry than seen in the normal subjects ($n = 51$). The degree of asymmetry was significantly different between the two groups ($p < 0.001$). (Reproduced with permission from Hides et al 1994, p. 169.)

with acute first-episode unilateral low back pain and demonstrating unilateral segmental inhibition of the multifidus muscle participated in this clinical trial (Hides et al 1996b). Patients were randomly allocated to a control (non-active treatment) or treatment group. Outcome measures for both groups included weekly assessments of pain, disability, range of motion and measurement of multifidus cross-sectional area over the 4-week intervention period. Patients were reassessed at 10 weeks; 39

subjects were interviewed at 1 year and 36 subjects were interviewed at 3 years to establish long-term recurrence rates for low back pain (Hides et al 2001).

The decrease in multifidus size was localized to specific vertebral levels (Fig. 11.6). Subjects in the treatment group performed specific localized multifidus exercises (see Ch. 14) aimed at restoring the stabilization function of this muscle. Low back pain subsided in virtually all subjects, regardless of group (Fig. 11.7a,b), and there were no differences

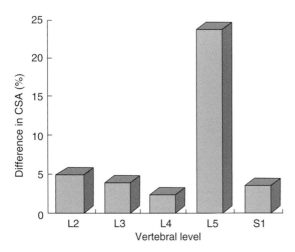

Figure 11.6   Ultrasound imaging results showing the between-side percentage difference in multifidus cross-sectional area (CSA) for vertebral levels L2–S1 in 34 patients who demonstrated multifidus asymmetry at the L5 vertebral level. Note the greatest difference in CSA between sides at the affected vertebral level (L5), with minimal asymmetry between sides demonstrated at the other lumbar vertebral levels. (Reproduced with permission from Hides et al 1996b, p. 2767.)

in disability scores (Fig. 11.7c) between the two groups at 4 weeks. The measures most commonly used in low back pain outcome trials demonstrated a return to normal function in 4 weeks, reflecting the well-known natural recovery of an acute episode of low back pain.

In the back pain group who underwent standard medical management (control group), the reduced size of the multifidus in the symptomatic side notably remained almost unchanged over the 4-week period of the trial (Fig. 11.8). In these control subjects, multifidus muscle recovery was not spontaneous with the relief of pain. In contrast, the exercise intervention resulted in restoration of the multifidus cross-sectional area within the 4-week treatment period. Therefore, despite relief of pain and general muscle use in returning to normal activity levels, patients in the control group still displayed decreased multifidus muscle size at 4 weeks that persisted to the 10-week follow-up.

Long-term results revealed that subjects from the specific exercise group experienced fewer recurrences of low back pain than subjects from the control group. One year after treatment, recurrence in the specific exercise group was 30% compared with 84% in the control group ($p < 0.001$). Two to three years after treatment, recurrence in the specific exercise group was 35% compared with 75% in the control group ($p < 0.01$). Subjects in the control group were 12.4 times more likely to suffer recurrences of low back pain than subjects in the specific exercise group in the first year following the initial episode, and nine times more likely to suffer recurrences in years 2–3. In year 1, approximately one patient in the specific exercise group reported pain for every three subjects who did not, while approximately four patients in the control group reported recurrences for every one that did not. In years 2–3, the likelihood of reporting recurrences of low back pain in the exercise group increased slightly to approximately 2:5, while the likelihood of recurrences in the control group reduced to 10:3. Reanalysis of the years 2–3 data using best case analysis revealed that subjects in the control group were still 5.9 times more likely to suffer recurrences of low back pain than subjects in the specific exercise group. The most likely explanation is that persistence of the segmental multifidus muscle inhibition, still evident in the control group at the 10-week follow-up, exposed the injured segment to decreased muscle support and a predisposition to further injury.

This study highlights the importance of identifying and measuring the specific dysfunctions in the muscle system that are directly associated with the pain or injury. Possession of this knowledge directed very specific treatment to the dysfunctional muscle and provided a direct measure of the impairment on which to evaluate the effectiveness of the rehabilitation approach. The other commonly used outcome assessments (pain, range of motion and disability assessments) do not seem to relate to the recurrence rate of symptoms in the first year following the initial injury.

The effects of different exercise approaches on the cross-sectional area of the multifidus of patients with chronic low back pain has been examined using CT scanning (Danneels et al 2001). Patients were divided into three groups; all performed stabilization exercises but group 2 also performed dynamic resistance training and group

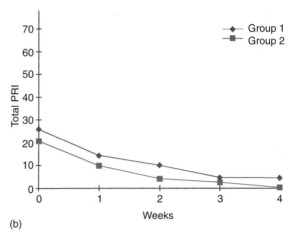

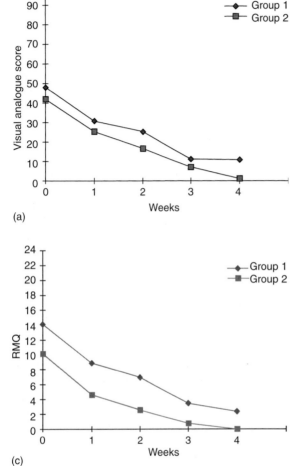

(a)

(b)

(c)

Figure 11.7 Pain and disability scores obtained for patients in group 1 (control group) and group 2 (specific exercise group) for the baseline measurement (week 0) and at weeks 1–4 of the study. (a) Using visual analogue scales, no significant difference was observed at any time between pain scores for the two groups. (b) There was no significant difference between pain scores on the total pain rating index (PRI) of the McGill Pain Questionnaire. (c) There was no sigificant difference in disability scores obtained on the Rowland Morris Disability Index (RMQ). (Reproduced with permission from Hides et al 1996b, p. 2765.)

3 also performed dynamic-static resistance training. While positive outcomes were seen in subjects of all three groups, comparison between pre- and posttraining multifidus cross-sectional areas revealed a significant increase in group 3 subjects only. The static holding component, between the concentric and eccentric phase, was thought to be essential for inducing hypertrophy of the multifidus in patients with chronic low back pain. This study highlights an important issue. It is important to activate the multifidus and to restore normal control of the muscle. In patients with chronic low back pain, it will be necessary to progress to loaded activities to achieve hypertrophy of the muscle. This would seem to be a logical approach to reverse the long-standing changes

seen in the multifidus as a result of a chronic problem (see Chs 15 and 16).

Summary

There is a significant body of evidence illustrating that the lumbar multifidus muscle is adversely affected in patients with low back pain and that dysfunction occurs with the first episode of back pain. As the multifidus muscle provides local segmental stability of the lumbar spine in normal function, dysfunction of the multifidus could be assumed to have substantial adverse effects in patients with low back pain. Evidence of long-term sequelae has already been provided in postsurgery patients. Dysfunction of the multifidus has been

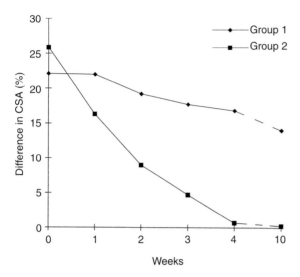

Figure 11.8 Ultrasound imaging results showing multifidus muscle recovery for patients in group 1 (control group) and group 2 (exercise group) for the baseline measure (week 0), weeks 1–4 of the study and the 10-week follow-up examination. Muscle size is presented as the difference between sides (expressed as a percentage) in cross-sectional area (CSA) at the most affected vertebral level. (Reproduced with permission from Hides et al 1996b, p. 2767.)

demonstrated in patients with low back pain in muscle activation, fatiguability, composition, size and consistency. Information pertaining to the specific nature of dysfunction of the multifidus muscle in patients with low back pain has provided a basis for the development of effective rehabilitation programmes.

CLINICAL RELEVANCE

Prescription of therapeutic exercise for the patient with low back pain should be based both on the normal function of the paraspinal muscles and on the presence and nature of impairment. Evidence of impairment of the multifidus in patients with low back pain has been detected through measurement of multifidus activation, fatiguability, composition and size and consistency.

As measurements of muscle activation can discriminate between patients with back pain and asymptomatic controls, rehabilitation should aim to normalize the activation of the multifidus.

Surgical studies have reported the long-term sequelae of muscle dysfunction associated with surgery. Abnormalities of the internal structure of the type I muscle fibres was one of the key dysfunctions identified at initial biopsy. In subjects who improved, these dysfunctions were reduced at the long term follow-up. Reversal of pathological changes should be the aim of rehabilitation, and an approach aimed at restoring the normal function of the multifidus is warranted.

Studies that have measured multifidus size and consistency have provided evidence of decreased multifidus cross-sectional area in patients with low back pain. Atrophy was selective for the multifidus in patients with chronic low back pain (Danneels et al 2000), and was specific to the L5 vertebral level. Further evidence of segmental decreases in multifidus cross-sectional area in patients with chronic low back pain has been recently provided (T. Wallwork et al 2003 unpublished data, S. Kelley et al 2003 unpublished data). In patients with acute unilateral low back pain, multifidus atrophy was localized to the painful segment and side (Hides et al 1994, 1996b). The implication for rehabilitation is that techniques must be precise and localized to the affected segments to be effective, as multifidus size was not restored in control subjects who resumed full normal work, sport and leisure activities. For subjects with chronic low back pain, low-level activation of the multifidus alone did not reverse multifidus atrophy (Danneels et al 2000). Reversal of chronic multifidus atrophy, therefore, requires progression to loaded exercise. Examination of multifidus activation data using ultrasound imaging (T. Wallwork et al 2003 unpublished data) also showed that changes in the control of the multifidus are segmental and specific and, therefore, require specific re-education.

The use of imaging techniques has provided a wealth of information for both the research and clinical perspectives. Ultrasound imaging is currently used in routine clinical practice to examine the size and consistency of the multifidus and is used to provide feedback of activation of the synergy muscles in rehabilitation (see Appendix to Ch. 5, pp. 89–92). In clinical practice, changes in consistency of the multifidus can be easily observed using ultrasound imaging. The ultrasound appearance of muscle is usually dark because of its high fluid content (blood). The presence of fatty infiltration, fibrous changes or scar tissue (non-contractile tissue) leads to a change in appearance, as non-contractile tissue is white in appearance (greater echogenicity). These changes can be seen at specific vertebral levels and are not difficult for the clinician to detect using ultrasound imaging. In contrast, measurement of the multifidus cross-sectional area requires extensive training and practice to become proficient. While it would seem advantageous to be able to measure the multifidus in clinical practice, this measurement should not be performed until repeatability and reliability studies have been performed by the operator. This is an important point, as serial measures are required to ascertain the effectiveness of rehabilitation (muscle hypertrophy). If the measurement error is greater than the changes seen in rehabilitation, any true changes during rehabilitation will be masked. That is not to say that real-time ultrasound imaging is not useful for examination of multifidus atrophy in patients with low back pain in clinical practice. The clinician can observe for atrophy and report that it exists; however, figures should not be ascribed until repeatability and reliability have been established. For the clinicians that do not have access to ultrasound imaging, use should be made of the patients' CT and MR scans when available. The size and consistency of the multifidus muscles can be observed at each vertebral level, and these changes can be shown to the patient. This will help to convey to the patient that impairment exists, and it also offers incentive to comply with a rehabilitation programme. On CT scans, normal muscle appears grey and uniform. Consistency changes will present as dark areas. In contrast, on MRI, fatty infiltration and fibrous changes will appear white. Normal muscle consistency can be demonstrated by showing the patient the psoas muscle, which rarely shows consistency changes. An axial MRI of the lumbar spine and muscles is shown in Figure 4.5 (p. 64). Figure 11.9 shows a MRI of a subject with acute low back pain. This image shows a decrease in cross-sectional area, but no alterations in consistency. Consistency changes may be more common in subjects with chronic low back pain. Figure 11.10 shows a MRI of a patient with chronic low back pain and here

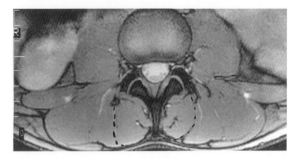

Figure 11.9 Magnetic resonance image of the multifidus in a patient with acute low back pain. The multifidus on the patient's left side (right side of image) is atrophied compared with that on the patient's right side. Note that there is no alteration of muscle consistency in the acute situation.

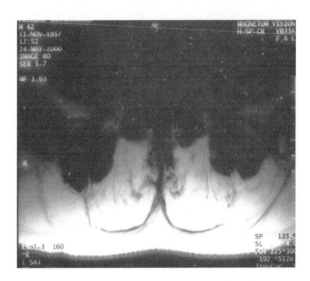

Figure 11.10 Magnetic resonance image of a patient with chronic low back pain, showing almost complete fatty infiltration of the multifidus muscle. The normal muscle is dark in appearance, and the fat layer and fatty infiltration of the multifidus is white in appearance.

there is almost complete fatty infiltration of the multifidus. A CT scan of the same patient is shown in Figure 11.11. A CT scan showing patchy (more usual) changes in consistency is shown in Figure 11.12. Whether MR and CT images, and/or the use of ultrasound imaging, are used to educate the patient of the existing impairment, and its specific nature, or are used by the clinician in conjunction

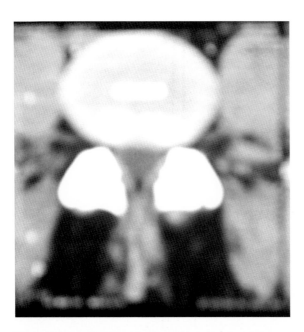

Figure 11.11   Computed tomographic scan of a patient with chronic low back pain demonstrating almost complete fatty infiltration of the multifidus. The normal muscle is seen as grey in colour; the fatty infiltration appears black.

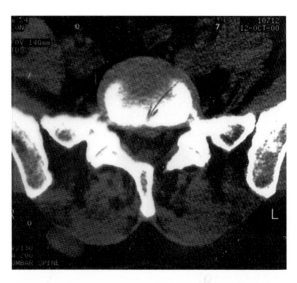

Figure 11.12   Computed tomographic scan of a patient with chronic low back pain showing patchy changes in the deep ventrolateral corners of the patient's multifidus muscles, with greater changes on the patient's left side (right side of image) than on the right. The normal muscle tissue appears grey in colour; the non-contractile tissue appears black (as a result of fatty infiltration, fibrotic changes or scar tissue).

with clinical assessment, they are useful additions to the clinical picture. Certainly, the clinician's learning curve increases rapidly by having visual confirmation of muscle palpation skills available.

By being able to localize the impairment to the specific vertebral level/levels involved, muscle rehabilitation should be streamlined and more effective.

Chapter 12

Impairments in muscles controlling pelvic orientation and weightbearing

Carolyn Richardson

INTRODUCTION

As with Chapters 10 and 11, this chapter will focus on the impairments in the joint protection mechanisms in relation to patients with low back pain. It is important to emphasize that it is the impairments in joint protection mechanisms, rather than impairment in the movement patterns (explained in Ch. 1), which will be the focus of the motor control dysfunction that is related to the orientation and weightbearing function of the pelvis.

Both local and global muscles play an important part in determining the orientation and weightbearing function of the pelvis. Chapters 5 and 6 describe the integration for local and global muscles for weightbearing and contain the background information for this chapter. Here we deal with the specific problems that develop in the deep muscle corset (i.e. the antigravity function of the deep muscle synergy) and its ability to stiffen the pelvic joints (Ch. 5), as well as the differential changes in the weightbearing and non-weightbearing muscles (Ch. 7) that affect the orientation and weightbearing function of the pelvis in relation to the hips and spine.

The impairments that have been described for the abdominal and paraspinal muscles would affect all postures and movements of a patient with low back pain. However, in considering the antigravity function of these muscles and its close relationship with the function of the other antigravity muscles of the pelvis and lower limb, there is another aspect of impairment of the joint protection mechanisms related to the 'deep muscle corset' that needs to be addressed.

DEEP MUSCLE CORSET: PROBLEMS IN LOW BACK PAIN

Patterns of dysfunction in the transversus abdominis and multifidus have been studied for several years in our clinics where real-time ultrasound is used in the assessment and treatment of the deep muscle synergy in patients with low back pain. The main problem observed in the transversus abdominis muscle in low back pain has been an inability to develop the corset action on the instruction to draw in the abdominal wall. Problems involve either no contraction of the muscle, asymmetry of contraction or, in the most severe motor control problems, a lengthening (eccentric) contraction as the transversus abdominis contracts (and thickens) against increasing intra-abdominal pressure.

It is difficult to measure the contraction pattern of transversus abdominis in relation to whether each side of the muscle shortens, remains static or lengthens. Magnetic resonance imaging (MRI) is one of the few ways in which the bilateral corset (muscle and fascia) can be measured in its entirety. In addition, MRI can also measure the transversus abdominis muscle length before and after the instruction to draw in the abdominal wall. An MRI study to validate the dysfunction in transversus abdominis, detected through the clinical use of real-time ultrasound, is nearing completion at the University of Queensland. Figure 12.1a is a diagrammatic representation of an MRI of a resting corset contraction and Figure 12.1b shows the resultant corset contraction after instruction to draw in the abdominal wall in a low back pain patient with severe motor control problems.

The neurophysiological explanation for this lengthening contraction, which results in a 'pushing out' and 'bracing' of the abdominal wall in patients with low back pain, is extremely complex and relies on the interaction of the diaphragm, pelvic floor, transverses abdominis as well as the abdominal obliques muscles. This MRI study should shed some light on abdominal muscle function in patients with low back pain and on the

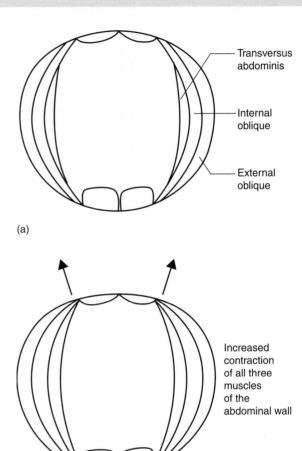

(a)

(b)

Figure 12.1 Diagrammatic representation of an MRI, demonstrating the three abdominal muscles (a) during relaxation of the abdominal wall and (b) during an attempt to draw in the abdominal wall in a patient with significant motor control problem.

relationship of these muscle impairments to the movement of the abdominal wall.

The end result (i.e. impairment in the ability to form a corset action) would affect joint stiffness at the sacro-iliac joints and, more importantly, lessen the normal sensory input resulting from compression of the joints through the corset action (Ch. 5).

In line with this, it is important to consider the impairment problems found in the thoracolumbar fascia of patients with low back pain. While it is recognized that the thoracolumbar fascia has a significant role in biomechanics, it is its sensory role that many believe is the key to its involvement in the control of the lumbopelvic region (Yahia et al 1992). In patients with chronic low back pain who were undergoing surgery, Bednar et al (1995) found no sign of the mechanoreceptors usually present in the fascia. This loss would cause a deficiency in the proprioceptive role of the fascia and would adversely influence the ability to form the corset action.

Lack of sacro-iliac joint stiffness, as well as decreased sensory input through poor corset function in patients with low back pain, would likely affect the weightbearing function of the pelvis. In addition, impairments develop in the global muscles controlling the orientation and weightbearing function of the pelvis. The significance of the effects of the different types of impairment in the one-joint and multijoint muscles that attach to the pelvis can only be realized by establishing models of pelvic control in the two planes of movement that come under the influence of gravity (i.e. weightbearing postures).

GLOBAL MUSCLES INVOLVED IN CONTROL OF PELVIC ORIENTATION AND WEIGHTBEARING

The complex muscle recruitment patterns required to control the supporting and moving functions of the lumbopelvic region (lumbar spine, pelvis and hip joints) in three planes is extremely difficult to assess, especially as many of the most important muscles lie deep within the pelvis. When any muscle or combination of muscles becomes dysfunctional, either unilaterally or bilaterally, there is an infinite combination of movement impairments that could result, depending on the individual.

The relationship between the spine and the pelvis is usually studied clinically through focusing on lumbopelvic rhythm during a forward flexed movement of the trunk with the knees straight. This movement task is regularly used by physiotherapists to determine trunk range of movement. Lumbopelvic rhythm, including the effect of additional trunk loading on the patterns of movement, has also been the focus of research studies (Nelson et al 1995). While this technique of assessment

would give an indication of the movement impairments present in low back pain, it would be difficult to determine the degree of loss of lumbopelvic stability from such a task. Therefore, many clinicians and researchers in low back pain have used a different model of assessment for determining the degree of loss of lumbopelvic stability.

A model for weightbearing: a neutral lumbopelvic unit

In order to assess and treat the physical problems in the clinic, physiotherapists have taken the view that the resultant supporting role of all the muscles attached to the pelvis can be assessed indirectly by a patient's ability to support and control a static, mid or neutral position of the lumbopelvic unit in response to a variety of external and internal loads.

To explain the biomechanical effects of the impairments that develop in the muscles responsible for pelvic orientation in relation to weightbearing, it is important to establish a neutral, standard pelvic position, from which the biomechanical effects (e.g. tilting and torsion) resulting from individual muscle impairments can be readily assessed. The model also serves as a standard for clinical muscle testing procedures, where the function of individual muscles can be determined in relation to a maintained neutral position of the pelvis and lumbar spine.

For the standard neutral weightbearing position, the pelvis needs to be controlled in a mid position, with the anterior and posterior superior iliac spines level and in line, in relation to a neutral lumbar spine position, for all planes of movement (saggital, frontal and coronal). This static model of weightbearing function for the lumbar spine and pelvis is shown in Figure 12.2, where functional movement in all planes would normally occur in the joints of the thoracic spine or at the hip joints, with the lumbopelvic region maintaining a static, isometrically controlled position whether in upright, lean forward positions or in single leg stance.

To understand the dysfunction that occurs in low back pain, it is first important to review the functional synergies that control pelvic position in

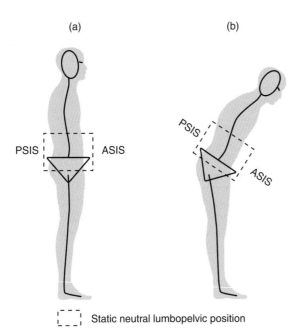

Static neutral lumbopelvic position

Figure 12.2 The neutral lumbopelvic unit during erect standing (a), and in a forward lean position (b). PSIS, posterior superior iliac spine; ASIS, anterior superior iliac spine.

this static model in the two planes of movement (saggital and frontal) that come under the influence of gravity (i.e. weightbearing postures).

Pelvic control in the saggital plane

Two functionally coupled groups of synergists work together to control (a) posterior pelvic tilt and (b) anterior pelvic tilt. A working model for lumbopelvic stability and weightbearing would be that the group muscle synergists involved in control in one direction of pelvic rotation (e.g. posterior pelvic tilt) should be in equilibrium with the group muscle synergists involved in control of the opposite direction of pelvic rotation (e.g. anterior pelvic tilt) in any particular trunk inclination (Fig. 12.2). That is, two antagonist muscle groups work together (in differing ranges of muscle length) in the sagittal plane to maintain static position of the pelvis relative to the spine, with trunk flexion/extension safely occurring at the hips rather than at the lumbar spine and pelvis as a whole.

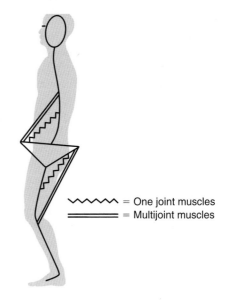

= One joint muscles
= Multijoint muscles

Figure 12.3 Muscles involved in posterior pelvic tilt.

For practical reasons of presenting these concepts for rehabilitation, muscles have been allocated to weightbearing and non-weightbearing categories even though many of the lumbopelvic muscle categories have not been validly determined as yet through microgravity, deloading research.

Posterior pelvic tilt Two functionally coupled groups of synergist muscles control the degrees of concentric posterior pelvic tilt (and eccentric anterior pelvic tilt) (Fig. 12.3):
- posterior hip muscles: gluteus maximus (weightbearing), hamstrings (non-weightbearing)
- abdominal muscles: rectus abdominis, internal oblique, external oblique (non-weightbearing).

Anterior pelvic tilt Two functionally coupled groups of synergists control the degrees of concentric anter-ior pelvic tilt (and eccentric posterior pelvic tilt) (Fig. 12.4):
- anterior hip muscles: iliacus (weightbearing), psoas, rectus femoris, tensor fascia lata (non-weightbearing)
- lumbar and thoracic erector spinae: lumbar erector spinae (weightbearing, one area of the spine), thoracic erector spinae (non-weightbearing).

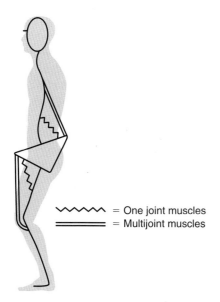

Figure 12.4   Muscles involved in anterior pelvic tilt.

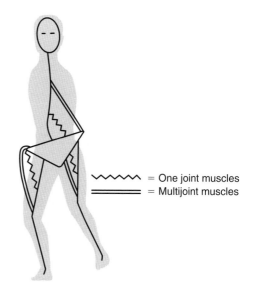

Figure 12.5   Muscles involved in lateral pelvic tilt.

Pelvic control in the frontal plane

A similar situation of equilibrium between lateral pelvic tilt to the right and lateral pelvic tilt to the left would occur in the frontal plane, as was described for the saggital plane for anterior and posterior pelvic tilt.

Lateral pelvic tilt upwards to the left   Three functionally coupled groups of synergists control degrees of concentric (left) pelvic tilt (and eccentric (right) lateral pelvic tilt) (Fig. 12.5):

- right lateral hip muscles: gluteus medius (weightbearing), tensor fascia lata (non-weightbearing)
- left medial hip muscles: adductor magnus, adductor brevis (weightbearing), adductor longus (non-weightbearing).
- left side flexors of the trunk: lumbar erector spinae (weightbearing, one area of the spine), thoracic erector spinae, external oblique muscle, quadratus lumborum (non-weightbearing).

Lateral pelvic tilt upwards to the right   Two functionally coupled groups of synergists control degrees of concentric (right) pelvic tilt (and eccentric (left) lateral pelvic tilt); The pattern of muscle activation would be as above but on the opposite side of the body.

IMPAIRMENTS IN MUSCLES CONTROLLING PELVIC ORIENTATION AND WEIGHTBEARING

Each group of synergists controlling one direction of tilt consists of both one-joint (predicted weightbearing) and multijoint (predicted non-weightbearing) synergists, which are differentially affected in deloading, injury and pain. This will have a marked effect on pelvic loading and movement patterns, especially if changes are unilateral. The predicted changes in each synergistic muscle would be different for the one-joint and multijoint muscles.

Weightbearing muscles attached to the pelvis

Weightbearing muscles have large attachments to the pelvis, controlling one direction of movement at a joint (or one area of the spine). Such muscles would be more involved in stabilization of pelvic position for weightbearing rather than in movement of the hips (Ch. 6). Examples would include gluteus maximus, gluteus medius, iliacus, adductor magnus and lumbar erector spinae.

Based on the development of impairments after deloading, injury or pain, as argued in this text, some of these muscles in patients with low back pain are likely to be atrophied, have reduced endurance (increased fatiguability), increased length and with the normal recruitment required for tonic holding patterns changing to more phasic, erratic patterns.

Non–weightbearing muscles attached to pelvis

The non-weightbearing muscles have smaller attachments to the pelvis, influence several directions of movement at more than one joint and would likely be more involved in moving the trunk and limbs rather than pelvic stabilization for weightbearing. Examples would include hamstring, external oblique/internal oblique, thoracic erector spinae, quadratus lumborum, rectus femoris, tensor fascia latae and adductor longus.

Again based on the development of impairments as argued in this text, some of these musles in patients with low back pain are likely to have increased activation levels, increased endurance (reduced fatiguability), decreased length and with normal phasic recruitment during movement changing to more tonic, holding recruitment patterns.

Evidence of dysfunction in selected pelvic muscle synergists in low back pain

While the one-joint and multijoint synergists of the pelvis have been implicated in low back pain, few studies have addressed the function/dysfunction of these individual muscles, because of difficulties in measuring such parameters. Electromyography (EMG) to study functional tasks or clinical muscle testing procedures have been used to assess the function of individual muscle synergists (Palmer and Epler 1998).

Gluteus maximus

Few studies have been undertaken on the function of gluteus maximus, as its function is difficult to measure separately from the hamstrings. Dysfunction (weakness) in gluteus maximus has been reported by many clinicians treating low back pain and it is known that hip–spine interaction

(lumbopelvic rhythm) is disturbed in low back pain during sagittal trunk flexion–extension (Paquet et al 1994) although the precise reason is unclear.

More concrete evidence has come from EMG studies performed on patients with low back pain. Reduced gluteal activation was reported by Bullock-Saxton et al (1993), and Kankaanpaa et al (1998) showed increased fatiguability of gluteus maximus during trunk and hip extensor endurance testing. The authors suggested that the cause was likely to be deconditioning, but it could be the result of deloading or injury/pain linked to dysfunction of the lumbopelvic joints. Leinonen et al (2000) also used EMG to examine gluteus maximus during sagittal plane flexion and extension and demonstrated a relative change in activation time of gluteus maximus in patients with low back pain, with no change in the paravertebral muscles or hamstrings.

Hamstrings

Hamstring tightness is one of the most common findings in low back pain (reviewed by Nourbakhsh and Arab 2002). Tight, overactive hamstrings have also been implicated in the development of ligament strains associated with the sacro-iliac joint (Vleeming et al 1997). In addition, a recent EMG study on back pain subjects (with sacroiliac pain) has demonstrated that, in addition to a delayed activation of gluteus maximus, low back pain patients displayed significantly earlier onset of the hamstring muscles (i.e. biceps femoris) (Hungerford et al 2003).

Iliacus

Intramuscular EMG research studies have demonstrated that, while iliacus and psoas both have a role in hip flexion, iliacus has the supporting role of controlling the femoral head in relation to the pelvis, while psoas has more of a trunk-positioning role (Andersson et al 1997). Although studies have demonstated that iliacus functions in a separate way to psoas in relation to joint stability, most clinical studies on patients with low back pain have necessarily taken iliopsoas as a single functional entity.

In a review on the mechanical factors linked with low back pain, Nourbakhsh and Arab (2002) reported studies that demonstrated decreased length and strength in iliopsoas in low back pain. However, Aspinall (1993), in a review that focused on length-associated changes in the muscle, predicted that iliopsoas is either lengthened or shortened as a result of postures and activity patterns. Dysfunction in this muscle may depend on individual lifestyles and postures, hence there is a need, as with other pelvic muscles, to test each patient to ascertain any presenting problems.

Tensor fascia lata

It has been reported that stretching the iliotibial band is often used in the treatment of low back pain but no studies have measured muscle length (reviewed by Nourbakhsh and Arab 2002).

Quadratus lumborum

Clinically, tightness of quadratus lumborum unilaterally or bilaterally is often present in patients with low back pain. The muscle is the most common source of trigger points in low back pain (Simons and Travell 1983), and if specific therapy (e.g. manual pressure, relaxation techniques) is applied to this muscle, many clinicians claim substantial relief of low back pain (Graber 1997). In studying the relationship between low back pain and quadratus lumborum, some clinicians (Bryner 1996) have attempted to study the pain patterns evoked by palpation of the muscle, in an effort to demonstrate that these are the cause of the patient's pain. However, because of the difficulty in establishing suitable research protocols, it will be some time before the precise relationship between problems in quadratus lumborum and low back pain can be resolved. In any case, this is a muscle which is generally seen as being overactive in low back pain.

Lumbar erector spinae

In a study of mechanical factors associated with low back pain in 600 subjects, Nourbakhsh and Arab (2002) found that it was only back extensor endurance that related to the back pain problem. Several EMG studies by Roy et al (1989, 1990) have confirmed that it is the loss of endurance of the lumbar erector spinae which is highly correlated

with low back pain. In an EMG study involving trunk rotation, Ng et al (2002a) demonstrated significantly less activation of the lumbar erector spinae in subjects with low back pain in rotation, which was also associated with an increase in fatiguability. This group of muscles are definitely affected in patients with low back pain. Importantly, this coincides with the lumbar erector spinae likely having an important antigravity role in upright postures.

Because it has been reported that the thoracic erector spinae are likely to become overactive with reduced fatiguablity (Ch. 11), finding a clinical test that reflects lack of endurance of the lumbar muscles without the influence of the thoracic erector spinae has been a challenge to clinicians. A forward lean with maintenance of neutral spine and pelvic position can be used to test coordination and endurance of the lumbar back extensors (Fig. 12.6). Hamilton and Richardson (1995) demonstrated that patients with low back pain could not hold the neutral spinal curve in 15 degrees of forward flexion. This test and exercise strategy is described in detail in Chapter 15.

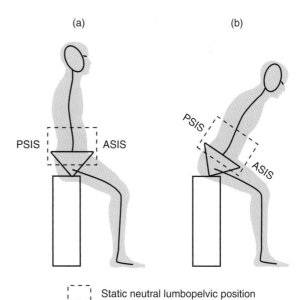

Figure 12.6   The neutral lumbopelvic unit during (a) erect high sitting and (b) in a forward lean position. PSIS, posterior superior iliac spine; ASIS, anterior superior iliac spine.

External oblique/internal oblique

Several EMG studies by Ng et al (2002a,b) demonstrated another important result that furthered our understanding of muscles influencing pelvic position and control. Subjects with low back pain had increased activation levels and increased endurance (i.e. reduced fatiguability) of the external obliques (the right side was significant) during fatiguing trunk rotations. Interestingly the internal obliques demonstrated similar dysfunctional patterns but this did not reach statistical significance. Overactivity of internal obliques is reported to be a major problem in patients with low back pain at our back clinic. Reasons for this are not understood. It could be that with dysfunction of gluteus maximus, increased activation of internal obliques is used to compensate for the loss of control of posterior pelvic tilt.

Adductor magnus and brevis

The adductors form a large muscle mass that secures the pelvic position for lateral stability. Importantly, adductor magnus, which is a major extensor of the hip in weightbearing (i.e. sit to stand), would also contribute significantly, with gluteus maximus, in pelvic support of the lumbopelvic region in the saggital plane (Pohtilla 1969). In a recent study, in which clinical muscle tests of antigravity function of the adductors were assessed, runners without low back pain could perform the test, but runners who had experienced low back pain had a definite weakness of these muscles (T. Rowe, R. Toppenberg and C. A. Richardson 2003, unpublished data). This would suggest that further research is required in patients with low back pain to determine if weakness and lack of endurance of adductor magnus (and brevis) could be a predisposing factor in the development of loss of pelvic control and low back pain.

Relationship between joint range of movement, muscle dysfunction and low back pain

Impairments in range of movements of various joints could also influence the development of lumbopelvic control problems.

Trunk range of movement

Many studies have demonstrated that trunk range of movement does not differ between patients with low back pain and healthy controls (reviewed by Ng et al 2002c). However, there is some evidence that asymmetry of rotation and lateral flexion range of movement could be a problem in patients with back pain (Gomez 1994). This asymmetry in range could result from many factors, most importantly asymmetry of quadratus lumborum length.

At a segmental level, increased intersegmental movement in the upper lumbar spine and thoracolumbar junction is often reported in low back pain and has been linked to a shortening of muscle length of iliopsoas (Jorgensson 1993).

Range of movement at hips and thoracic spine

Lack of range of the hip and thoracic spine (i.e. the adjacent joints to the neutral lumbopelvic region (Fig. 12.2)) is often observed in patients with low back pain. It is considered that mobility in these joints is important, especially for rotation, so that damaging rotation stress to the lumbar spine is avoided and injury prevented. A decrease in hip range of motion (mainly hip rotation) has been reported by Chesworth et al (1994). In a recent study undertaken in our laboratory, asymmetry of hip range of movement was detected in runners with low back pain compared with runners without low back pain (T. Rowe, R. Toppenberg and C. A. Richardson 2003, unpublished data). This measure could also have been influenced by tight muscles (e.g. tensor fascia lata) in the region.

CLINICAL RELEVANCE

Assumptions to assist in clinical practice

There are several standard physiotherapy assessment procedures that can be used to assess indirectly a dysfunction in lumbopelvic muscle control. Standard postural assessments involving observation of relaxed stance and then single leg stance would give some indication of lumbopelvic control. Assessments of the spine and pelvic deviation in forward trunk lean while controlling a static, neutral position of the lumbopelvic region is usually completed from a high sitting position (Hamilton and Richardson 1995), illustrated in Fig. 12.6, from a standing position (Sahrmann 2002), illustrated in Figure 12.2, or from a standing position with flexed hips and knees.

Impairments in individual muscle synergists could be quantified through specific muscle testing of individual muscle synergists.

1. Antigravity inner range hold for the one-joint (weightbearing) muscles, adapted from the grade 3 antigravity muscle tests described by Palmer and Epler (1998). This would test the ability of the weightbearing synergist to hold in their fully shortened position (explained in Ch. 7).

2. Specific muscle length tests for the multijoint (non-weightbearing) muscles, adapted from the length tests described in Palmer and Epler (1998). This would test the degree of overactivity in an indirect way (explained in Ch. 7).

Range of movement (passive and active), particularly the hip and thoracic spine, would be important to assess. Low back pain has been associated with a decrease in range of hip motion, especially rotation (Chesworth et al 1994), as well as a decreased range of motion/stiffness in the thoracic spine (especially rotation). These aspects would need to be assessed for both preventative and rehabilitative exercise for low back pain.

The future

An approach that focuses on joint protection mechanisms and load transfer is particularly important when considering the problems in the control of mechanical tissue loading related to the pelvis. A large number of muscles attach to the pelvis and are capable of producing many different directions of muscle force at various types and levels of contraction. As individual muscle dysfunction would relate to many aspects of an individual's lifestyle factors, associated with deloading (Ch. 7), injury (Ch. 8) or pain (Ch. 9), it is likely that individuals would display a large variety of muscle impairments. Dysfunction could affect any number of muscle synergists bilaterally or unilaterally, creating many permutations and combinations of resultant joint loading and torsions involving the pelvic bones themselves. This situation would, in turn, lead to a variety of tissue loading problems associated with joints or ligaments in the region.

Therefore, there are many difficulties for researchers in producing quantitative evidence of dysfunction in lumbopelvic muscle control for evidence-based research studies. This has been the main reason for lack of research results in the area.

A possible future direction could be to combine clinical tests with biomechanical models. A biomechanical model has already been devised and tested by Hoek van Dijke et al (1999) that is based on detailed lumbopelvic anatomy and is a 'tool for analyzing the relation between forces in muscles, ligaments and joints in the transfer of gravitational and external load from the upper body via the sacroiliac joints to the legs in normal situations and in pathology'. The model involves 94 muscle parts, six ligaments and six joints. Our continuing collaboration with Professor Snijders and Erasmus University will allow the joint protection model of a neutral lumbopelvic unit, and the individual clinical muscle impairments described in this chapter, to be incorporated into this biomechanical model to give an indication of the changes in forces and load transfer associated with low back pain. Hopefully, this will result in a far better understanding of the aetiology of low back pain and will assist in demonstrating the benefits of prescribed prevention exercises.

SECTION 5

Treatment and prevention of low back pain

Chapter 13

Principles of the 'segmental stabilization' exercise model

Carolyn Richardson, Julie Hides and Paul Hodges

INTRODUCTION

The applied science of 'maintaining and promoting musculo-skeletal health' can only be developed by devising principles based on the systematic formulation of knowledge gained from clinical experience, experimental studies and the process of induction. Understanding the principles underlying the therapeutic strategies is necessary to allow development of both optimal treatment and evidence-based research.

This expanded 'segmental stabilization training' (SST) management approach is guided by principles that have been devised from extensive clinical experience in the area of low back pain, together with an increased understanding of the complex neurophysiological processes involved in joint protection and the impairments that are involved in the development of painful symptoms. These issues have been discussed in detail in the earlier chapters.

The first consideration in developing principles is to establish testing procedures. Many experimental assessment procedures have been described in previous chapters that give essential information about the joint protection mechanisms, especially in the lumbopelvic region. However, there is a need for simple clinical tests to estimate the level of impairment in the general population as well as in patients with low back pain. In this way, client profiles can be collated that would give an indication of the specific type and level of exercise required to re-establish the optimum joint protection mechanisms.

It should be emphasized that we believe that these described principles may have important implications for the prevention and management of other conditions such as osteoarthritis of the weightbearing joints of the lower limb. In addition, it is envisaged, that some aspects of the SST model of exercise could assist in the refinement of exercise programmes for osteoporosis and stress incontinence, breathing exercises for chest conditions, as well as health-care exercise programmes for the elderly.

THE SEGMENTAL STABILIZATION MODEL OF EXERCISE

Earlier chapters have emphasized that joint protection mechanisms involve both open loop strategies, which are independent of sensory feedback, and closed loop strategies, which are dependent on sensory feedback. There is evidence that both strategies are disrupted in patients with low back pain, most likely the result of pain, injury to joint structures and through the process of 'deloading' (lack of weightbearing) resulting from lifestyle factors.

Therefore, for each individual patient with low back pain, many changes occur in the elements of motor control required for joint protection, and these need to be addressed in therapeutic exercise if back pain is to be treated and prevented successfully.

Many therapeutic exercise strategies for rehabilitation have been presented, including those based on training muscle performance and re-education of control by the central nervous system. As presented in the preceding chapters, a range of changes in terms of control and muscle performance have been identified (these are summarized below) and the challenge has been to identify optimal methods to train or retrain the capacity of the system to meet the demands imposed by external and internal factors. As a major factor in the dysfunction present in low back and pelvic pain relates to control of the muscle system, it is logical to draw on motor learning principles. The nervous system has considerable potential for plasticity and learning. Motor learning refers to the acquisition and refinement of movement and coordination that leads to a permanent change in movement performance.

Two key theories of motor learning have been developed. One popular model, first presented by Fitts and Posner (1967), considers that learning involves three main stages: cognitive, associative and autonomous phases. In the cognitive phase, the focus is on cognitively oriented problems. All elements of the movement performance are organized consciously with attention to feedback, movement sequence, performance and instruction during repetition and practice. This phase is characterized by frequent large errors and variability. The second stage is the associative phase, in which the fundamentals of the movement have been acquired and the cognitive demands are reduced. The focus moves from simple elements of performance of the task to consistency of performance, success and refinement. Correspondingly, the frequency and size of errors are reduced. The final stage of motor learning, the autonomous phase, is achieved after considerable practice and experience. The task becomes habitual or automatic and the requirement for conscious intervention is reduced. Although the features of each phase are distinct, it is important to consider that there is a smooth transition between phases and it may not be obvious when a person moves between phases. Other models of motor learning have similar features to this three-phase process with differences in the emphasis placed on elements of the progression of learning. For instance, Gentile (1987) divided learning into two phases based on the goal of the learner. In the first phase, the goal of the learner is to 'get the idea' of the task. The second phase involves fixation or diversification of the skill, that is improved consistency in stable environments and improved transfer to new contexts. Irrespective of the specific features of each model, the basic elements of motor learning are similar.

A rationale for the management of motor control changes in low back and pelvic pain may lie in these conventional motor learning theories. Clearly, this must be based on accurate identification of the deficit in movement performance that needs to be addressed. Once identified, strategies can be implemented to re-educate the control of these components. In other words, the goal is to give the patient the 'idea' of the correct performance. This could occur through cognitive attention to the task with specific feedback, as is common in skill learning, or through guided experience of the correct performance via sensory inputs such as sensorimotor integration techniques. Therefore, a range of exercise options are available to meet the demand of re-education of movement performance that fall within the spectrum of motor learning.

The key to effective motor learning lies in identification of the nature of the deficits in performance and utilization of optimal strategies to induce change in performance that are tailored to the individual patient's needs. The changes in the joint protection mechanisms, it has been argued, include both the local and global muscle systems.

For the local muscle system:

- loss of feedforward response of the local muscles;
- loss of independent control of the local muscles from the global (especially non-weightbearing) muscles;
- reflex inhibition of the lumbar multifidus;
- loss of the ability to form a 'shortening' contraction of transversus abdominis (bilaterally or unilaterally); and
- altered position sense in the lumbopelvic region and inability to maintain a neutral spinal position.

For the global muscle system:

- division of function of global muscles (i.e. weightbearing and non-weightbearing muscles) at the extremes of the motor control continuum; with weightbearing muscles closely associated with closed loop motor function and non-weightbearing muscles closely linked to open loop motor function;
- deloading (lack of weightbearing) as well as injury to joint structures results in a loss of joint protective function of the weightbearing muscles (as well as the local muscle system), with consequent changes in joint loading; this is compounded with increased contribution of the non-weightbearing muscles to the joint protection role.

The consequences of deloading/injury in the global system can be considered from a neurophysiological point of view.

Weightbearing muscles   Recruitment of the weightbearing muscles could be affected by reduction in support for muscle contraction from the muscle spindle system through lower levels of activation of gamma motoneurons and a subsequent reduction in spindle afferent discharge (and reduced tonic activity), potentially in response to decreased afferent input from the joint mechanoreceptors. Thus weightbearing muscles would display a reduced sensitivity to the stretch, most particularly in gravity, weightbearing conditions. This situation would gradually lead to changes in muscle fibres (towards fast twitch) and resultant atrophy of the muscle.

Non-weightbearing muscles   It is likely that the opposite occurs in the non-weightbearing muscles. An increase in gamma support for muscle contraction through increased spindle sensitivity (and increased tonic activity) would result in the non-weightbearing muscles displaying an increased sensitivity to the stretch. This situation would gradually lead to changes in muscle fibres (towards slow twitch) and resultant hypertrophy of the muscle.

Implications for practice for the local muscle system

There are a number of implications for practice:

- develop the skill of an independent contraction of the local muscle synergy;
- decrease the contribution of the overactive global muscles (mainly non-weightbearing muscles);
- use a motor relearning approach to reteach the skill of developing a 'corset' action of transversus abdominis and multifidus in response to the cue to draw in the abdominal wall;
- use specific facilitation and feedback techniques to ensure each segment of multifidus (especially deep parts) is activated;
- use specific feedback techniques to develop kinaesthetic awareness of local muscle contractions;
- develop ability to hold the 'corset' action tonically over extended periods of time; and
- use repeated movements of the lumbopelvic region, in non-weightbearing positions initially, to improve position sense (position sense will improve as the local muscle synergy is activated).

Implications for practice in integration of the local with the global muscle system

This approach also has implications for practice in terms of successfully integrating the local global muscle systems:

- treating the local and weightbearing muscles is likely to reverse impairments in the non-weightbearing muscles;
- initially use specific facilitation techniques for the dysfunctional weightbearing muscles, with emphasis on increasing weightbearing load cues;
- use optimal weightbearing postures (neutral lumbopelvic region) to re-establish recruitment of both the local and weightbearing muscles;
- weightbearing muscles should be trained under the stretch from gravity in flexed and more upright postures (both eccentric and concentric contractions);
- use static weightbearing postures with increasing holds and/or very slow and controlled weightbearing exercise to enhance the feedback mechanisms;
- increase gravitational load cues (e.g. uneven, unstable surfaces) gradually, ensuring local and weightbearing muscles are responding to the increases in load; and
- at a later stage, may need to add in specific muscle-lengthening techniques for non-weightbearing muscles, especially if the muscle tightness is in the passive rather than the active elements of the muscle.

Stages for exercise management

The SST model of exercise includes the principles of motor learning theory. As the process necessarily needs to restore several levels of impairments in joint protection, involving dysfunction of many different local, weightbearing and non-weightbearing muscles, the training model needs to involve a problem-solving approach, where clinical tests, reflecting the dysfunction mechanisms, are used to decide the best type of treatment approach for an individual client. In order to achieve this, assessments and their related treatments have been simplified by dividing them

into progressive stages, where one stage of assessment and treatment is ideally completed prior to proceeding to the next stage.

The process of 'segmentation', that is breaking functional posture and movement up into its component parts, is used for each progressive stage. According to motor learning theory, segmentation can be used to train the components of functional posture and movement that are in deficit, which can then be integrated into function. The segmental approach which we have devised develops through three stages of segmental control, with each stage exposing the individual client to increasing challenges to their joint protection mechanisms.

Stage 1: local segmental control

The simplification here refers to re-establishing directly the simultaneous contraction of the deep muscle synergy (i.e. transversus abdominis, deep multifidus, pelvic floor and diaphragm) independently of the global muscles (i.e. both weightbearing and non-weightbearing muscles). This simultaneous contraction of the synergy, independent of the global muscles, should occur with the postural cue to 'draw in the lower abdominal wall'. Another important simplification is that throughout this initial stage, the weight of the body is minimized in order to allow the patient or client to focus on this specific skill involved in joint protection.

Training 'local segmental control' involves activating and facilitating the local muscle system, while using techniques (e.g. feedback) to reduce the contribution of the global muscles, most particularly the non-weightbearing global muscles. Instructional cues, body position and various feedback techniques (including palpation, electromyography and real-time ultrasound) are used simultaneously to facilitate the local synergy and inhibit and/or relax the more active global muscles. The ability to hold this pattern through developing specific muscular control (without the addition of any load) may serve also to help to restore kinaesthetic awareness and lumbopelvic position sense, usually found to be impaired in the patient with low back pain.

This basic segmental element of posture and movement forms the foundation on which to build an integrated system capable of protecting the joints of the lumbopelvic region from high forces and high loads.

Stage 2: closed chain segmental control

The next component or segment of posture and movement that should be addressed is the entity of local segmental control (stage 1) combined with the weightbearing function of the trunk, girdles and limbs. This stage addresses the next level of impairment in the joint protection mechanisms occurring in patients with low back pain (i.e. the antigravity muscle support system).

The aim is to maintain the local muscle synergy contraction (on the cue to draw in the lower abdominal wall), while gradually progressing load cues through the body using weightbearing closed chain exercise. Weightbearing load is added very slowly, ensuring all weightbearing muscles from each segment of the kinetic chain are activated to give effective antigravity support and provide efficient and safe load transfer through the segments of the body. The focus is especially to ensure activation of the local and weightbearing muscles of the lumbar spine and pelvis, and the ability to maintain a static lumbopelvic posture for weightbearing. These muscles are likely to be dysfunctional in patients with low back pain. In addition, lifestyle factors of many individuals, which could have led to a dysfunction in these muscles, need to be addressed, as they may place them at risk of sustaining further low back injury.

Stage 3: open chain segmental control

With weightbearing patterns in hand (stage 2), there is a third segmental or simplified model that needs to be addressed prior to functional, skill-specific movement tasks becoming the focus. The aim is to continue to maintain local segmental control while load is added through open kinetic chain movement of adjacent segments (e.g. movement between the lumbopelvic region and lower limb through the hip joint). This final step is to direct progression so that all muscles (i.e. the local, weightbearing and non-weightbearing) are integrated into functional movement tasks in a formal way.

This third stage allows any loss of local segmental control during high loaded open chain tasks to be detected, as well as ensuring that there is no compensation by the more active (i.e. non-weightbearing) muscles. In addition, loss of range or asymmetry of joints adjacent to the lumbopelvic region needs to be addressed to ensure that loss of movement range does not interfere with the ability of the individual to maintain lumbopelvic stability during movement.

GENERAL PRINCIPLES FOR THE SEGMENTAL STABILIZATION MODEL

There are many general principles that apply to most therapeutic exercise programmes for low back pain. The principles are particularly important for this SST model of exercise.

The close relationship between stabilization exercise and pain relief

The close association between segmental stabilization and pain can be used for both prevention and treatment purposes. A theoretical construct (Richardson and Jull 1995a) has described how exercise, which aims to influence muscle control and joint protection, should ultimately lead to pain control. However, our contention is that pain relief and joint protection rely on the specific nature of the segmental exercise programme, and general exercises used to retrain functional movement may not address the specific impairments in the joint protection system and, therefore, may not be as effective for long-term pain relief.

The effects of the exercise intervention will be enhanced if other treatment modalities that relieve pain, inflammation and oedema are used in conjunction with segmental stabilization. These treatments may include anti-inflammatory medication, electrophysical agents and mobilization or manipulation techniques.

Keep tissue loading as low as possible for testing and training exercise strategies

As the relief of pain is the main goal of treatment, all exercise should proceed with the target joint in a mid or neutral position. The aim is to keep the tissue loading as low as possible while the joint protection mechanisms are being developed through stages. Ergonomic advice is appropriate at this stage to reduce tissue loading. Pain should remain at a minimum.

Use clinical measures of the muscle dysfunction to profile the level of musculo-skeletal health in relation to joint protection mechanisms

The division of skeletal muscles from a motor control perspective into local, weightbearing and non-weightbearing categories has resulted in an expanded view of the function of muscles and their role in joint protection, and of the type of dysfunction which occurs in the muscles as a result of deloading (Ch. 7), injury (Ch. 8) or pain (Ch. 9). Most measures explained in the following chapters rely on basic clinical knowledge. Measures of muscle function that do not require high levels of clinical skill are currently being developed.

In relation to low back pain, clinical measures of the dysfunction of the muscle control system give an indication of what type of therapeutic exercise is required to restore the muscle control for joint protection. In addition, clinical measures allow profiling of some aspects of musculo-skeletal health in relation to joint protection, so specific exercise can be prescribed appropriately to prevent future pain and injury.

Exercise should be focused on tonic holding contractions rather than fast phasic contractions

It has been argued that it is the tonic function of the local and the weightbearing muscles which is likely impaired in the patient with low back pain. It must be remembered that, in the early stages, a tonic contraction would be no more than 30% of the maximum voluntary contraction. Throughout all the exercise stages, the emphasis is on isometric holding contractions in static positions or exercise via very slow and controlled movement. Individuals with poor control will usually attempt fast or phasic contractions.

Care must be taken with exercise progression

Both type and level of load are important. Too much load may lead to fatigue of the muscles involved in joint protection. Further joint injury may occur if load is added too quickly and the muscles fail to respond to the level of load owing to a loss of proprioception. Therefore, load needs to be carefully controlled and training movements are initially slow and controlled and must not proceed to the point of muscle fatigue. This is the major difference between this approach and strength training, as the changing patterns of motor control with fatigue can lead to poor joint control and exacerbation of painful symptoms. Load is added initially through the use of closed chain exercise.

Treatment outcomes will be influenced by several factors

The findings of the patient interview and physical examination need to be taken into account as they will influence treatment outcomes. Some factors which may be particularly important to outcome, are:

- amount and extent of pathology;
- classification of low back pain (acute, subacute, chronic, recurrent episodic);
- pain location, quality and intensity;
- presence of respiratory conditions;
- skeletal deformities (e.g. scoliosis, increased thoracic kyphosis);
- leg length discrepancies;
- postural deviations (e.g. sway back, flat back, lordotic posture); and
- continence.

Lifestyle activities that would be detrimental to the segmental training should be identified

Chapter 7 outlines the activities that may cause impairments in joint protection mechanisms.

AIMS FOR EACH STAGE OF SEGMENTAL CONTROL

The three stages of the exercise model form the building blocks for the development of the joint protection mechanisms, for both low- and high-load functional situations. Each stage includes clinical assessments of the level of impairment in the joint protection mechanisms, followed by the suggested

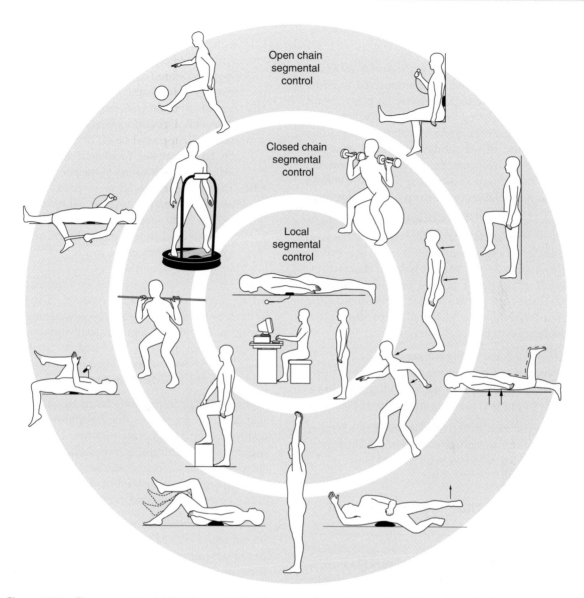

Figure 13.1 The segmental stabilization model for the prevention and treatment of low back pain. (Adapted from Richardson and Jull 1995b.)

exercise techniques. The exercise principles, in addition to the general principles of the SST model, are given for each of the stages and are illustrated in Figure 13.1.

Stage 1: local segmental control (Ch. 14)

The aim in stage 1 is to train the local muscles to provide segmental protection of joints in the lumbopelvic region without the addition of load or antigravity weightbearing function.

1. *Assess the level of impairment in the joint protection mechanisms* The cue to 'pull in the lower abdomen' is used to assess the automatic activation of the co-contraction pattern (i.e. local muscle synergy). This is assessed through a supine test as well as a prone test with the pressure biofeedback unit. The ability to perform an

isometric multifidus contraction (at each segmental level) is also assessed.

2. *Clinical problem solving and implication of test results* The test results need to be interpreted to allow for precise exercise prescription. It is important that, during testing procedures, the substitution strategies are observed and interpreted. It is this recognition of substitution strategies that signals to the clinician the postures, movements and instructions which may be best avoided during facilitation of the deep muscle synergy.

3. *Rehabilitation of the joint protection mechanisms* Facilitation of the independent control of the local muscle synergy is promoted with the aim of developing low-level tonic holding contractions while maintaining normal breathing patterns. Strategies are presented that will minimize the non-weightbearing global muscles during the facilitation of the local synergy.

4. *Progression into sitting and standing positions* In preparation for more functional weightbearing positions, activation of the local muscles is gradually progressed to sitting and standing positions.

5. *Implementation of the activation strategies* Further suggestions are added to assist in the implementation of the exercises in a practical way.

Stage 2: closed chain segmental control (Ch. 15)

Stage 2 involves the integration of the local muscles into segmental, antigravity weightbearing function. Integration of the local and weightbearing muscles is best achieved through weightbearing (closed) kinetic chain exercises with gradually increasing gravitational (i.e. gravity-related) load cues.

The treatment aims are as follows.

1. *Train individual parts of the antigravity weightbearing holding posture* There are many different muscle groups at many individual segments (i.e. joints) that need to be co-ordinated to hold the flexed weightbearing posture effectively. The focus initially is on individual parts of the antigravity posture.

   (i) *Begin loading the neutral spine/pelvic position in sitting* The aim is to maintain a neutral spine/pelvic position in upright sitting with gradual added antigravity muscle activity using two different methods: upper quadrant closed chain exercise and trunk forward lean.

   (ii) *Activate dysfunctional weightbearing muscles of the pelvis* Traditional muscle testing techniques (Palmer and Epler 1998) are used as the basis for the functional tests of the weightbearing muscles of the pelvis.

   (iii) *Train quadriceps holding in partial weightbearing* Isometric holding achieved with body weight against wall (i.e. wall squat) could be used to test and train the quadriceps muscle endurance in preparation for closed chain activities.

2. *Train the weightbearing muscles in weightbearing (closed chain) exercise in flexed postures* The type of exercise techniques used at this treatment stage includes the slow lunge or semi-squat, with weightbearing muscles stretched to facilitate their contribution to weightbearing, with non-weightbearing muscles relaxed.

3. *Train the weightbearing muscles in weightbearing (closed chain) exercise in flexed postures with the addition of unstable, moving surfaces* In order to facilitate the weightbearing muscles further, under increasing gravitational load cues, unstable and moving surfaces (balance boards, rubber discs, trampolines) can be used.

4. *Train the weightbearing muscles in weightbearing (closed chain) exercise on more challenging surfaces and in more upright postures* Progress is made to more upright positions, for example walking on unstable, uneven or sloping surfaces such as soft sand, grassy slopes or rough ground. The most challenging surface in a formal setting for closed chain exercise comes through the use of a new exercise tool – whole body vibration.

Stage 3: open chain segmental control and progression into function (Ch. 16)

The aim in stage 3 is to continue to develop segmental control at individual joints in relation to open kinetic chain movement of adjacent segments (while maintaining neutral lumbopelvic posture).

In addition to the formal open chain exercise programme, steps are taken to progress into function, which involves movement of the trunk with higher loads and speeds. Maintaining local segmental control is required prior to all exercise techniques, whether formal or functional. Specific aims are as follows.

1. Open chain segmental control:
   - decrease compensatory movement of the lumbopelvic region during movement of adjacent segments;
   - reduce tightness/overactivity in the non-weightbearing muscles if necessary; and
   - treat problems of trunk muscle strength and endurance in open chain exercise.
2. Progression into function:
   - progress to functional activites (sporting and occupational) that use a combination of open and closed chain tasks, which include trunk movement as well as higher loads and higher speeds;
   - develop countermeasures to prevent loss of joint protection; and
   - maintain and check segmental control regularly.

Relation to other exercise programmes for prevention and treatment of low back pain

There are a huge number of exercise programmes that are reported to improve low back pain. These include pilates, thai chi, yoga and ball programmes. These exercise programmes include some excellent exercise techniques that would be very suitable for prevention and rehabilitation of low back pain under the SST model. Chapters 14–16 give some examples of exercises that would fulfil the principles of SST, but they are only a guide; many other exercises would be very suitable.

Chapter 14

Local segmental control

Julie Hides, Carolyn Richardson and Paul Hodges

INTRODUCTION

Achieving local segmental control involves activation and training of the muscles of the local synergy. This phase of training involves development of the most basic element of segmental stabilization training, joint protection. It is essential that local segmental control is mastered prior to progression to the next stage of rehabilitation, closed chain segmental control. This initial stage relies on facilitating the independent control of the local muscle synergy in non-loaded situations where there should be minimum contribution of the global (weightbearing and non-weightbearing) muscles.

This chapter begins with the assessment of the level of impairment in the joint protection mechanisms with a focus on the local muscle system. This is followed by clinical problem solving and interpretation of test results and mechanisms for rehabilitation of the joint protection.

ASSESSMENT OF THE LEVEL OF IMPAIRMENT IN JOINT PROTECTION MECHANISMS

Impairments are assessed in two ways: checking the ability to achieve the normal spinal curves (position sense), tests of the corset action (Ch. 5). The corset relies on co-activation of four separate synergists. We have developed formal tests for multifidus and transversus abdominis. These are tested separately even though they should always contract together.

The ability to achieve the normal spinal curves (position sense)

It is ultimately important that the patient can attain normal spinal curves for optimum and efficient distribution of load and joint protection. For this reason, a baseline assessment of the patient's normal unsupported sitting posture and their ability to correct it is required. Patients will often sit in a position of lumbar flexion and posterior pelvic tilt and will have difficulty achieving a normal lumbar lordosis and thoracic kyphosis. This clinical visual assessment can be repeated throughout the rehabilitation process, and should improve as muscle function improves.

Prone and supine tests of the corset action

The assessment of the corset action is based on the instructional cue to 'pull in the lower abdomen' to estimate if an automatic activation of the co-contraction pattern (i.e. local muscle synergy) occurs (see Ch. 5).

Prone test with the pressure biofeedback unit

The patient lies prone with the arms by the side, head in the midline and the pressure biofeedback unit (Appendix 14.1) is placed under the abdomen with the navel in the centre and the distal edge of the pad in line with the right and left anterior superior iliac spines (Fig. 14.1). The pressure pad is inflated to 70 mmHg and allowed to stabilize. This pressure inflates the pad sufficiently to detect changes in position of the abdominal wall but is comfortable and does not press into the abdominal contents. At rest, small deviations of the indicator on the pressure dial will be evident with abdominal movement during normal respiration, and, therefore, it is essential to identify the point about which the level fluctuates.

It is important to instruct the patient to relax the abdomen fully prior to attempting the test. The cue to pull in the lower abdomen must be preceded by the instruction to take a relaxed breath in and out and then, without breathing in, draw the abdomen in towards the spine without taking a breath. It is optimal when testing to dissociate

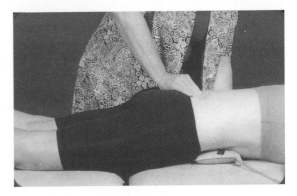

Figure 14.1 The muscle test for the transversus abdominis muscle, performed in the prone position using the pressure biofeedback unit. (Reproduced with permission from Northwater Publishing, Australia.)

breathing from the performance of the contraction since the patient may simulate the abdominal movement simply by reducing the pressure in the thorax, drawing the diaphragm up and the abdominal wall in, in the same manner as when a person breathes in to squeeze through a narrow space. However, if the patient is unable to do this, the test can be modified by allowing the patient to draw in the abdominal wall without altering their breathing pattern.

When a patient is asked 'Draw in your abdominal wall without moving your spine or pelvis', there should be a co-contraction of the local synergy muscles (i.e. the corset action described in Ch. 5), with each side of transverses abdominis contracting and shortening into its inner range in this position. The action of the transversus abdominis is to draw in the abdominal wall and also narrow the waist. The most successful way to emphasize activation of the transversus abdominis is to instruct the patient to concentrate on the lower part of the abdomen. Recent evidence suggests that when attention is focused on the lower abdominal wall, the contraction of transverses abdominis is more independent of the superficial muscles (Urquhart et al 2003). The drawing in of the lower abdomen is illustrated in Figure 14.2. If the patient experiences difficulty initiating this action, additional assistance can be provided by the clinician placing his or her hands on their own abdomen and demonstrating the movement of the lower abdomen towards the spine.

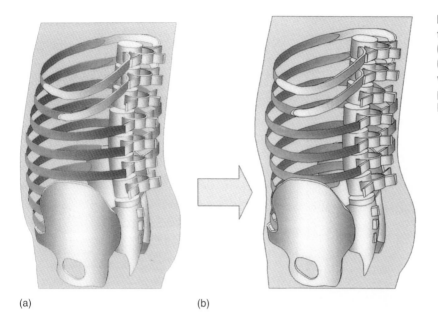

Figure 14.2 The action of transversus abdominis. (a) Relaxed abdominal wall. (b) The drawn in abdominal wall. (Reproduced with permission from Northwater Publishing, Australia.)

(a)   (b)

Once the contraction has been achieved, the patient should recommence relaxed normal breathing. The clinician should perform three tasks while completing the test. These include observation of the dial of the pressure biofeedback unit, observation of the pelvis and trunk for spinal or pelvic movement and palpation of the abdominal wall during the test. The abdomen is palpated (on each side) medially and inferiorly to the anterior superior iliac spine (Hides et al 2000). With a correct activation of the transversus abdominis, a slowly developing deep tension may be felt in the abdominal wall. In contrast, if a global pattern of activation is used, the abdominal wall will be felt to bulge.

Once satisfied, the action is repeated and the pressure change noted. If the patient can perform the test well, the contraction can be held for 10 seconds. The procedure can be repeated up to 10 times to test the endurance of the muscles.

Test results The pressure biofeedback unit provides important information about the relationship between the local and global muscles of the anterior abdominal wall. The three elements of testing should all be recorded for meaningful interpretation of test results. There are three possible test results.

1. An optimal performance of the test reduces the pressure by approximately 4–10 mmHg in the absence of spinal or pelvic movement and without bulging of the abdomen. This pressure change indicates that the patient is able to contract the transversus abdominis into its shortened (inner) range, independently of the other abdominal muscles (Fig. 14.3a,b). The three elements should all be recorded, to allow improvement to be monitored in subsequent sessions, e.g. pressure fall, 6 mmHg; spinal movement, nil; bulging of the abdominal wall, nil.

2. If the patient performs the test without spinal movement or bulging of the abdomen, but the pressure in the dial falls 0–4 mmHg, the patient may have contracted the transversus abdominis but with insufficient shortening to decrease the pressure adequately. The other possibility is asymmetry of contraction of transversus abdominis. Both of these situations need to be reviewed in the light of the supine test (below). Bilateral palpation of the abdominal wall can be used to detect asymmetry and presence of contraction of the transversus abdominis. Ultrasound imaging can be used to provide confirmation. The prone test using the pressure

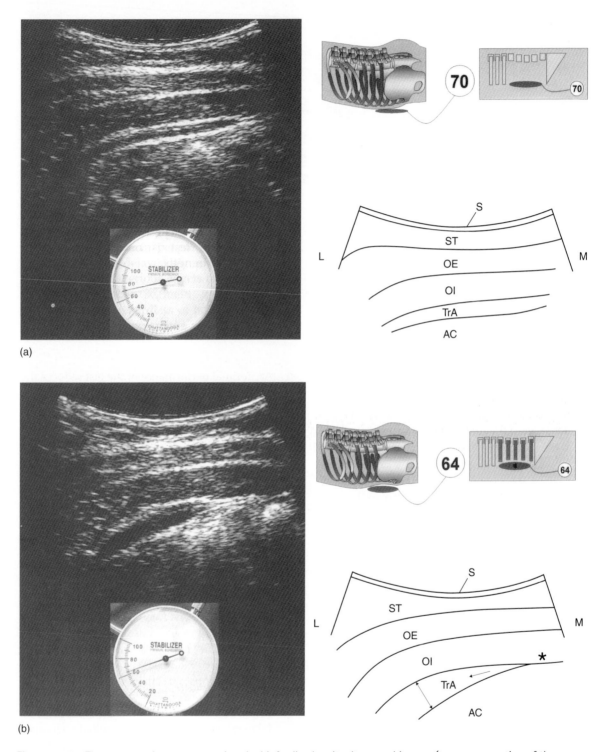

(a)

(b)

Figure 14.3 The pressure changes seen using the biofeedback unit, ultrasound images (transverse section of the anterolateral abdominal wall) and schematic representations of the clinical muscle test for the transversus abdominis

(*continued*)

biofeedback unit should be performed at subsequent sessions to monitor for improvement, which would be indicated by the patient now being able to achieve a greater reduction in pressure.

3. A pattern of global activation is seen in Figure 14.3c. If the patient uses the global muscles, then there are two possible test outcomes depending on whether or not the spine or pelvis has moved.

   (i) If a global contraction of the abdominal wall is performed, and the spine is kept immobile, then the pressure in the biofeedback unit should increase. This will be confirmed by palpation of the abdominal wall, which will reveal bulging. An example of recording would be, pressure increase, 8 mmHg; spinal movement, nil; bulging of the abdominal wall, detected.

   (ii) If the patient moves the spine, then the pressure in the biofeedback unit will decrease. Using the other two elements of assessment rather than observation of the dial alone will ensure that a false-positive test result is avoided. If the subject has moved the spine, palpation will often reveal flexion of the thoracolumbar junction (Fig. 14.4). This may be accompanied by depression of the rib cage (Fig. 14.5). The other common movement is posterior pelvic tilt (Fig. 14.6). Spinal movement can often be subtle, however. If it has occurred and is undetected by palpation, bulging of the abdominal wall

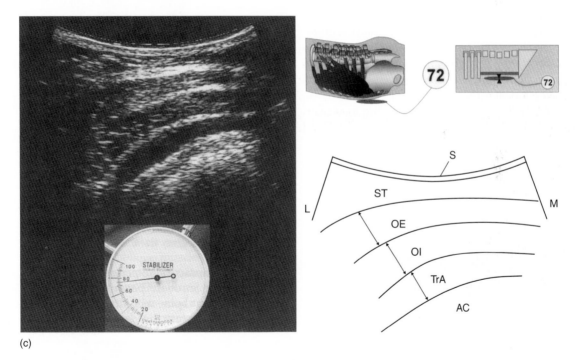

(c)

Figure 14.3 (*Continued*)
(TrA). (a) At rest before the test; the baseline pressure is 70 mmHg. (b) On correct performance of the abdominal drawing-in action. The pressure reduces by 6 mmHg. The contraction of the TrA can be seen on the ultrasound image. Note the corset-like appearance and the tensioning on the fascia medially (*). On contraction, the width of the TrA increases. (c) On incorrect performance of the abdominal drawing-in action, the pressure is increased slightly. The ultrasound image shows contraction of all the muscles of the abdominal wall simultaneously. The obliquus externus abdominis (OE) and obliquus internus abdominis (OI) have contracted together and each has increased in depth. There is no corset action of the TrA. AC, abdominal contents; L, lateral; M, medial; S, skin; ST, subcutaneous tissue. (Schematic representations reproduced with permission from Northwater Publishing, Australia.)

should be detected, allowing correct interpretation of the test. This could be recorded as pressure change, decrease 4 mmHg; spinal movement, movement of pelvis/thoracolumbar junction; bulging of the abdomen, detected.

It is important to record all three elements of the muscle test, as each element should change as the patient's performance of the test improves with treatment. For example, an initial improvement of the global activation pattern presented above (pressure increase, 8 mmHg; spinal movement, nil; bulging of the abdominal wall, detected) may be: pressure increase, nil; spinal movement, nil; bulging of the abdominal wall, nil. As inner range contraction of the transversus abdominis improves over time, another improvement may be: pressure change, decrease 4 mmHg; spinal movement, nil; bulging of the abdominal wall, nil. Further reductions in pressure may be seen and recorded over time.

In addition to three elements of clinical assessment, surface electromyography (EMG) electrodes can be placed on the likely overactive global muscles (i.e. the oblique abdominal muscles) to give an additional means of quantifying their overactivity and repeated to confirm test results and

interpretation. Electrode positions are described below in the section on EMG biofeedback. In addition, ultrasound imaging can be used. The transducer is placed on the patient's lateral abdominal

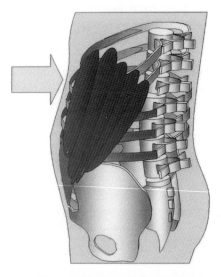

Figure 14.5 Rib cage depression observed when a patient attempts to use the global muscles in the muscle test for the transversus abdominis. (Reproduced with permission from Northwater Publishing, Australia.)

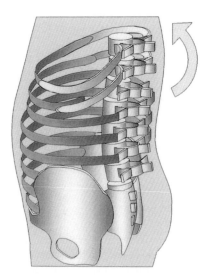

Figure 14.4 Flexion of the thoracolumbar junction observed when a patient attempts to use the global muscles in the muscle test for the transversus abdominis. (Reproduced with permission from Northwater Publishing, Australia.)

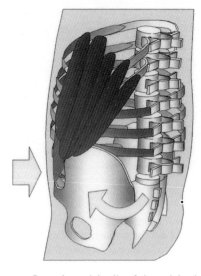

Figure 14.6 Posterior pelvic tilt of the pelvis observed when a patient attempts to use the global muscles in the muscle test for the transversus abdominis. (Reproduced with permission from Northwater Publishing, Australia.)

wall, approximately in line with the umbilicus. Although the anterior fascia cannot be viewed in the prone position, the three layers of the abdominal wall are evident. On ultrasound imaging, the clinician should observe for narrowing of the waistline (contraction of the transversus abdominis) and minimal contraction (thickening) of the oblique abdominal muscles. The quality of the contraction should be smooth and controlled. Features of a global pattern of activation may include widening of the waistline, a rapid speed of contraction and thickening of all of the three layers of the abdominal wall. The contraction may also be poorly controlled and erratic. Again, repeated imaging allows changes with treatment to be assessed.

Note on testing Many people with low back pain will find it difficult to perform this muscle test and will have a poor test result. Some people with no history of low back pain may also have difficulty, initially, in performing the contraction. In a recent study, 30 subjects without low back pain were screened to see if they could attain an optimal pattern of muscle contraction. The inclusion criteria for the study included being able to decrease the pressure on the dial by 4–10 mmHg (in the absence of spinal movement and bulging of the abdomen), and confirmation of the correct pattern using real-time ultrasound imaging. Only 13 of the 30 had an optimal pattern (Richardson et al 2002).

It may be impractical to perform the test in the prone position in obese patients, in those with impaired lumbar spine mobility, in patients with significant respiratory disease or for subjects who are in the later stages of pregnancy. In these cases, the abdominal drawing-in action can be assessed in either supine lying or by observation of the abdominal wall in four-point kneeling, standing or supported standing. Alternatively, ultrasound imaging with or without surface EMG may be used to observe the pattern of activation. However, whenever possible, the prone muscle test should be performed, as this allows recording of outcomes that can be compared during the course of treatment.

Relationship between low back pain and the prone test Several studies have been undertaken to evaluate whether the ability to perform the clinical test of the corset action of the transversus

abdominis can identify people with low back pain. The first of these involved the assessment of 37 people presenting to a medical practice for problems other than low back pain (Richardson et al 1995); of these 54% had a history of low back pain. The examiners were blinded to the presentation of the subjects. Subjects undertook the abdominal drawing-in test in the prone position, and the examiner recorded any pressure reduction. Using the criterion that a fall in pressure of less than 6 mmHg or an increase in pressure indicates poor transversus abdominis activation, the examiners could correctly classify 90% of subjects for their history of low back pain.

Relationship between clinical and laboratory tests An important question is whether the delayed contraction of the transversus abdominis in people with low back pain, as determined in laboratory motor control studies, is related to the clinical tests of the ability to perform a relatively independent contraction of this muscle. This was examined in a study in which subjects with and without low back pain were assessed using the clinical test and by evaluation of the timing of onset of contraction of the transversus abdominis in a limb-movement task (Hodges et al 1996). In this study subjects were classified into poor function, good function and intermediate groups on the basis of their ability to reduce pressure and the time of onset of EMG activity. Although the measures were not linearly correlated, there was good agreement between those subjects with a poor ability to decrease the pressure and those with a delay in transversus abdominis contraction, and between subjects who could decrease the pressure and those who had early activation of transversus abdominis. Therefore, the quality of motor control of the transversus abdominis, which can be measured directly by using fine-wire electrodes (which are not readily available in clinical practice), can be estimated indirectly from the performance shown in the clinical assessments.

Supine test

Additional information may be gained by repeating the test for the transversus abdominis in the supine position. In this position, the abdominal wall is more accessible for observation, palpation and ultrasound imaging. It is also usually easier for the patient to contract the transversus abdominis in the supine position. Supine lying is a good position to assess for symmetry of activation of the muscles of the abdominal wall.

Instructions are the same as for the prone test with the same initial breathing pattern. The test necessitates assessment of the pattern of the transversus abdominis contraction. The resulting contraction of transversus abdominis can be checked with palpation and/or real-time ultrasound imaging.

Palpation to test individual activation patterns of transversus abdominis and isometric holding ability (in shortened range) The abdominal palpation test has been described in Hides et al (2000). The ideal position for tactile cues is medially and inferiorly to the anterior superior iliac spines and lateral to the rectus abdominis. In this region, the transversus abdominis is overlaid by the internus obliquus abdominis. The thumbs or middle three fingers are used to sink gently but deeply into the abdominal wall (Fig. 14.7). Either the clinician or the patient can use the technique. This position cues the patient to the lower abdomen. With a correct contraction of the transversus abdominis, the clinician feels a slowly developing deep tension in the abdominal wall (Fig. 14.8a,b). With an incorrect action, the clinician may find one of three conditions on palpation. First, there may be no activity. Second, a dominance or substitution by the oblique abdominals may occur, which can be detected via a rapid development of tension in the abdominal wall (a superficial muscle contraction). Third, the palpating fingers are pushed out of the abdominal wall by a bracing action by the oblique abdominal muscles and subsequent increase in intra-abdominal pressure (Fig 14.8c). Alternatively, the clinician can place his/her hands around the patient's waist during the contraction. With a correct pattern of activation, the waistline will narrow. With an incorrect pattern of activation, the waistline will widen.

Another anomaly is palpation of an abnormal left/right asymmetry in activation of the muscles of the abdominal wall. This may be very subtle and is usually perceived on palpation as increased

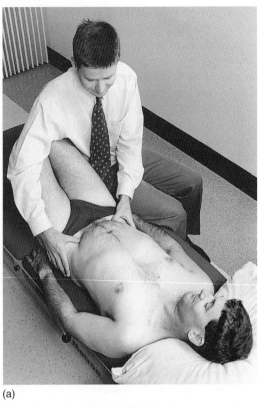

(a)

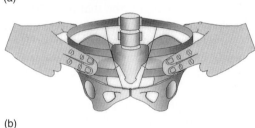

(b)

Figure 14.7 Palpation during transversus abdominis activation. (a) The hand position for palpation. (b) How to feel if the correct contraction is occurring. (Schematic representation reproduced with permission from Northwater Publishing, Australia.)

activation of the oblique abdominal muscles (or more bulging of the abdomen) on one side more than the other.

Real-time ultrasound to test individual activation patterns of transversus abdominis isometric holding ability (in shortened range) The ultrasound features of a correct pattern of activation of the transversus abdominis are described in

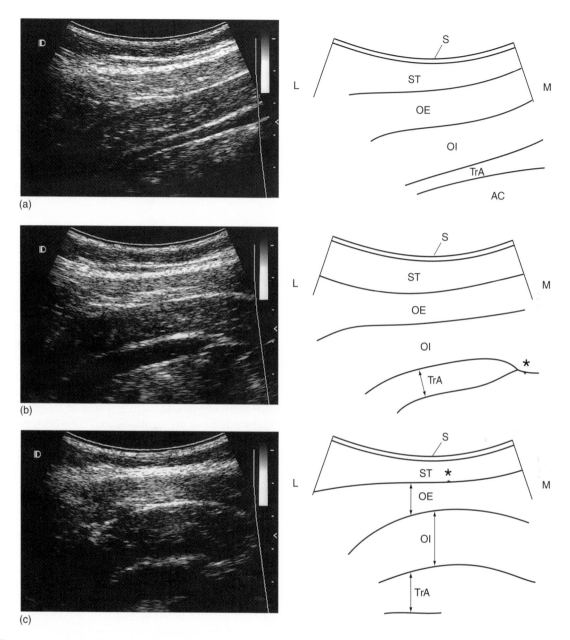

Figure 14.8 An inside view of the palpatory cues. Ultrasound images of the abdominal wall in transverse section (transducer placed anterolaterally). (a) Relaxed abdominal wall. Note the curved skin (S) line owing to the convex shape of the transducer. (b) Abdominal wall following performance of the correct drawing-in action (palpation: deep tension in the abdominal wall). On contraction of the transversus abdominis (TrA), the muscle increases in depth (↕) and tensions the fascia, which attaches to rectus abdominis (*). There is little change in the superficial muscles (obliquus externus abdominis (OE) and obliquus internus abdominis (OI)). On palpation, deep tension is felt in the abdominal wall as the TrA pulls the lower abdomen in. (c) Abdominal wall following incorrect performance of drawing-in action (palpation: pushing-out action of the abdominal wall). Note the increased depth of the OE, OI and TrA (↕) as the isolated activation of the TrA is lost. The distance from the superior border of the OE to the skin is decreased as the patient pushes out (*). On palpation, the fingers are pushed outwards. AC, abdominal contents; L, lateral; M, medial; ST, subcutaneous tissue.

detail in Chapter 5. A key feature of the correct pattern of activation is that the contraction can be performed in a slow, smooth and controlled manner. The key elements of dysfunction are that all three muscles of the anterolateral abdominal wall thicken and contract, but the contraction of the transversus abdominis does not tension the anterior fascia, and the transversus abdominis does not wrap around the waistline (corset action) (see Fig. 5.5, p. 83). If the control of the activation is poor, the quality of the contraction may be seen to be fast and more erratic in nature.

Holding time   It should be possible to hold this contraction of the synergy through drawing in the lower abdominal wall while normal breathing is maintained for at least 10 seconds, without phasic erratic contractions occurring. If it is difficult for a patient to breathe in this manner, and he or she substitutes rapid and shallow upper chest breathing, it should be noted, as this gives an indication of how well the patient can perform the test. Ideally, the contraction of the muscle should be held with minimal volitional effort and with maintenance of normal respiration. If the patient performs the test poorly, there is no point holding the contraction. At the completion of the test, the contraction should be released in a slow and controlled manner. If the patient performs the muscle test poorly, the clinician may reinstruct the patient and retest to check that the result was accurate and not just caused by a failure to understand what was required. However, the clinician should bear in mind that fatigue has a significant influence on the contraction of the transversus abdominis and many patients may not be able to hold for the 10 seconds. Record the number of seconds achieved.

Substitution (i.e. excessive activation) of the global (non–weightbearing) muscles during this low-load testing procedure   It should be possible to achieve the contraction of the local synergy with minimal contribution (i.e. without domination) of the other, more superficial muscles of the abdominal wall. EMG has been used to assess the accompanying contraction of the oblique abdominal muscles during the transversus abdominis muscle test. It was shown that the contraction of the oblique abdominal muscles during the test

was less than 15% of their maximal voluntary contraction (Richardson et al 2002). EMG can, therefore, be used in conjunction with the supine test to quantify the activation of the superficial muscles.

Testing the segmental lumbar multifidus

This test assesses the ability to perform an isometric multifidus contraction (check if deep fibres are activated at each lumbar level) in co-contraction with transversus abdominis.

Testing the segmental lumbar multifidus in the prone position

Screening assessments of the segmental lumbar multifidus are difficult for unskilled testers, as they rely on sensitive palpation or use of real-time ultrasound. However, the experienced clinician can make a clinical judgement through palpation of the muscle contraction at the segmental level. The clinical assessment of the lumbar multifidus is conducted in the prone position, as in the abdominal drawing-in test. While it would be expected that the lumbar multifidus would contract together with the transversus abdominis in the prone position test, specific commands and techniques are used to improve the focus of the clinician and patient on the lumbar multifidus, in order to test its activation and tonic holding ability separately at each segmental level.

Assessment of the lumbar multifidus begins with palpation of the muscle at each segment, with the patient relaxed and in the prone position (Fig. 14.9). The muscle is palpated adjacent to the spinous process and a side-to-side comparison is made at each lumbar level; in addition, a comparison is made of the segments above and below. The clinician feels for any loss in muscle consistency at the segment; this is in line with the segmental inhibition at the symptomatic segment detected by Hides et al (1996) in their study of patients with acute/subacute low back pain, and localised segmental multifidus atrophy in chronic low back pain (Danneels et al 2001, S. Kelley et al 2003 unpublished data, T. Wallwork et al 2003 unpublished data). If the clinician has access to ultrasound imaging, the consistency of the multifidus can be examined

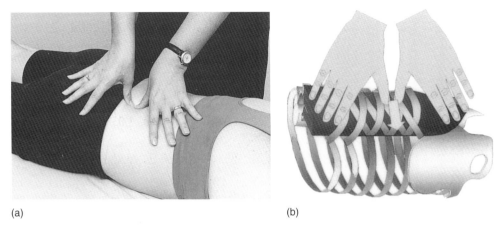

(a)   (b)

Figure 14.9   Palpation for muscle consistency of the multifidus muscle at each vertebral level. (a) The hand position for palpation. (b) Palpating feels for differences between sides and between vertebral levels. (Schematic representation reproduced with permission from Northwater Publishing, Australia.)

segmentally. The multifidus usually appears black on ultrasound imaging because of its excellent perfusion. When fibrous changes, scar tissue or fatty infiltration are present, the multifidus at that segment will appear whiter (increased echogenicity) or have patchy changes. The clinician can scan each segment of the multifidus and then compare this visual inspection with palpation findings. Computed tomography and magnetic resonance imaging (MRI) can similarly be used to assess segmental changes in consistency, and the scans can be shown to the patient (see Ch. 11).

For stabilization and joint protection, it is the activation of the deep multifidus fascicles that particularly needs to be tested. They contract isometrically and segmentally and do not generate movement of the spine as they are close to the centre of rotation of the lumbar segments. The superficial multifidus fibres contribute to spinal extension. Therefore, to test the stabilization and protection role of the multifidus, rather than its torque-producing role, an isometric, segmental contraction test has been developed. Furthermore, testing the multifidus in an inner range, antigravity contraction into inner range of extension of the lumbar spine, is inappropriate as, apart from this not being commensurate with its stabilization role, it would be impossible to differentiate the activity of the multifidus from the other muscles that produce extension of the lumbar spine.

The test of the specific activation of the lumbar multifidus at the segmental level can be considered as a specific motor skill. Recent research has confirmed the clinical finding that isometric contraction of the multifidus should occur at each vertebral level (Van et al 2003 unpublished data, T. Wallwork et al 2003 unpublished data), that subjects with a history of low back pain are less able to activate the segmental muscle than control subjects, and that the loss of multifidus activation is a segmental response (T. Wallwork et al 2003 unpublished data). As indicated, the prone position test is used to perform the muscle activation test.

This test measures the ability of the patient to activate the segmental multifidus in response to the command 'Gently swell out your muscles under my fingers without moving your spine or pelvis. Hold the contraction while breathing normally' (Fig. 14.10). There is no focus by the subject on the individual muscle actions, only on the tester's fingers gently compressing the muscle at a local segmental level and the instruction to swell out without spinal or pelvic movement. A variety of hand positions can be used to perform the test. The clinician can use the thumbs, the index or middle fingers of each hand, or the thumb and index fingers of one hand to palpate each segmental level. The fingers are gently but firmly sunk into the muscle belly in preparation for the test (Fig. 14.11), but it is important for the clinician to

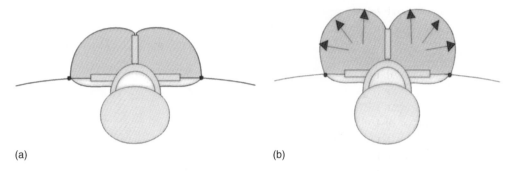

Figure 14.10   Activation of the multifidus muscle. (a) The relaxed muscle in transverse section. (b) The swelling out action of the multifidus; it is constrained within its own fascia. (Reproduced with permission from Northwater Publishing, Australia.)

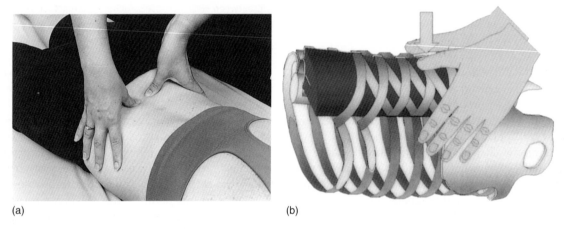

Figure 14.11   Palpation for the contraction of the right and left muscles at each segment of the lumbar multifidus. (a) The hand position for palpation. (b) Palpating feels for differences between sides and between vertebral levels. (Schematic representation reproduced with permission from Northwater Publishing, Australia.)

release the pressure gently as the patient contracts the muscle, otherwise, the compressive force could inhibit the contraction.

As for the test of the transversus abdominis corset action, the subject is asked to breathe in, then out and to hold the breath out. The patient is instructed to swell out the muscle gently and slowly into the fingers, and then to resume normal breathing. The clinician concentrates on feeling for a deep development of tension in the muscle, which indicates the activation of multifidus at that segment. The patient's ability to hold the contraction indicates the muscle's tonic holding capacity.

An inability to activate the segmental multifidus is indicated by palpating no or little muscle tension development under the fingers. A rapid and superficial development of tension is unsatisfactory, and indicates that either the patient is using only the superficial fibres in an extension action or the clinician is palpating the stiffness in the long tendons of the thoracic portion of erector spinae, which traverse the area. If the patient uses the superficial multifidus fibres, this may cause an anterior pelvic tilt. Often, the patient may remark that this action is painful. Of all of the substitution strategies, this is perhaps the most concerning. The correct activation should not induce pain. The action of the thoracic erector spinae muscles instead of lumbar multifidus may also be observed directly by changes in the shape of the muscle bellies in the thoracic region. Alternatively, the amount of unnecessary muscle activity in these global muscles during the testing manoeuvre can be monitored using EMG. The other common strategy that the patient may use to simulate the correct action is a posterior pelvic tilt, in an attempt to push the muscle back into the clinician's fingers.

The clinical assessment of the segmental lumbar multifidus is, therefore, made by the tester palpating the multifidus activation at each lumbar level, including whether a controlled tonic hold can be achieved. More objective evidence can be obtained through the use of real-time ultrasound imaging as the patient attempts the testing manoeuvre (Hides et al 1996b). The depth of the multifidus changes during the isometric holding contraction, and this can be viewed using real-time ultrasound images (Van et al 2003 unpublished data, T. Wallwork et al 2003 unpublished data). Repeatability and reliability of the measure have been demonstrated (Van et al 2003 unpublished data, T. Wallwork et al 2003 unpublished data). Figure 14.12 illustrates a longitudinal section of the multifidus at the L5 level when in a relaxed state (Fig. 14.12a) and when the muscle has contracted isometrically (Fig. 14.12b). An increase in depth of the muscle can be observed; this is the contraction measured by palpation of the segmental levels of the multifidus by the clinician. During the test for segmental activation of the multifidus, the anterior abdominal wall can also be palpated. If bulging of the abdominal wall is palpated and the flexors have contracted, this would indicate that the patient is trying to overcome an extension moment in order to keep the spine in a static position. In other words the abdominals are contracting in order to overcome the extension moment of the more superficial fibres of multifidus and the erector spinae.

Relationship between clinical tests and other measures

Real-time ultrasound imaging has been used to confirm both the palpation and the activation tests for the multifidus. Imaging has been conducted formally for patients with acute/subacute low back pain (Hides et al 1994, 1998, 2001) and for those with chronic low back pain (T. Wallwork

et al 2000 unpublished data). In the former group, the changes in the muscle are specific to the affected vertebral level and to the symptomatic side in unilateral pain (Hides et al 1994, 1998). This localized response in the multifidus has been demonstrated using real-time ultrasound imaging and confirmed using MRI (Hides et al 1995). Furthermore, in 26 patients with acute/subacute low back pain, joints were examined manually to determine if the most affected vertebral level (as assessed by a blinded examiner) corresponded with the location of the changes in size of the multifidus. The results of the two independent tests corresponded in 24 of 26 (Hides et al 1994). In patients with chronic low back pain, palpation correlated well with decreased cross-sectional area and decreased activation of the segmental multifidus, when performed by three blinded assessors (T. Wallwork et al 2003 unpublished data). The change in depth of the multifidus muscle, which the clinician palpates as a deep tensioning in the muscle, can be seen in the parasagittal section of the multifidus. The change in depth of the muscle from the relaxed to the contracted state can be seen in Figure 14.12. Interestingly, the closest correlation was between clinical assessment of atrophy or clinical assessment of multifidus activation and activation testing on ultrasound. Cross-sectional area measurements may, in fact, represent changes over several past episodes of low back pain; for example, if the pain is on the right side at present but has previously been in the left side, atrophy may be present on both sides of the spine at the affected vertebral level. However, if the pain is currently on the right side, both the activation testing on ultrasound and the clinical testing of activation were closely correlated. This is a positive finding in that activation testing on ultrasound and clinical assessment are probably more reflective of the presenting signs and symptoms at the time of assessment than cross-sectional area measurements, which may reflect evidence of atrophy from previous episodes of low back pain.

Various patterns are emerging in the nature of multifidus muscle dysfunction in different patient groups, which we have been able to view using real-time ultrasound imaging. Patients with acute low back pain commonly seem unable to activate the multifidus at the affected vertebral level. Patients

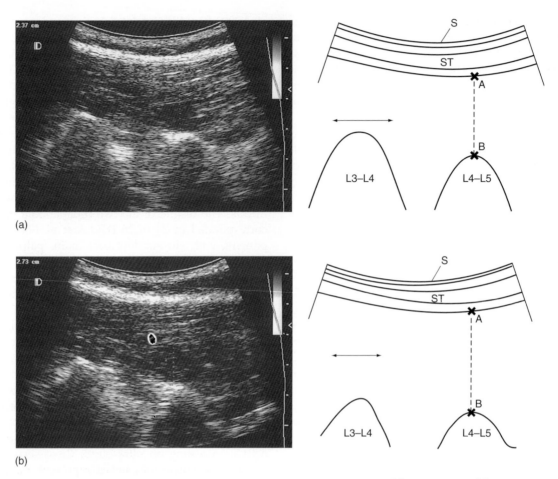

Figure 14.12 Ultrasound images of the lumbar multifidus in longitudinal section: (a) relaxed state; (b) after isometric contraction. The line AB represents the depth of the muscle from its superior aspect to the superior aspect of the L4–L5 zygapophyseal joint. In the relaxed state (a) this is 2.37 cm; on contraction (b) this depth increases to 2.73 cm. S, skin; ST subcutaneous tissue. The multifidus fibres run in the direction of the arrow (↔).

with chronic low back pain exhibit different patterns. Some are unable to activate the multifidus, while others may perform quick, phasic contractions that are poorly controlled. Often there is a predominance of activity in the superficial fibres of the multifidus. With practice, the palpation test can be used by the clinician to detect these differences.

CLINICAL PROBLEM SOLVING AND IMPLICATIONS OF THE TEST RESULTS

Clinical examination and research have revealed that patients with low back pain are unable to perform an isometric continuous co-contraction of the transversus abdominis and the lumbar multifidus independently of the action of the global muscles. There is a process of clinical problem solving that is undertaken in preparation for prescribing the exercise and facilitation strategies, a process that must continue throughout the whole rehabilitation period. The individual nature and extent of the global muscle overactivity, detected as unwanted global muscle activity during attempts to perform the skill, directs the selection of the most expedient treatment for the individual patient.

The clinical presentation of the patient with low back pain, in terms of muscle dysfunction, seems to fall into a continuum. At one end of the continuum is the patient with lack of control in muscles of the local system but minimum compensation by the global muscles. In fact, these patients may exhibit lack of strength and endurance of their antigravity and even global muscles. At the other end is the patient with low back pain with lack of control in muscles of the local muscle system, and maximum compensation and overactivity in the global muscle system. The presentation of most patients with low back pain probably lies somewhere in between these two extremes. Clinical practice suggests that patients with maximal compensation in the global muscle system offer the greater challenge to the therapeutic skills of the practitioner, as these patients appear to have greater problems.

In approaching treatment, the clinician must answer two basic questions.

1. Does the patient present with unwanted global muscle activity?
2. If so, which muscles are problematic?

These questions need to be answered in order to institute best-practice therapeutic exercise. For patients without unwanted overactivity in the global muscles, the clinician can simply choose the best ways of activating the local muscle system before progression onto the next stage of rehabilitation. However, in patients with unwanted global muscle overactivity, the clinician must choose strategies that simultaneously reduce the unwanted global muscle activity while activating the co-contraction in the local muscles for spinal segmental support. To this end, the clinician must undertake an additional process to analyze the nature and extent of the unwanted global muscle activity. Elements of this process for recognition of individual presentations is described separately and in some detail in this text. Once the clinician becomes skilled, the process is not time consuming, as the analysis and treatment proceed together.

Signs of unwanted global muscle activation

Careful analytical observation of the trunk manoeuvres can give an indication of any marked substitution by the global muscles, and these observations can be made either during the tests or on other occasions of convenience where the abdominal wall can be viewed in its entirety. The most commonly overactive global muscles identified to date that substitute for the transversus abdominis and lumbar multifidus are the obliquus externus abdominis and obliquus internus abdominis. The rectus abdominis and thoracic portions of the erector spinae may also present problems. The following discussion is not exhaustive and the clinician should be aware that other unique strategies may present in an individual patient and should be corrected. Substitution can be detected by observing aberrant trunk movements and contours, by palpation and by surface electromyography.

Spinal movement

It must be noted that the specific co-contraction of the transversus abdominis and deep portions of the lumbar multifidus does not produce spinal movement.

Contraction of the obliquus externus abdominis, obliquus abdominis internus and rectus abdominis may produce backward pelvic tilting and flexion of the trunk. In the prone position test, any observed slight flexion of the thoracolumbar and lumbopelvic area could be caused by the action of these muscles instead of the transversus abdominis. The movement at the thoracolumbar junction is often very subtle, and palpating for movement is a useful adjunct to observation. In addition, a quite rapid reduction in pressure (as indicated by the pressure biofeedback unit; see Appendix at the end of this chapter) during the test could signal flexion of the spine and indicate a dominance in these muscles.

A slight backward pelvic tilting action can be substituted for the correct swelling-out action during the isometric test of the segmental lumbar multifidus. This is the most common substitution seen clinically. The patient attempts to push too hard posteriorly and flexes the lumbar spine. Another substitution strategy involves a slight anterior pelvic tilt at the lumbosacral junction. This occurs when the patient predominantly uses the more superficial multifidus fibres in the contraction, causing the spine to extend. Patients often report this type of contraction to be painful. Maximal contraction of all the multifidus fascicles in concert with the lumbar erector spinae muscles can generate an anterior shearing force at the lumbosacral junction (Bogduk et al 1992b). Even though the contraction is not maximal in the test attempt, this substitution must be detected. If the patient performs the lumbar multifidus contraction incorrectly, too vigorously and without co-activation of the transversus abdominis, there is a potential to aggravate the patient's pain.

The rib cage

Further indications of substitution strategies can be gained by observing the movement of the rib cage during the abdominal drawing-in action with the patient in a standing or supine crook-lying position. The muscle fibres of the obliquus externus abdominis originate from the external surface of the lower ribs, unlike those of the transversus abdominis, which originate from the internal surface. Contraction of the anteromedial fibres of the obliquus externus abdominis produces a downward and inward movement of the rib cage, which is observed as a subtle depression in its ventral aspect.

The abdominal wall

Observation of the entire abdominal wall during the contraction can also give a good indication of any predominance of the obliquus externus abdominis and obliquus internus abdominis. When teaching the abdominal drawing-in action in the four-point kneeling position, in the prone test or in other positions such as supine crook lying or standing, dominant activity in the obliquus externus abdominis can be observed when movement of the abdominal wall is initiated or predominates in the upper quadrants rather than the lower quadrants below the navel. The formation of a transverse fold in the upper abdomen is another indication of an overactive obliquus externus abdominis, and contraction of the muscle fibres at their origin on the rib cage may be observed (Fig. 14.13). Another sign that the obliquus externus abdominis may be overactive is an increase in the lateral diameter of the abdominal wall commensurate with a subtle abdominal bracing manoeuvre, and this can be identified by palpation of the lateral abdominal wall bilaterally during the performance of the contraction. In addition, tightness in longitudinally directed fibres in the anterolateral abdomen on palpation is a common sign of obliquus externus abdominis substitution. It can also be useful to palpate over the muscle fibres of the rectus abdominis anteriorly during the performance of the contraction in order to assess any contribution of this muscle to the drawing-in action, which may be subtle.

Breathing pattern

We have observed clinically that the breathing pattern can be altered in patients with chronic low back pain. The oblique abdominals are sometimes active during both inspiration and expiration. These muscles should normally be relaxed during the breathing cycle, except during forced expiration (DeTroyer et al 1990, Hodges et al 1997b). Clinically, overactivity of the oblique abdominal muscles may cause depression of the ribcage and flexion through the thoracolumbar junction.

Recent research has confirmed a difference in rib cage mobility in patients with chronic low back pain and poor control of the transversus abdominis (Scott and Deeg 2003 unpublished data). The excursion of the ribcage was measured (6 degrees of freedom) in patients with chronic low back pain and control subjects without a history of low back pain. Exclusion criteria for the patients with low back pain included previous surgery, thoracic spine abnormalities, history of pulmonary disease or a musical background that would have involved training of diaphragmatic control. It was confirmed using ultrasound imaging that subjects with low back pain had poor control of the transversus abdominis. Results showed that lateral excursion of the rib cage was significantly decreased in the patients with low back pain compared with the control subjects ($p < 0.05$). These research findings support our clinical observations that patients with low back pain find it difficult to activate the transversus abdominis appropriately if the oblique abdominal muscles are active during the breathing cycle. Further ongoing research using ultrasound imaging on the diaphragm and surface EMG of the oblique abdominals will help to explain the mechanism involved.

On a clinical note, it is important when teaching patients to breathe in, and then out, hold the breath out and draw in the abdominal wall, that

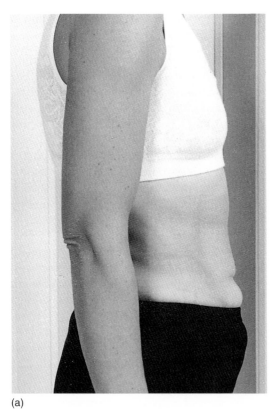 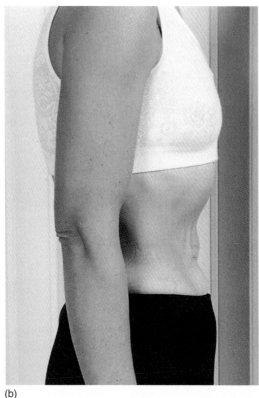

(a)   (b)

Figure 14.13   Contraction of the abdomen. (a) The relaxed state. (b) Dominant contraction of the obliquus externus abdominis is indicated by a transverse fold or skin crease just superior to the umbilicus.

they do not force the air out in the expiratory phase. If they do this, they will activate the transversus abdominis and oblique abdominal muscles together in their forced expiratory role, and they will then be unable to perform the required contraction of the transversus abdominis. We have also observed that some patients with low back pain are able to draw in their abdominal wall successfully but are then unable to maintain the contraction once they try to resume breathing. It, therefore, seems important to try to establish a diaphragmatic pattern of breathing and to decrease activity in the oblique abdominal muscles before attempting to train the patient in activation of the muscles of the local muscle synergy. An altered breathing pattern seems to be an indicator of patients who will be more difficult to facilitate and train. Perhaps this is because the control of at least two of the four synergy muscles is disturbed (diaphragm and transversus abdominis), with

the additional complication of overactivity of the global muscles. Ultimately, patients should be able to integrate the stability and respiratory functions of the diaphragm, in that they should be able to stabilize the spine in the presence of normal respiration.

Unwanted activity in the back extensors

An increase in activity of the thoracic portions of the erector spinae, observed in prone lying or standing in either the abdominal drawing-in test or the test of isometric segmental lumbar multifidus contraction, can be another sign of muscle substitution. The presence of this contraction with the obliquus externus abdominis, obliquus internus abdominis and rectus abdominis may be observed as a global co-contraction pattern in patients with low back pain. This pattern demands a lot of energy from the patient and is inefficient.

It is important to consider the effects of over-activity of the global muscles on spinal orientation. It appears that the response of the spine is to buckle at vulnerable points. For example, if the oblique abdominal muscles are overactive, the patient with low back pain will remain upright but will flex at the thoracolumbar junction. This deviation from the correct alignment of the spinal curves in the upright position may affect the ability of the spine to distribute loads effectively. The relevance for the clinician is that the clinician must be able to observe the deviations from the normal alignment owing to overactivity of the global muscles. This will help in retraining; ultimately these deviations should change in response to treatment, unlike changes in spinal alignment owing to spinal pathology.

This relationship is similarly important in the presence of spinal pathology, as this will affect the clinician's predictions of outcomes from intervention. A good example is the patient with low back pain with Scheuermann's disease. A fixed thoracic spine will have enormous impact on control of the lumbar intervertebral segments. For example, the patient with limited mobility of the thoracic spine may compensate by increasing their motion of the lumbar spine. If this patient then suffers low back pain, the aim of intervention may be to increase segmental control of the spinal segments, commonly the lumbosacral junction. There are two important clinical considerations in this case. First, even if good segmental control at the lumbosacral junction is achieved, this may not be enough to alleviate the patient's symptoms if too much movement is imposed on this level to compensate for the deficiency and lack of normal movement at the thoracic spine. Second, any small amount of increase in motion that can be achieved at thoracic spine level will have a big effect in reducing load and strain on the lumbar spine. This, in combination with activation of the local stabilizing muscles, would be the first step in rehabilitation.

Summary

In summary, recognition of physical signs of unwanted global muscle activity signals to the clinician which postures, movements and instructions to avoid during the facilitation and training of the deep muscle activation.

Rehabilitation of the joint protection mechanisms

Strategies are presented here that will minimize the non-weightbearing global muscles of the trunk while facilitating the local muscle synergy. This means activating without allowing the substitutions of the global synergists, which occurred in the testing procedures.

For normal function, the transversus abdominis, the deep fibres of the lumbar multifidus, the diaphragm and the pelvic floor must be modulated continuously to control the lumbopelvic region independently of the contractions of the global muscles, which produce the trunk and pelvic movements. The first step is to give formal exercises to train the patient to contract the deep muscles cognitively and to ensure that the muscles of the local synergy can contract independently of the global muscles. To allow the patient to learn the correct deep muscle activation skill as efficiently as possible, the most suitable instructions, body positions and techniques of facilitation are chosen for the individual patient.

Instructions and teaching cues

The patient must be provided with a clear explanation of the nature of muscle activity required for joint support, the need for particular muscles to be performing this task and, therefore, the precision required in training. Since the level of contraction required is minimal in comparison with the conventional images of exercise for strength training or cardiovascular fitness, it is necessary continually to impress on the patient concepts of motor control and skill training. An explanation of the need to change the way the brain is using the muscle rather than increasing the muscle strength is helpful. A description of the effort required in the muscle to support the joints (e.g. less than 10–15% of maximum effort) helps to convey the aims of precision and control of muscle activity and the need for endurance.

The other major system that requires some form of explanation for the patient is the gamma system. This can be put into relatively simple terms if it is described as 'muscle tone'. It can be explained to the patient that we want to optimize the 'muscle tone of their lumbopelvic corset'. 'Tone' is also a good word to use, as most patients would accept and understand why the exercises are very different from strengthening exercises, and why low-level continuous activation of these muscles is important. It is, in fact, the neurophysiology that is the critical element, and the sensitivity of the gamma system is one aspect we are aiming to alter. Further explanation could include that the system which controls these muscles is fragile, and that the same patterns of loss of control of the tonic muscles are seen in injury, immobilization and deloading situations.

The use of diagrams and models is effective at this stage. A demonstration by the clinician of the correct contraction of the transversus abdominis and lumbar multifidus, with the patient observing or palpating the correct action is also very useful. The patient then perceives from the outset the subtlety and precise nature of the contractions involved. The sequence used in the testing procedure is still followed in training: the patient takes in a relaxed breath, breathes out gently, ceases breathing while he or she attempts to activate the deep muscles, and then resumes a relaxed breathing pattern while holding the contraction. It is a matter of trial and error to find the instruction that correctly cues the patient.

Tactile cues assist in teaching the isometric contraction of the lumbar multifidus at the segmental level. This can be provided by the clinician or patient (Fig. 14.14). Care should be taken to sink the thumb and/or fingers gently but firmly deeply into the muscle bellies adjacent to the spinous process in order to facilitate the contraction. This is similar to the testing procedure. Accurate feedback on correct performance can be gained by feeling a deep and slowly generated tension developing under the fingers as the muscle swells out in response to the resistance. Feeling a rapid or superficial contraction may indicate either contraction of the longer superficial fibres of the multifidus or tension in the tendinous portion of the thoracic erector spinae, which span the lumbar area.

Tactile cues and use of palpation skills for teaching and training the contraction of transversus abdominis are very useful and have been described in the testing procedures. The breathing procedures that were instigated prior to testing are

also important for rehabilitation strategies. This is because the action of the transversus abdominis can also be mimicked by sucking in the abdominal wall and reducing the intrathoracic pressure without contracting the transversus abdominis. When a deep breath is taken by increasing the lateral diameter of the rib cage or by increasing the upper chest volume through the use of the accessory respiratory muscles (e.g. the scalenes and sternocleidomastoid), the volume of the thorax is increased. This has the potential to elevate the diaphragm, in addition to producing inward movement of air. The consequence of this upward diaphragm movement is inward movement of the abdominal wall, giving the appearance of contraction of transversus abdominis (Fig. 14.15). Since the abdominal wall movement is performed passively, no palpable contraction or tightening of any muscle of the abdominal wall will be perceived.

Body position

Because of the orientation and mechanics of the muscle fibres of the transversus abdominis and, in particular, the deep fibres of the multifidus, the actions of these muscles are independent of spinal posture and their length–tension relationship is not affected by spinal position (McGill 1991). This could imply that, for patients with back pain, any spinal or lumbopelvic posture could theoretically be chosen to teach and train the muscle contractions in the first instance. However, in reality, there are sound reasons why rehabilitation should be commenced in a non-weightbearing position. For this exercise approach, the deep local muscle synergy must be activated in preparation for weightbearing. The biomechanical model of Snijders et al (1995) predicts that the action of the transverse fibres of pelvic muscles such as transversus abdominis stiffen the sacro-iliac joints (i.e. force closure) and stabilize the pelvis. While one of the key functions of these transverse muscles is most likely the control of weightbearing through the lumbopelvic region, the biomechanical model predicts that this horizontal force is independent of the gravitational load. Therefore, training in non-weightbearing prior to weightbearing is likely to be an advantage when specific training of the lumbopelvic stability mechanism is required, and

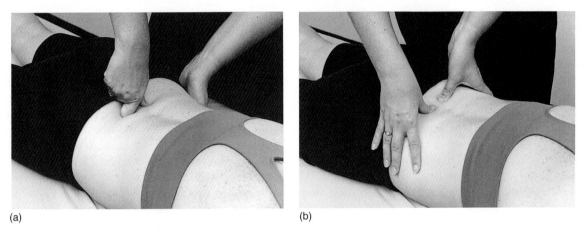

(a) (b)

Figure 14.14 Two hand positions for tactile facilitation of the segmental lumbar multifidus.

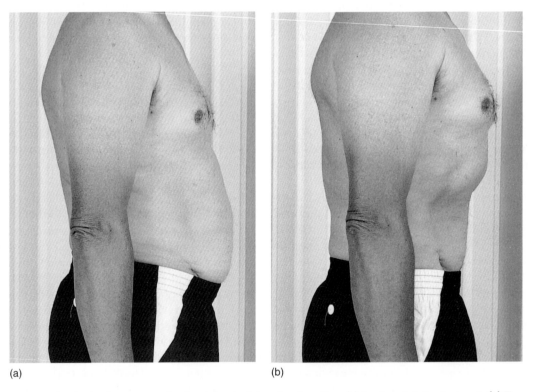

(a) (b)

Figure 14.15 A substitution strategy for the abdominal drawing-in action. (a) A relaxed abdominal wall. (b) The action of the transversus abdominis is mimicked by sucking in the abdominal wall.

retraining should occur before the forces of gravity are imposed.

Another key reason why a non-weightbearing position is chosen in the initial instance is that these positions allow the global muscles to minimize their activity by decreasing their role in supporting the body against gravity. It may, therefore, allow relaxation of the global muscles if overactivity is present, and it will be easier to facilitate independent activation of the muscles of the local synergy. Various options are available, including side lying, supine crook lying, prone lying, three-quarters from prone lying and high-supported sitting.

The one exception to this rule is training or re-education of the lumbar lordosis in the sitting position. Although described later in this chapter (see progression to sitting and standing positions), patients will commonly spend a great deal of their day in the sitting position, especially those who work on computers. For this reason, discussion of spinal position, passive supports and control of the lordosis using the multifidus may be conducted concurrently with the rest of the facilitation strategies described here. The neutral spine position is facilatory in itself for the multifidus muscle, and another advantage of initiating this aspect early is that it will help the patients with poor proprioception and kinaesthetic sense to be able to start to activate the multifidus in a slightly easier, less-specific way.

The choice of initial position for facilitation is by trial and error. It is based on controlling factors that could otherwise be detrimental to performance (e.g. unwanted global muscle activity) or, conversely, helpful to the patient to achieve the local muscle action. Body positioning alters the load on the spinal structures. The patient should be pain free in the position chosen, as pain during the muscle activation strategy may invoke muscle inhibition. The effects of gravity combined with the weight of the abdominal contents (e.g. in side lying) might be useful in providing a stretch stimulus to transversus abdominis activation. Side lying is also a position in which the lumbar spine can be positioned in neutral. Control of spinal position may be crucial for activation of the local muscles. The study of Williams et al (2000) placed the lumbar spines of cats into moderate sustained flexion and recorded the multifidus with intramuscular EMG. Prolonged flexion of the lumbar spine resulted in tension–relaxation and laxity of the multifidus viscoelastic structures and loss of protective reflexive muscular activity within 3 minutes, followed by spasms in the multifidus and other posterior muscles that could be detected by EMG. Although performed on cats, this study holds implications for humans. It is important to train the co-contraction of transversus abdominis

and multifidus in positions where the lumbar spine position can be controlled. Non-weightbearing postures allow this to occur more easily. The position chosen must also help to promote good and relaxed breathing patterns. The side lying or three-quarters prone position may also be useful for the facilitation of the lumbar multifidus. In this position, the patient may be able to relax the thoracic components of the erector spinae muscles. All clinicians can probably relate to the situation in prone lying where they are unable to palpate the segments of the multifidus. This has erroneously been mistaken in the past for multifidus spasm. If the patient is positioned in side lying or three-quarters from prone lying, this will often relax the thoracic components of the erector spinae and take the tension off the thoracolumbar fascia. This will allow palpation of the segmental multifidus, verifying that spasm in the multifidus is not the cause.

Facilitation through activation of individual muscles of the synergy

When a patient is unable to activate the transversus abdominis or segmental lumbar multifidus correctly with a simple instruction of the required action, or if the patient is having difficulty controlling a substitution strategy, the next step is to facilitate this contraction. The key to facilitation of transversus abdominis and lumbar multifidus contraction is careful teaching of the actions, with specific attention to the correction of compensations. If a substitution is allowed to persist, then the correct activation of the transversus abdominis or lumbar multifidus will not be achieved, and training of the optimal strategy for trunk control will not occur at the same rate or with the same success. There are several techniques that can be used to assist with this activation and the correction of substitutions. These techniques are based on principles of motor control and neuromuscular physiology and represent the culmination of various research projects and clinical expertise. The principle of these techniques is essentially to allow the patient to achieve the best possible contraction in the early stages. As soon as possible, the clinician should aim to have the patient gain cognitive control of the transversus abdominis and lumbar multifidus without needing to rely on any facilitation technique. Thus, facilitation provides an intermediate but essential step in the path to achieving cognitive control. As with any manual therapy technique, a high level of skill and precision is required by the clinician to master these facilitation techniques, and the clinician must be willing to practise the techniques in order to gain proficiency in their use.

The patient needs to gain a perception of the contraction prior to performing precise repetitions of the action. In the beginning, most patients cannot perceive or appreciate the deep muscle contraction and require facilitation. While the outcome is to facilitate the co-activation of the synergy muscles, strategies often focus the patient's attention to particular elements for easier learning. There are several facilitation techniques that have been demonstrated to be useful clinically in treating patients with back pain. The clinician must appreciate that treatment needs to be tailored to the individual patient in order to find the strategy (or strategies) to which the patient best responds.

Four key muscle groups work in synergy: the transversus abdominis, lumbar multifidus, the pelvic floor and diaphragm (see Chs 2–4). An explanation to patients of the cylinder-like effect that these muscles have in their supporting role in the lumbopelvic region helps them to understand the use and interplay of the activation of these muscles in facilitatory strategies (see Chs 2 and 3). In fact, any one of the four muscles can be used to help to facilitate another.

Transversus abdominis and lumbar multifidus

The co-activation of the transversus abdominis and the lumbar multifidus can be utilized quite successfully in facilitation. If the patient cognitively achieves the contraction of either the transversus abdominis or the lumbar multifidus more readily, then the successful muscle contraction can be used to facilitate the other one. Very simply, if the patient cannot consciously activate the transversus abdominis, then the clinician tries to achieve activation through facilitation of the lumbar multifidus or, conversely, focuses on the activation of transversus abdominis to facilitate lumbar multifidus. Logically, the contraction of the primary muscle must be performed well to achieve the desired result. For example, a phasic and poorly executed multifidus contraction may result in co-activation of the oblique abdominal muscles rather than the transversus abdominis. The clinician may need to experiment with patient position to find the ideal combination for the individual patient.

Pelvic floor   Use of contraction of the muscles of the pelvic floor is one of the most effective methods of achieving activation of the transversus abdominis. In order for the transversus abdominis to contribute to stabilization of the spine, it is essential for the contraction of the diaphragm and pelvic floor muscles to occur concurrently in order to maintain the abdominal contents within the abdominal cavity. Research has shown that contraction of the pubococcygeus occurs concurrently with that of the transversus abdominis, and activity of the pelvic floor changes the activity of the transversus abdominis (Ch. 3). Several researchers have also noted that contraction of the abdominal muscles, in particular the transversus abdominis, is associated with contraction of the pelvic floor muscles in retraining the pelvic floor muscles for the management of urinary stress incontinence (Sapsford et al 1998). Other clinical evidence has emerged of a relationship between transversus abdominis and the pelvic floor. This has arisen from claims from patients that their stress incontinence problem has reduced following a course of exercises for the transversus abdominis and, conversely, people managed for stress incontinence reporting a reduced incidence of low back pain. The use of contraction of the pelvic floor muscles to facilitate contraction of the transversus abdominis is particularly useful in patients who are having difficulty understanding the movement that is required to contract the transversus abdominis. It is also a primary technique for those who cannot relax their obliquus externus abdominis and obliquus abdominis internus in the abdominal drawing-in task.

Contraction of the pelvic floor can be utilized in a number of ways. It can be used either in isolation without the addition of a cognitive transversus abdominis contraction, or combined with a cognitive contraction of the transversus abdominis or other facilitation techniques. With the implementation of this facilitation strategy, it is important first to teach an effective contraction of the pelvic floor muscles. Many methods are available to do this, although the principles of slow, gentle and low effort of contraction should be employed. A clear description of the anatomy as a muscular sling between the tail bone and the front of the pelvis is essential to assist the patient to visualize the contraction. The reader is referred to Sapsford et al (1998) for a more detailed description of methods of achieving contraction of the pelvic floor muscles. The clinician is advised to use whatever techniques they have within their competence and they deem necessary to achieve the correct contraction.

Supine crook lying or side lying seem to be the better positions for initial teaching of the pelvic floor contraction, although the strategy can certainly be used later in standing or sitting. The clinician and/or patient gently, but deeply, palpates the lower quadrant of the abdomen. The sequence used is identical to that described before, where the patient takes in a relaxed breath, breathes out gently and then draws the pelvic floor up slowly and gently. It is important that the patient is directed to contract the anterior aspect of the pelvic floor to activate the pubococcygeus. It is important that the patient does not contract the posterior part of the pelvic floor and the puborectalis. This is achieved by instructing the patient to slowly and gently draw up the anterior aspect of the pelvic floor, as if stopping the flow of urine. It is important that the subject does not feel any contraction around the back passage. The clinician feels for the deep tension developing in the abdominal wall as the transversus abdominis co-activates with the pelvic floor. A rapidly developing or superficial tension in the abdominal wall usually accompanies a fast or inadequate attempt at contraction of the pelvic floor and signals substitution with the global muscles. The feedback provided to the patient by self-palpation of the abdominal wall can be quite potent towards their understanding of the synergistic muscle facilitation strategy.

With the aim of this stage of management being to train transversus abdominis activation without domination by the other global abdominal muscles, activation via the pelvic floor alone is often sufficient in the early stages of rehabilitation. This is so when the obliquus externus abdominis and/or the obliquus internus abdominis are overactive and any attempt to extend the synergistic contraction into the abdomen results in this global muscle activity. As soon as possible, the patient is taught to extend the contraction consciously up into the lower abdomen and draw in the lower abdominal wall. Self-monitoring with palpation for the desired response in the abdominal wall is essential in the learning process for cognitive control of the transversus abdominis.

Conscious interplay between initiation of a pelvic floor contraction followed by a gentle reinforcement of the transversus abdominis contraction and then back to focus on the pelvic floor can increase awareness of both muscles. If the patient has trouble achieving a pelvic floor contraction, other methods with which the clinician is familiar should be tried to assist with activation.

Pelvic floor contraction can also be used to teach and facilitate an isometric contraction of the segmental multifidus. It is particularly helpful when the patient has a poor awareness of the multifidus muscle, the lumbar segment as well as the desired muscle contraction. Facilitation can be attempted in side or prone lying initially, or later in standing. While the clinician palpates the targeted vertebral level, the patient is asked to draw up the pelvic floor slowly. A slow and gentle deep tensioning of the multifidus muscle is the desired response. The contraction should slowly build in intensity and is, therefore, subtle to detect. If a quick contraction is palpated, it is likely that contraction of the superficial fibres has occurred. The subject should be encouraged to try again with less effort. Ultrasound imaging may be used to verify all of these patterns of activation.

Breathing patterns (diaphragm) The role of transversus abdominis in the production of expiration could theoretically be utilized to activate the diaphragm. Ideally, the only possible way to achieve isolation of the transversus abdominis is during involuntary increases in expiration by techniques such as by hyperoxic hypercapnia (rebreathing carbon dioxide, DeTroyer et al 1990, Wakai et al 1992) or by the provision of an inspiratory load, which produces an involuntary increase in expiratory airflow (DeTroyer et al 1990, Hodges et al 1997b). Both produce an involuntary and selective increase in transversus abdominis activity during expiration to increase the expiratory airflow. However, it is observed in research and clinical practice that all the abdominal muscles are commonly activated with voluntary increases in expiratory flow (DeTroyer et al 1990, Hodges et al 1997b), and a global pattern of activation is, therefore, the most likely outcome in the clinical situation. Future research may identify strategies that use the contraction of the diaphragm to facilitate directly transversus abdominis contraction. We have observed clinically that relaxed breathing can decrease global muscle activation, which, in turn, can allow activation of a transversus abdominis contraction.

Verbal and visual feedback

It is vital to provide adequate verbal and visual feedback to the patient of their performance. In the motor control literature, this principle is known as the 'knowledge of performance' and 'knowledge of results' (Schmidt 1988). Studies have reported reduced kinaesthetic acuity in people with low back pain (Parkhurst and Burnett 1994), which may compound learning problems. Irrespective of whether or not the patient's kinaesthetic sense has been affected by the back injury, provision of enhanced feedback appears to be a critical factor required to achieve an isolated contraction of the transversus abdominis and segmental lumbar multifidus (Van et al 2003 unpublished data).

Direct visual feedback of the correct deep muscle contraction through the use of real-time ultrasound imaging is proving to be a very effective form of feedback in both teaching and learning of the action for the transversus abdominis and lumbar multifidus (Hides et al 1996b, Stokes et al 1997, see Appendix to Ch 5, pp. 89–92). Imaging the muscles in real-time gives a guarantee of the success, or otherwise, of a particular facilitation strategy. Opportunities exist for real-time ultrasound imaging techniques to be developed and used for each of the four deep muscles targeted in the rehabilitation of lumbopelvic control. The diaphragm can be imaged intercostally, a technique that has been validated. Alternatively, the diaphragm has been

imaged subcostally on the right side of the body through the liver. Diaphragmatic ascent and descent can be observed and then monitored after the patient draws in the transversus abdominis and recommences normal respiration. Diaphragmatic descent can also be observed when the other muscles of the local synergy are activated. For the pelvic floor, researchers have imaged the bladder neck with the transducer placed translabially in the female patient (Schaer et al 1995). The transducer is placed in the midline, in sagittal alignment, until the appropriate image is observed. Measurements are taken from the symphysis pubis, ideally in two planes, to measure both elevation of the bladder neck in a cephalad direction and ventral shift of the bladder neck. Movements can be described as cranioventral displacement of the bladder neck relative to the symphysis pubis on pelvic floor muscle contraction and dorsocaudal or posteroinferior displacement of the bladder neck on straining. In addition, clinicians are also currently reporting use of ultrasound imaging to monitor pelvic floor activation with the transducer placed suprapubically. This technique has been investigated by Murphy et al (2001). Ultrasound imaging of the pubocervical fascia was conducted in transverse and sagittal planes during contractions of the pelvic floor, which was verified manually by digital vaginal palpation. Two ultrasound units could thus be used to provide simultaneous feedback of two muscles of the synergy.

The contraction of the transversus abdominis and any substitution, especially by the obliquus internus abdominis or obliquus externus abdominis, can be observed by placing the transducer over the anterolateral abdominal wall to view the three muscle layers in transverse section (Fig. 14.16). Ultrasound feedback is more reliable for obliquus internus abdominis than obliquus externus abdominis. In fact, obliquus internus abdominis thickness can be recorded but there is little relationship between obliquus externus abdominis activity and ultrasound changes, which may be caused by architectural factors, such as the extensibility of the fascial attachment or the placement of the transducer (Hodges et al 2003d). EMG biofeedback can easily be used for the obliquus abdominis externus as it is a superficial muscle, so this combination can successfully be used to provide feedback

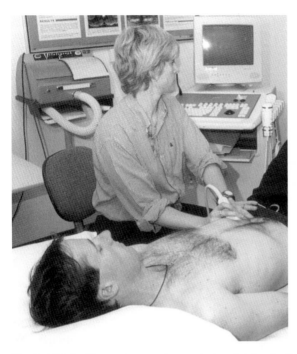

Figure 14.16   The patient receives real-time feedback of the muscles of the anterolateral wall from the real-time ultrasound.

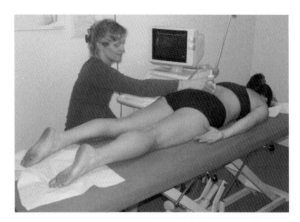

Figure 14.17   Imaging the lumbar multifidus in the parasagittal plane.

of activation. To allow understanding of the ultrasound image, the patient is orientated to the ultrasound image of the three muscle layers. The action to be observed with a correct transversus abdominis contraction is explained as the slow and controlled drawing in of this muscle in its corset-like action and appearance. This should occur with relative relaxation and little movement of the obliquus externus abdominis and obliquus internus abdominis. Simultaneous contraction of the three muscle layers as a single entity should not occur. When this does occur, the patient can realize his or her poor pattern of control and how the transversus abdominis has lost specific independent function (see Ch. 5). The effectiveness of various facilitation methods can be assessed until one that cues the patient successfully is observed. Meanwhile, the patient, in trying these methods to facilitate transversus abdominis activation, watches the real-time image of the muscle and palpates their lower abdominal wall to learn the correct muscle action. In addition, their ability to hold the contraction can be observed and monitored, as can the time at

which the muscle becomes fatigued and the localized contraction is either lost or is joined by the contraction of obliquus externus abdominis or internus abdominis in substitution. An additional use of the ultrasound is that patients can observe when the oblique abdominal muscles are overactive and use it to give feedback of when they contract the overactive muscles. If there is tonic activation of the global oblique abdominal muscles, they will appear 'thicker' on ultrasound imaging. This will allow the patient to evaluate the effectiveness of strategies to decrease their activity, such as change of position, adoption of a neutral spine position and use of relaxed diaphragmatic breathing strategies. The muscles will appear 'thinner' once they relax.

A parasagittal section is used for direct observation of the activation of the lumbar multifidus for facilitation purposes (Hides et al 1998, Van et al 2003 unpublished data, T. Wallwork et al 2003 unpublished data). The ultrasound transducer is placed lateral to the spinous processes, allowing a longitudinal image of the multifidus, including the dysfunctional segment (Fig. 14.17). Particular interest should be centred on watching the deep fibres of the muscle adjacent to the zygapophyseal joints (Fig. 14.18). The patient can observe the muscle contraction while consciously trying to 'swell out' the muscle at the segmental level or trying to activate the muscle with the contraction of the transversus abdominis or the pelvic floor. Simultaneously, the patient can palpate the lower abdomen to feel the co-activation of the transversus

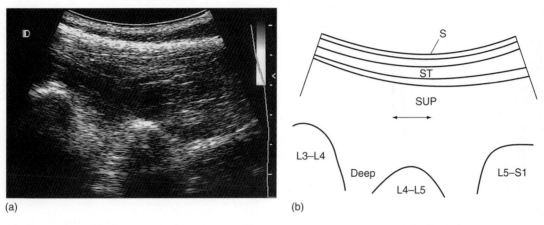

(a)   (b)

Figure 14.18 The multifidus in longitudinal section. (a) Ultrasound image. (b) The skin (S) and subcutaneous tissue (ST) are superiorly, with the multifidus fibres running in the direction of the arrow (↔). Inferiorly are the zygapophyseal joints L3–L4, L4–L5 and L5–S1. The deep fibres of the multifidus are seen surrounding the zygapophyseal joints. Deep, deep multifidus fibres; SUP, superficial.

abdominis. Precise feedback is given, which ensures that the patient is activating the multifidus at the affected segment. The quality of the contraction is appreciated as a slow increase in vertical depth of the multifidus, including the deep fibres, and the ability to hold the contraction can also be monitored as the maintenance of this vertical dimension. Sidelying is a good position to view the contraction of the multifidus and the transversus abdominis. To assess whether co-contraction is occurring, the patient can contract the segmental multifidus while the clinician images the transversus abdominis and vice versa.

The use of ultrasound imaging as a feedback tool in rehabilitation provides a notable advance in the rehabilitation of deep muscles. The effectiveness of ultrasound feedback on motor learning has been evaluated for subjects without a history of low back pain (Van et al 2003 unpublished data) to determine if the use of ultrasound imaging as visual feedback enhances learning the motor skill of contracting the multifidus muscle isometrically. Normal subjects were randomly allocated to either a control or an intervention group. The ability of subjects to perform an isometric multifidus contraction was determined using ultrasound imaging. The depth of the multifidus was measured both at rest and during voluntary contraction. To enhance the learning effect, the control group received instruction on how to perform the contraction plus verbal feedback. The intervention group received the same intervention with the addition of visual feedback using real-time ultrasound imaging. Subjects were taught how to perform the multifidus muscle contraction over 10 contractions (acquisition phase) using the two different forms of feedback. One week after the learning phase, multifidus contraction was reassessed in both groups to determine the extent to which the skill had been acquired by each group. For both groups, an improvement in the depth of multifidus was demonstrated during voluntary contraction. However, subjects in the intervention group performed significantly better in the acquisition phase ($p < 0.001$) and demonstrated greater retention 1 week later than subjects in the control group, indicating greater learning effects.

In practice, other external visual facilitatory techniques may be used, including the use of a mirror placed obliquely at the side of the patient so that he or she can monitor the appearance of the abdominal wall for their own practice at home. The provision of specific guidelines to the patient indicating the external appearance of the abdominal wall in their specific substitution strategy and how they may recognise this is vital. This visual feedback is best accompanied by palpation for either the gentle contraction in the lower abdomen or for deep tension development in the segmental multifidus (Fig. 14.19).

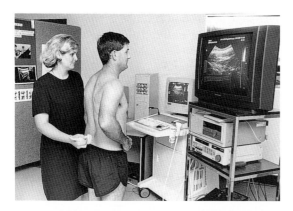

Figure 14.19 Visual and tactile feedback for the patient when practising the deep muscle co-contraction.

In some cases, when the patient performs the transversus abdominis or the lumbar multifidus contraction independently of the other trunk muscles, they may claim that they feel they are doing nothing. This is generally because the contraction is subtle, and the normal perception of an abdominal muscle contraction, for example, is the performance of a trunk movement such as a sit-up or posterior pelvic tilt. Verbal reassurance that this is normal and reiteration of the functional role of the muscles is always required. It also highlights the importance of the patient understanding the whole concept of deep muscle support and control, and supports the potential advantage of the more routine use of ultrasound imaging in future rehabilitation.

Lumbopelvic position

Although any of the techniques described above may be used in many different body positions, the precise position of the lumbopelvic region may itself be facilitatory for activation of the muscles of the local synergy. In support of this relationship, we have research evidence that better co-activation of the transversus abdominis occurs when the pelvic floor is contracted with the lumbar spine placed in a more neutral position (Sapsford et al 1997b). Biomechanical research has shown that the spine will be unable to distribute forces optimally if it is not positioned in a neutral position (Keifer et al 1997, 1998). There is a consensus that the local

muscles are involved in segmental support and, therefore, contribute to the precise positioning of the lumbosacral curve. The antithesis of this situation is overactivity of the global muscles, which may cause flexion of the thoracolumbar junction and upper lumbar spine. Therefore, positioning the spine in a precise neutral lumbosacral curve may be successful in assisting the patient to achieve a co-contraction of the local synergy muscles.

Direct strategies to decrease overactivity of muscles

Many of the techniques already described incorporate body positions or strategies to decrease overactivity of global muscles. As mentioned, the muscles of primary concern with respect to overactivity are the oblique abdominal muscles and/or the thoracic components of the erector spinae muscles. If the patient has difficulty relaxing these or other global muscles and the strategies already described are unsuccessful, then the clinician can explore other measures to gain relaxation of the overactive muscle(s).

Dealing with asymmetry of activation Evidence of asymmetry of activation of the transversus abdominis has been provided by neurophysiological studies in patients with chronic low back pain (see Ch. 10). Treating patients with this presentation can prove challenging. Ultrasound imaging is useful both in demonstrating the asymmetry and in re-education. Patients can usually feel the asymmetry of activation using palpation. What is detected on palpation is bulging on one side of the abdomen, as the oblique abdominal muscles overlying the transversus abdominis that is not performing the corset action are overactive. It is imperative that the activity of the overactive muscles are minimized, and this will usually entail a strategy of gently activating the transversus abdominis only to the point before the oblique abdominal muscles on that side are activated. This highlights another important clinical feature. One of the most useful clinical techniques is delivery of precise instructions. In this situation, it is instructing the patient to stop contracting the muscles prior to the point where overactivity becomes evident. As this overactivity decreases, the transversus abdominis below the overactive muscles will gradually improve and will start to tension the fascia again. Progression must be gradual to ensure that the overlying oblique abdominals do not become dominant again. Eventually, symmetry of action of the transversus abdominis will be restored. Self-palpation must be well taught to the patient if this strategy is to succeed. If patients are unable to detect the deep tensioning of the transversus abdominis, a useful instruction is to get the patient to focus on the release of the contraction (Hides et al 2000). This can be described to the patient as a sensation of 'melting away' and may be easier to detect than the contraction itself. The clinician must ensure that the patient can feel something on either the contraction or its release to allow self-palpation to be effective.

Restoration of normal breathing We have observed clinically that breathing patterns are sometimes altered in patients with chronic low back pain. In normal inspiration, the most important muscle is the diaphragm. The abdominal muscles are not involved. In forced expiration, the abdominal muscles act both to depress the thoracic cage and to elevate the diaphragm by raising the intra-abdominal pressure (DeTroyer and Estenne 1988). The abdominal muscles should only take part in the respiratory cycle when expiratory flow is increased or in positions where the abdominal contents are dependent and activity is required to restore the diaphragm to the ascended position; they should remain relaxed in normal quiet breathing.

In some patients with chronic low back pain, the activity of obliquus externus abdominis and/or obliquus abdominis internus has been observed clinically during quiet inspiration and expiration. We have also observed the use of accessory muscles of inspiration in these patients, and patterns of upper chest breathing. The cause of this change in breathing pattern may well relate to the change in thoracic cage dimensions owing to overactivity of the global muscles adversely affecting excursion of the diaphragm. In patients with this challenging presentation, there are two aims.

1. *To decrease overactivity of the global muscles.* This may be achieved, as discussed above, by change in position and use of relaxation techniques. In addition, massage of the oblique abdominals can be trialed, as can mobilization of the thoracolumbar region. Ultrasound imaging can be used to provide feedback. As the muscles relax, they will appear 'thinner' in dimension on ultrasound imaging.

2. *To restore normal diaphragmatic breathing patterns and excursion.* The use of positioning (as in postoperative and respiratory patients) should be remembered for patients who are having difficulty in establishing the appropriate relaxed breathing pattern. The reader is referred to respiratory physical therapy texts for the many alternatives. Diaphragmatic breathing involves both an increase in the anteroposterior dimensions of the abdomen and bibasal expansion of the rib cage. In clinical practice, when trying to restore normal breathing patterns, it may be useful to instruct the patient to make inspiration the active component and relax through expiration. Manual facilitation and other strategies may help to change the breathing pattern.

Overactivity of the global muscles requires increased effort and is inefficient. From clinical experience, even before their pain improves, patients will feel significantly improved once they have restored a normal breathing pattern and position of the spine. As the patient learns to control the diaphragm and relax the muscles of the abdominal wall, re-education of the local synergy muscles can begin. If the oblique abdominal muscles are active in breathing, it is our experience that it will be challenging to facilitate the local muscle synergy until this pattern is rectified. On a clinical note regarding respiration, the aim of treatment is to restore eventually tonic activation of the local muscle synergy combined with normal respiration. At this stage, the clinician may wish to check that, while the activation of the local synergy of muscles is maintained, both components of normal respiration can be performed, including bibasal expansion and rise and fall of the abdomen ('abdominal breathing').

EMG biofeedback Biofeedback from EMG has traditionally been used on the target muscle of the rehabilitation exercise to provide evidence of its contraction (Soderberg and Cook 1984). In retraining the transversus abdominis, electrodes placed over the lateral abdominal wall will detect EMG activity from all muscles and, therefore, provide little useful information. Placement of an electrode over the triangle formed between the anterior superior iliac spine, navel and pubic symphysis will detect activity of both the obliquus internus abdominis and the transversus abdominis, making this placement unsuitable when attempting to train a more specific activation of the transversus abdominis. It also appears that EMG is of little value for providing feedback for the multifidus contraction. While the muscle becomes superficial in the lower regions of the lumbar spine, it is the deep fibres that are most involved in segmental support. Nevertheless, in the training of the deep muscle co-contraction, biofeedback from EMG has become a most successful adjunct to treatment. Instead of being used to monitor the activation in contracting muscles, it is used to ensure relaxation in the global muscles while training the independent activation of the deep muscles.

The use of biofeedback from EMG has proved particularly helpful in assisting patients to relax excessive activity and avoid substitution by the oblique abdominal muscles and the rectus abdominis, as well as the thoracic portions of the erector spinae (Fig. 14.20). The most appropriate placement for the electrodes for viewing the obliquus externus abdominis is in parallel with the fibres of this muscle over the anterior end of the eighth rib (Ng et al 1998). For general observation of the oblique abdominal muscles, electrodes should be placed along a line connecting the most inferior point of the costal margin and the contralateral pubic tubercle (Ng et al 1998). For the rectus abdominis, the best position of the electrodes is below the navel, 2 cm lateral to the midline. With these electrode positions there is minimal interference from the adjacent abdominal muscles. The biofeedback from EMG can be used in conjunction with all the other facilitation strategies discussed and is used potently with feedback from ultrasound imaging. It is a method that is growing in use in the clinical situation because of its effectiveness in giving some objectivity to the effectiveness of the technique chosen.

For reasons identical to those described above, electrical stimulation is not an option when training isolated contraction of the transversus abdominis, since other muscles almost always overlie it.

Elevation of the rib cage   Since the action of obliquus externus abdominis on the rib cage is to draw the ribs downwards and inwards, it can be useful to use the intercostal muscles cognitively to elevate the rib cage prior to the performance of transversus abdominis contraction in an attempt to reduce obliquus externus abdominis substitution. To implement this technique, the therapist instructs the patient to perform a gentle bibasal expansion against either the therapist's or their own hands placed laterally on the rib cage. Once this has been performed, the patient then performs a contraction of the transversus abdominis, either directly or using one of the other facilitation techniques such as pelvic floor muscle contraction. It is essential that the therapist assesses and ensures that the rib cage elevation has been successful in reducing obliquus externus abdominis contraction before the transversus abdominis contraction is attempted.

Other inhibitory techniques and positions   For those skilled in them, there are many different techniques within physical therapy practice that can be used to decrease overactivity in muscles, and notably in this case the obliquus externus and internus abdominis muscles. Various neurological techniques such as proprioceptive neuromuscular

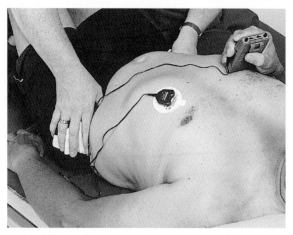

Figure 14.20   Placement of the electromyograph electrode over the eighth rib to monitor activity in the obliquus externus abdominis.

facilitation (Knott and Voss 1968) and Bobath techniques (Lennon 1982) provide useful methods of addressing the problems of overactive muscles. Other techniques such as myofascial treatment of the abdominal and lumbar trigger points (Travell and Simons 1983) or deep inhibitory massage may also be appropriate to achieve relaxation. Taping techniques may also be of use. These can be employed for any muscles around the lumbopelvic region that are assessed to be overactive in the individual patient, for example the quadratus lumborum, hamstrings, etc.

Progression into sitting and standing positions

In the clinical setting, progression into sitting and standing positions is commenced once the patient has achieved good control of the four synergy muscles in non-weightbearing positions. It is important that the patient can activate each of the four muscles well, and that co-contraction of the other synergy muscles occurs simultaneously. For example, in the side-lying position, transversus abdominis and the multifidus can be monitored for co-contraction while the subject activates the pelvic floor. Once good control is achieved, the patient can try the sitting or standing position.

It is more difficult for the patient to achieve activation of the muscles of the local muscle synergy in upright positions. One reason is that the patient may experience an increase in activation of the global muscles. This can be monitored by observing the thickness of the oblique abdominal muscles on ultrasound imaging. The patient should be encouraged to relax the abdominal wall and use diaphragmatic breathing patterns.

In sitting and standing, attention must be directed to the spinal curves. As mentioned earlier, the correction of the sitting posture is often commenced early in the rehabilitation process as patients often spend a considerable amount of time in the seated position. In this phase, patients should be instructed how to adjust the lumbar support in their chairs. Commonly, when patients are questioned regarding the location of the lumbar spine, they commonly point to the sacral area. Lumbar support is important as initially the multifidus will lack the endurance required to support the lumbar lordosis.

In addition to passive supports, patients should try during the day to correct the position of the lumbar spine actively and hold this for short periods. Attainment of a neutral spine position is facilitatory for the local muscles (Williams et al 2000). It has been shown that, when the pelvic floor contraction is used to activate the transversus abdominis in the sitting position, the best pattern of activation was achieved when the lumbar spine was placed in a neutral position (Sapsford et al 1997b). Patients with low back pain commonly sit in a position of posterior pelvic tilt. When asked to 'sit up straight', patients commonly extend at the thoracolumbar junction (Fig. 14.21). To teach the patient to achieve an upright position of the pelvis and restore a normal lumbosacral lordosis, correction should be initiated at the pelvis, by concentrating on slightly anteriorly tilting the sacrum (Fig. 14.22). As patients often tend to tilt further anteriorly than necessary, which can aggravate low back pain, it is helpful to instruct them to tilt anteriorly and then release slightly. Another cue for attaining a neutral lumbopelvic position is the pressure on the ischial tuberosities. As the patient moves into a position of posterior pelvic tilt, they will feel pressure on the ischial tuberosities. If they then anteriorly tilt, they will feel that the ischial tuberosities lift off the surface. A point midway between the two of these points is the correct neutral position. Another cue can be gained by observation of the shoulder girdle complex. In a position of posterior pelvic tilt, the shoulder girdle will feel elevated and protracted. In a position of anterior pelvic tilt, the patient will commonly extend at the thoracolumbar junction, and the shoulder blades will be placed in a retracted position. When a neutral lumbopelvic position is achieved, the shoulder girdle should feel relaxed because of the resultant correct alignment of the thoracic and cervical spines.

Ultrasound imaging can be used to highlight the role of the multifidus in achieving a normal lumbopelvic position (Fig. 14.23). If the ultrasound is placed in a parasagittal section, the multifidus can be viewed as the patient attempts the correction. If the patient extends the thoracolumbar junction, this will be achieved by the thoracic components of the erector spinae. Imaging of the multifidus will reveal that this pattern of activation

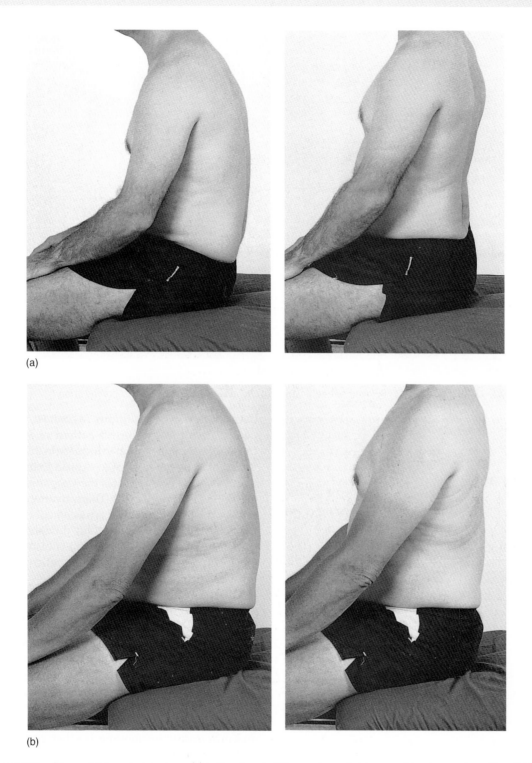

(a)

(b)

Figure 14.21   The upright neutral posture. (a) Left: relaxed sitting posture; right: normal lumbosacral position. (b) Left: relaxed sitting position; right: the upright trunk position attained through an incorrect extension in the thoracolumbar region, which leaves the lumbosacral junction in flexion.

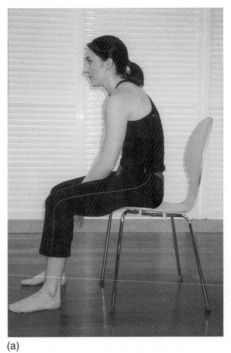
(a)

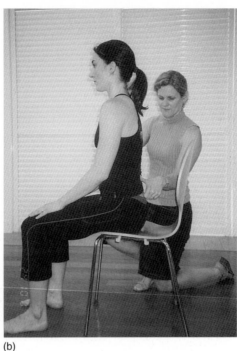
(b)

Figure 14.22 Sitting position. (a) Relaxed sitting posture. (b) Achieving a normal lumbosacral position.

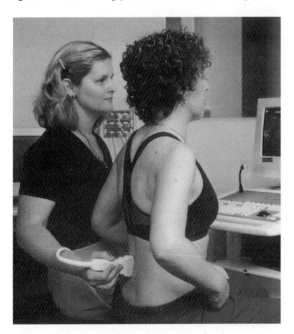

Figure 14.23 Using real-time ultrasound imaging to provide real-time feedback of multifidus muscle activation as the patient attempts to achieve a normal lumbopelvic position. (Reproduced with permission of Northwater Publishing, Australia).

does not recruit the multifidus. In contrast, when the patient performs the correct pattern of activation, the multifidus will be seen to increase in thickness as it contracts. It is important to explain to the patient that this correction activates the deep and superficial fibres of the multifidus. This activation does not replace the requirement for achievement of the isometric swelling of the multifidus described in this section and, in fact, may be used initially to focus the patient on the multifidus before the patient can perform the required isometric contraction.

Often the patient will master the activation of the local synergy muscles in the sitting position before the standing position. To aid progression to standing, a process of graduated weightbearing can be used. In the sitting position, the patient leans forward and takes weight through their arms on a surface placed in front of them. It is crucial that the normal spinal curves are maintained. The patient then activates the muscles of the synergy, and progression to standing is achieved by using higher surfaces until ultimately the patient can contract the muscles in the fully upright position, without upper limb support. An emphasis must be placed on maintaining the corset action and normal patterns of respiration. Palpation of the abdominal wall should be conducted to ensure that bulging does not occur, and that the pattern of activation remains symmetrical between sides.

IMPLEMENTATION OF THE ACTIVATION STRATEGIES

Many different techniques are available to assist in the facilitation of the muscles of the local synergy. Those described here are by no means all of them, and many additional techniques may exist that achieve the same goal. The clinician should keep in mind that the goal of the procedure is to regain tonic control and co-activation of these muscles so that the ability of these muscles to contract can be improved. The possibilities for facilitation are limited only by the creativity of the clinician. When trialling alternative techniques, it is essential to monitor closely for the appearance of substitution strategies. It is also important to remember that no one technique works for all people, and the clinician must stay aware of what is occurring so that a technique is quickly discarded if it is unsuccessful.

Each of the techniques described can be used in combination as well as separately. The clinician should be willing to try many different combinations until satisfied that the patient has achieved the best contraction. At first, the clinician may find this time consuming, but with practice and experience it is possible to identify patient presentations which suggest that a particular technique or combination of techniques may be the most appropriate. Logically, the most rapid rate of improvement can be expected if the best facilitation technique is identified for that patient. One useful technique, which seems obvious, is to use clear and concise instructions and to stop patients before they implement an incorrect pattern of activation. Even if patients can only perform a very small part of the contraction of the target muscle well, it is important that they limit the contraction before they adopt a poor pattern of activation.

Once a method has been found that results in contraction of the local synergy muscles without overactivity of the global trunk muscles, the effectiveness of the contraction is enhanced by repetition of the contraction. It is imperative that the patient can undertake the facilitation technique independently so that it can be practised at home between treatment sessions. In this phase of motor relearning, repetition is key, and the clinician and patient should plan times for practice. Furthermore, for motor relearning to be effective, it is imperative that the patient is repeating the correct action. The initial home programme must be clearly taught and documented so that both parties are confident that the programme is achievable. It is very useful to show patients strategies for self-detection of substitutions. Self-palpation of the abdomen medial to the anterior superior iliac crest can be used, with the patient instructed to avoid pushing out against their fingers, indicating an incorrect pattern of activation. It is useful to tell the patient that if they are having a bad day or are tired, or for any reason they are performing the activation poorly, they are better not to do it at all than to do it badly. This is because of the neurophysiology. The most likely mechanism of action, especially in the patient who has an almost immediate decrease in symptoms, is neurophysiological. Correct activation of the local muscles may lower the threshold of activation of the gamma system (i.e. bias the spindle towards an increased activation). The tonic activation of the appropriate muscles is then enough in some cases to decrease painful symptoms as the normal protective mechanism is restored. If the contraction is performed poorly, this effect is likely to be lost. The home programme should be tested in full at all treatment sessions with respect to the specific position, number of repetitions and contraction holding times.

It is essential that clinicians ask themselves three central questions before they permit a patient to go home to practice.

- What strategy works best to isolate the contraction of the local synergy muscles from contraction of the global muscles?
- How can the clinician and patient be sure that the correct contraction will be performed at home in each practice period?
- How many contractions can be performed and how long can a contraction be held before it is lost or another muscle has been substituted?

One of the main advantages of the patient being able to self-assess for substitutions or loss of holding is that they can to a certain extent self-direct progression by increasing the duration and number of contractions as their ability to activate the muscles improves. It is crucial that the patient develops endurance in the muscles of the local synergy. The length of time of this stage is variable and depends on the degree of a patient's motor control problems as well as their motivation and enthusiasm to practise. In controlled clinical trials, it has been demonstrated that this stage could be as long as 6–10 weeks in patients with chronic problems (O'Sullivan et al 1997) whereas in patients with acute first episodes of low back pain, activation and training of the local synergy in standing was achieved in 4 weeks (Hides et al 1996b).

Once activation and training of the local synergy muscles has been achieved in upright positions, the patient may wish to resume fitness activities that require integration of the local and global muscles. Before this can be considered, it will be necessary to assess closed chain (Ch. 15) and open chain (Ch. 16) segmental control. If the patient does not have impairments of control of the one-joint antigravity and global muscle systems, resumption of activities may be considered. Some activities (e.g. walking, running or swimming) will involve patterned activation of the global muscles, and this may challenge the control of the local muscle synergy. The aim is that the local synergy muscles will be activated automatically to control and protect the segments while the patient performs the activity. The patient at this stage should not have to focus on the synergy muscles while they perform the activity but should be concentrating on the skill at hand. From a clinical perspective, the patient may be encouraged to do two tests of the local muscle synergy. First, before participating in the activity, they should test that they can activate the synergy muscles. This should be performed in a position where the activation can be performed easily and well; this could be explained to the patient as a 'warm-up' of the local muscles prior to the activity. Initially, the activity should be resumed for a very limited period of time to allow assessment of the effect of the activity on low back pain and local muscle control. Second, after performing the activity, the patient should test if they can still activate the synergy muscles. If the patient is unable to activate the local muscles, this is a clinical indicator that

the control of the local synergy muscles is inadequate, and that progression to this level is not yet appropriate. Care should be taken with patients who have rehabilitated asymmetrical patterns of abdominal wall activation and then resume activities that load the trunk asymmetrically. A good example would be surf fishing, which requires asymmetrical activation of especially the oblique abdominal muscles. After the activity, the patient should check that they can activate the local synergy muscles and that they are still symmetrical in their activation pattern. Chapter 15 will discuss integration of local muscles into antigravity weightbearing function.

APPENDIX: DEVELOPMENT OF PRESSURE BIOFEEDBACK

During the development of the initial clinical tests of stabilization function, it was necessary to develop a device that could monitor the position (i.e. stable or unstable) of the lumbopelvic region during leg-loading tests performed with the patient in the supine position. A direct measure of the complex three-dimensional motion of the lumbopelvic region is not easy; therefore, an indirect method was developed for clinical testing (Stabilizer, Chattanooga USA). The pressure biofeedback unit (Richardson et al 1992) consists of an inelastic, three-section air-filled bag, which is inflated to fill the space between the target body area and a firm surface, and a pressure dial for monitoring the pressure in the bag for feedback on position (Fig. 14.24). The bag is inflated to an appropriate level for the purpose and the pressure recorded. Quite simply, movement of the body part off the bag results in a decrease in pressure, while movement of the body part onto the bag results in an increase in pressure.

The device has come into general use for stabilization exercises for all parts of the body. Its use in assessing the abdominal drawing-in action has, however, become its most important use in relation to the treatment of problems of the local muscle system in patients with low back pain. A method was needed to gain some quantification of the abdominal drawing-in action in the clinic, and the pressure biofeedback unit has met this need. As the transversus abdominis produces narrowing of

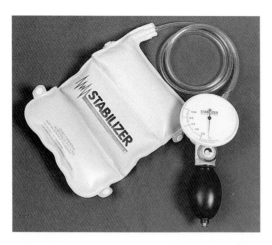

Figure 14.24 The pressure biofeedback unit consists of a three-section, inelastic inflatable pad with a pressure pump and dial.

the abdominal wall, measurement of the amount of movement of the abdomen that can be produced provides a method of identifying a patient's ability to perform the contraction. To understand this, it is necessary to consider the orientation of the abdominal muscles.

The majority of the muscle fibres of the rectus abdominis, obliquus externus abdominis and obliquus internus abdominis run either vertically or obliquely from the pelvis to the rib cage. When these muscles contract, they can flatten the abdominal wall but do not narrow the waist beyond this. In contrast, the fibres of the transversus abdominis are horizontal and can, therefore, produce a concavity of the abdominal wall without movement of the spine. Therefore, when the transversus abdominis contracts in isolation, concavity of the abdominal wall results, whereas substitution by the other abdominal muscles simply flattens the abdomen. Measurement of the elevation of the abdominal wall from the supporting surface using the pressure biofeedback unit, with the patient in the prone position, allows identification of both how well the transversus abdominis can be contracted and whether this action can be performed in isolation.

The principle underlying the use of the pressure biofeedback unit in this test is that the unit initially conforms to the patient's shape when it is placed under the abdomen. As the patient draws in the stomach off the pad, the pressure in the pad is reduced. The pressure reduction is proportional to the degree to which the patient can elevate the abdominal wall. The specific construction of this device has considerable advantages. First, since the material is inelastic it can accurately reflect abdominal wall motion without distortion. This is assisted by partitioning the device into three sections, which assists with the distribution of the air within the pad. When the device is positioned appropriately, the shape of the pad permits an evaluation to be made of the movement of the abdomen.

Chapter 15

Closed chain segmental control

Carolyn Richardson and Julie Hides

INTRODUCTION

The closed chain segmental control stage involves the integration of the local muscles into segmental, antigravity weightbearing function. Integration of the local and weightbearing muscles is best achieved through weightbearing (closed) kinetic chain exercises with gradually increasing gravitational (i.e. gravity-related) load cues. The pattern of muscle function at each segment of the kinetic chain is important. The basic posture used for this stage is a flexed working posture, so that the antigravity muscles are required to work optimally in eccentric contractions (Fig. 15.1a). While the semi-squat working posture, with the upper and lower limb flexed, is the starting position, exercises may involve the extension of the upper and lower limb to a fully extended antigravity position (Fig. 15.1b).

Before beginning this stage of the programme, it is important to assess the patient's ability to stretch the whole body fully against gravity, in case there is a loss of shoulder or hip flexion range. Performing this manoeuvre against a wall while maintaining a neutral lumbopelvic position will allow deficits in range to be detected (Fig. 15.2).

Most particularly this will give an indication of overactivity in the flexor muscles of the upper quadrant (e.g. latissimus dorsi, pectoralis major). importantly, this will give an indication of the effect of elevation of the upper limb on spinal position and direct the position for closed chain upper limb exercise while maintaining a neutral lumbopelvic position (see following section).

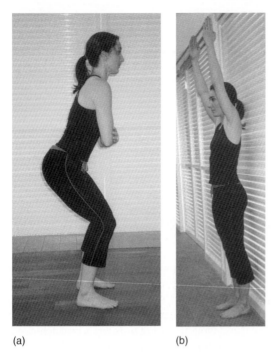

(a)   (b)

Figure 15.1   (a) The flexed weightbearing posture.
(b) The fully extended antigravity position.

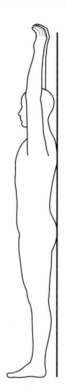

Figure 15.2   Assessing the extended antigravity position
against a wall.

Closed chain segmental control involves closed chain, weightbearing exercise to re-establish the role of the local and weightbearing muscles in joint protection. Because of the predicted reduced sensitivity of the local and weightbearing muscles to respond to gravitational load cues, this stage should progress slowly, depending on results of assessment, to ensure that both the local and the weightbearing muscles of the lumbopelvic region are recruited optimally in progressive weightbearing exercise. Most importantly, if the weightbearing load cues are too high, these muscles are likely to fail to respond to the load or, if they respond, fatigue quickly. In either situation, compensation by the non-weightbearing muscles would occur. The contribution by the non-weightbearing muscles should be minimized during this stage. This process should be viewed as reloading the local and weightbearing muscles while unloading the non-weightbearing muscles. For optimal achievement of this target, both the lower and upper girdle muscles should be involved, together with the trunk and spinal muscles.

No pain or discomfort should occur during the exercises, and care needs to be taken when progressing load or selecting the exercise endurance time. The progressive exercise described here serves only as a guide, many types of exercise would be suitable under the principles described in Chapter 13. As many of the suggested exercises are familiar to physiotherapists, as well as to many other health-care professionals, the details of the techniques, as have been described for local segmental control (Ch. 14), are not required.

TRAINING PROCEDURES: PROGRESSIVE STAGES

To increase compliance, explain to the patient the reason for each of the following stages of the progressive exercise programme.

1. Training individual parts of the antigravity weightbearing holding posture.
2. Weightbearing (closed chain) exercise in flexed postures.
3. Weightbearing (closed chain) exercise with addition of unstable, moving surfaces.

4. Weightbearing (closed chain) exercise on more challenging surfaces and in more upright postures.

These stages are preceded by assessments. For all treatment stages, the patient should first activate the local muscles to achieve a neutral spine and a neutral lumbopelvic unit in preparation for antigravity weightbearing exercise (this should have been achieved by the end of the local segmental control stage; pp. 214–217). Therefore, for all the following kinetic chain exercises, the patient should pull in the lower abdomen and hold, while breathing normally.

Training individual parts of the antigravity weightbearing holding posture

There are many different muscle groups at many individual segments (i.e. joints) that need to be co-ordinated to hold the flexed weightbearing posture effectively. The focus initially is on individual parts of the antigravity posture (Fig. 15.3), so three component parts are addressed. These are: loading the neutral spine in sitting, activating the dysfunctional weightbearing muscles of the pelvis, and ensuring that the quadriceps muscles are capable of holding (i.e. have efficient endurance) for weightbearing. Within each section, assessment procedures are included.

Begin loading the neutral spine/pelvic position in sitting

The aim is to maintain a neutral spine/pelvic position in upright sitting with gradual added antigravity muscle activity using two different methods: upper quadrant closed chain exercise and trunk forward lean.

Upper quadrant closed chain exercise The patient should begin to load the spine in upright sitting where body weight is partially supported and increase weightbearing through the addition of closed chain upper limb exercise. This could be achieved in the formal setting (Fig. 15.4a,b) or in home based exercise (Fig. 15.4c). It would be important to check that the spinal curves can be maintained.

Trunk forward lean First check the patient's ability to hold neutral spine and pelvis in trunk

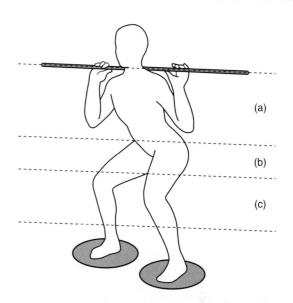

Figure 15.3 Individual parts of the antigravity posture: (a) the lumbopelvic region; (b) the hip region; (c) the knee region.

forward lean in sitting (i.e. ability to hold lumbopelvic position with the addition of gravitational load). This has been described by Hamilton and Richardson (1995) in a study in which both patients with low back pain and matched controls were assessed. The test involves leaning forward from the hips and noting the range of trunk flexion (forward lean) that the patient can achieve before substitution strategies occur (Fig. 15.5). Patients with low back pain cannot hold the spinal position beyond 15 degrees (Fig. 15.5b) and compensate in most cases with lumbar flexion (Fig. 15.5c). Sometimes substitution into extension can occur (Fig. 15.5d). Note the patient's hand position as well as the therapist's hand position to determine when substitution occurs.

In order to train the muscles to hold this position, a variety of facilitation techniques could be used. These include:

- add real-time ultrasound feedback, especially for the local muscles and the lumbar erector spinae;
- palpation of lumbar spine position (as for test);
- assist with pelvic position;
- with focus on inner range lumbar erector spinae, could use sweep tapping over the muscle or a 10 Hz minimal twitch contraction applied

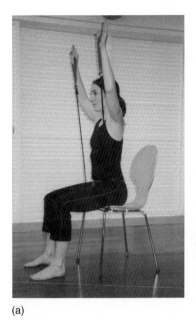 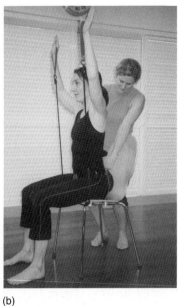 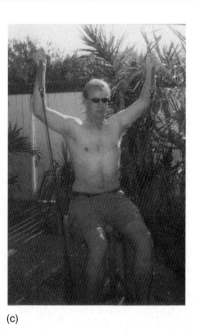

(a)   (b)   (c)

Figure 15.4 Closed chain upper limb exercise using elastic straps (Optimal Life Aus. Pty Ltd). (a) Spinal curves maintained in a formal setting. (b) Close monitoring in a formal setting. (c) Exercising in a home-based setting.

through a portable muscle stimulator (e.g. EMG Retrainer, Chattanooga, USA) directly to the lumbar erector spinae muscles, during the exercise training;

- use a mirror to assist in achieving and holding the position of the spinal curves;
- use biofeedback in the form of a posture biofeedback device placed in the lumbar curve to signal a change of position.

A posture biofeedback device gives feedback to the patient when a neutral spinal position is lost. New 'easy to use' models of postural biofeedback are currently being developed for formal exercise as well as for home use.

Activating the dysfunctional weightbearing muscles of the pelvis

Traditional muscle testing techniques (Palmer and Epler 1998) form the basis for the functional tests of the weightbearing muscles of the pelvis. It is the Grade 3 antigravity level of the tests that is important in detecting muscle dysfunction. For the one-joint antigravity muscles, these traditional muscle testing procedures have focused on testing the inner (shortened) range of muscle contraction. Inner

range has several advantages as a testing procedure for detecting dysfunction in the joint protection role of the weightbearing muscles:

- individual muscles are checked for their ability to hold against the force of gravity;
- individual muscles may be lengthened (i.e. added sarcomeres) because of poor posture, resulting in an inability to contract into their inner range (Ch. 12);
- high sensitivity of load receptors (i.e. influence of the gamma system) will be required in such shortened ranges of muscle length (earlier chapters have explained the likely potent negative effects of deloading (Ch. 7) and injury (Ch. 8) on the gamma system);
- allows detection of any opposing (antagonist) tight multijoint non-weightbearing muscles, which will be stretched during the inner range testing procedures for the agonist muscle.

The individual antigravity muscles of the lumbo-pelvic region are checked for inner range hold of limb load using the grade 3 antigravity muscle test with a 10 second hold. It is important that it is an isometric holding contraction without any phasic erratic limb movement. These tests are applied to muscles on each side of the body to note if any

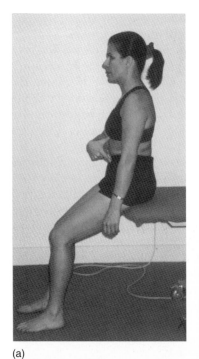

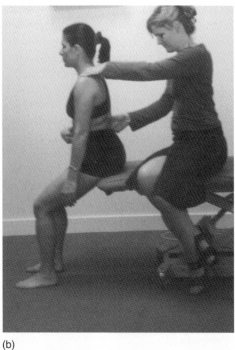

(a)

(b)

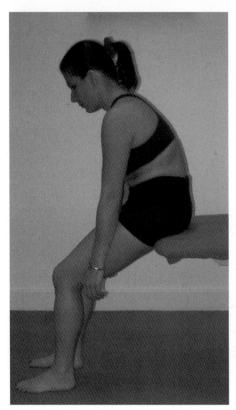

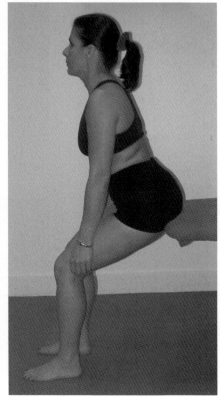

(c)

(d)

Figure 15.5   Spinal curves. (a) Spinal curves maintained in high sitting. (b) Spinal curves maintained in the trunk lean-forward task. (c) Spinal curves not maintained during the trunk lean-forward task (i.e. spinal flexion). (d) Spinal curves not maintained during the trunk lean-forward task (i.e. spinal extension).

assymmetry is present. The weightbearing muscles that are essential for weightbearing control of the pelvis need to be tested separately: gluteus maximus (Fig. 15.6), iliopsoas (Fig. 15.7), gluteus medius (focus gluteus medius posterior) (Fig. 15.8), and adductor magnus and brevis (Fig. 15.9).

Weightbearing needs to be progressed slowly to ensure that a dysfunctional antigravity system is responding to gravitational (sensory) load cues. The dysfunctions of the pelvic muscles detected through muscle testing procedures needs to be addressed in order to ensure that they are responding to weightbearing load.

Individual weak one-joint antigravity muscles with poor load control may need to be initially exercised in non-weightbearing or partial weightbearing positions and/or in more lengthened positions to begin to activate the correct patterns for loading. Then weightbearing cues are progressed with low-load simulated weightbearing with increasing isometric holds or with very slow movement. The therapist could provide hand pressure under the heel to provide a compression stimulus to the joints.

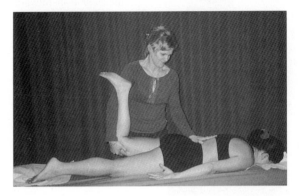

Figure 15.6 Antigravity muscle test for gluteus maximus.

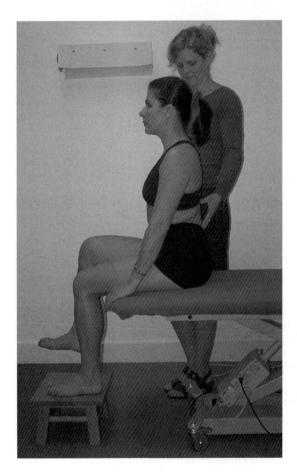

Figure 15.7 Antigravity muscle test for iliopsoas.

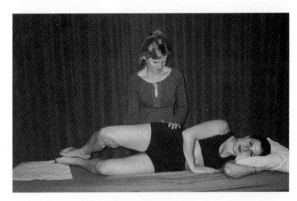

Figure 15.8 Antigravity muscle test for gluteus medius.

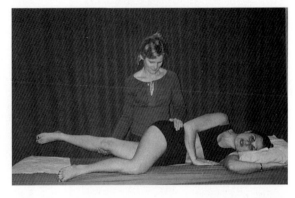

Figure 15.9 Antigravity muscle test for adductor magnus and brevis.

Palpation, electromyographic (EMG) biofeedback or ultrasound biofeedback could be used to check activation and give feedback to the patient.

Ensuring quadriceps holding in partial weightbearing

Isometric holding achieved with body weight against wall (i.e. wall squat; Fig. 15.10) could be used to test and train the quadriceps muscles in preparation for closed chain activities. This is to ensure that there is no lack of endurance in the quadriceps, which could limit the patient's ability to perform closed chain antigravity exercise (see next section).

Weightbearing (closed chain) exercise in flexed postures

The weightbearing (closed chain) exercise in flexed postures involves slow or isometric exercise incorporating the lower limb and, in many cases, including the upper limb in closed kinetic chain activity. The type of exercise techniques used include the slow lunge or semi-squat, with weightbearing muscles stretched to facilitate their contribution to weightbearing, and with non-weightbearing muscles relaxed.

Gradually gravitational load cues are increased, ensuring that the therapist can observe the patient's spine (i.e. suitably dressed). The patient should have bare feet to maximize sensory input through the soles of the feet. It must be ensured that the antigravity muscles are appropriately recruited (EMG, ultrasound, palpation) as in stage 1, and the endurance of the antigravity weightbearing muscle system is gradually increased during the closed chain exercises. Initially this could be achieved in simulated weightbearing (Fig. 15.11), including 'leg-press' exercise devices. An example of a weightbearing exercise in a flexed posture would be a squat with hip and knee flexion. This could be achieved in the formal setting (Fig. 15.12a) or as a home-based exercise (Fig. 15.12b). Similarly, a lunge with hip and knee flexion could be achieved in the formal setting (Fig. 15.13a) or in home-based exercise (Fig. 15.13b,c).

All exercise could progress from bilateral to unilateral weightbearing.

Weightbearing (closed chain) exercise with the addition of unstable, moving surfaces

In order to facilitate the weightbearing muscles further, under increasing gravitational load cues, unstable and moving surfaces can be used. Exercise tools, such as balance boards, rubber discs, trampolines or other equipment providing moving

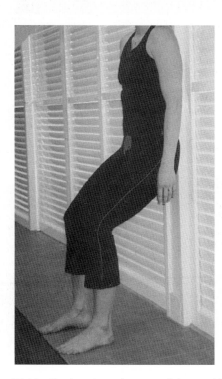

Figure 15.10 Testing the endurance of the quadriceps muscles.

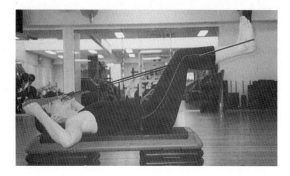

Figure 15.11 Simulated weightbearing with elastic straps.

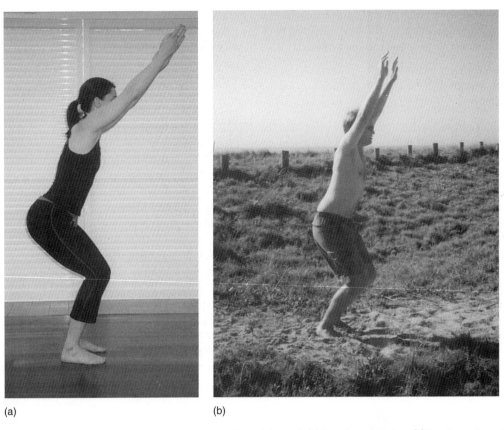

Figure 15.12   Closed chain exercise with arms elevated in line with trunk. (a) In a formal setting; (b) in a home based setting.

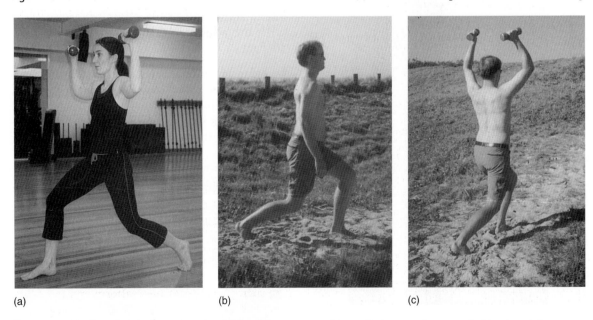

Figure 15.13   Closed chain lunge exercise. (a) Involving upper and lower limbs, ensuring a neutral lumbopelvic position. (b) Without the addition of hand weights. Note the neutral spinal curves. (c) With the addition of hand weights. Note the increased difficulty of maintaining the neutral spinal curves.

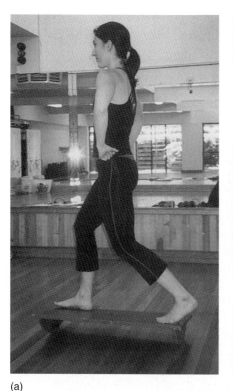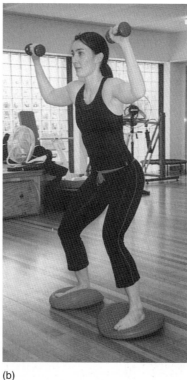

Figure 15.14   Closed chain exercise. (a) On a large balance board; (b) on uneven surfaces.

(a)   (b)

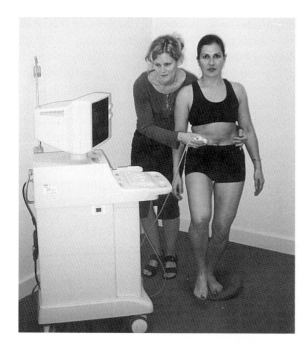

Figure 15.15   Monitoring the local muscle system during closed chain exercise on unstable surfaces.

surfaces, can be used as a platform on which to perform the closed chain exercises. It is important to watch for muscle fatigue and/or loss of the neutral posture. This type of exercise could be given more readily in the formal setting (Fig. 15.14b) or it could be a home-based exercise. Whenever possible the deep local system should be monitored during these activities in the formal setting (Fig. 15.15). Again, all exercise could progress from bilateral to unilateral weightbearing.

Weightbearing (closed chain) exercise on more challenging surfaces and in more upright postures

The most challenging surface in a formal setting for closed chain exercise comes through the use of a new exercise tool, whole body vibration (WBV). The patient stands on the platform and performs closed chain exercise (Fig. 15.16). The Appendix (p. 230) gives a detailed overview of the device and its use for patients with low back pain.

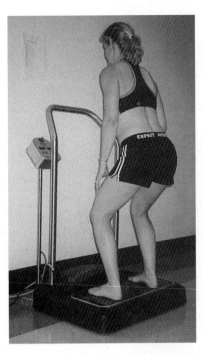

Figure 15.16 Closed chain exercise performed on the platform of a whole body vibration device.

Progression to unstable surfaces in more upright postures also provides a challenge for recruitment of the local and weightbearing muscle system. This could be achieved during walking on unstable, uneven, sloping or moving surfaces such as soft sand, grassy slopes or rough ground. Achieving joint protection through activation of the weightbearing muscles in an erect posture is more difficult as weightbearing muscles (e.g. gluteus maximus, adductor magnus) are in more shortened positions. Accurate detection of load cues would require more sensitive stretch receptors.

It is also important for the patient to change lifestyle activities and increase weightbearing through the skeleton in everyday activities: use knees to bend to do housework or gardening; increase the sensation of load and gravity through activities such as walking bare foot, walking on grass slopes or sand (Fig. 15.17); bush walking, windsurfing, skiing; if the patient is attending a gym, they should focus on closed chain exercise for resistance training (upper and lower limb).

APPENDIX: WHOLE BODY VIBRATION TO ENHANCE ANTIGRAVITY MUSCLE FUNCTION

WBV is a new tool to enhance the effects of exercise training that has been developed by biomechanical engineers in Europe. The device is manufactured by several companies (e.g. as Galileo™ and Power Plate™) and it is becoming popular with exercise enthusiasts, especially in the UK and Europe. This device was first developed by Russian space scientists, who recognized that this new concept for exercise had the potential to provide suitable countermeasures to prevent bone and muscle loss for astronauts in microgravity situations. It is our contention that carefully prescribed closed chain exercise performed on the vibrating platform could enhance the function of the antigravity muscle system for prevention and rehabilitation of many types of musculoskeletal injury, including, most importantly, low back pain.

The equipment variables that can be controlled in WBV are the frequency and amplitude of the vibratory stimulus. Frequencies of 1–50 Hz are usually available, with amplitude changes depending on whether the feet are placed at the centre (reduced amplitude) or to the outside (higher amplitude) of the vibrating platform. A timer is also included. Although most researchers concur that the physical effects of vibration on individual muscles can improve strength, power and flexibility (Issurin and Tenenbaum 1999), most agree that these physical changes occur through the effect of vibration on the pro-prioceptive system, that is through the stretch reflex (Ribot-Cisar et al 1998, Gollhofer et al 1998, Rittweger et al 2002). Interestingly Bosco et al (2000), while suggesting that vibration influences the proprioceptive feedback mechanisms, also suggest that increases in testosterone and growth hormone occur.

Roll et al (1980) showed that the effect of vibration changes, depending on whether the effect is specific to a muscle or not, is a more generalized effect. The effect of vibration on a single muscle gives an illusion of segmental movement. In contrast, a generalized vibration gives no movement sensation but induces a perception of a stabilized position. Importantly, to achieve this, the subject

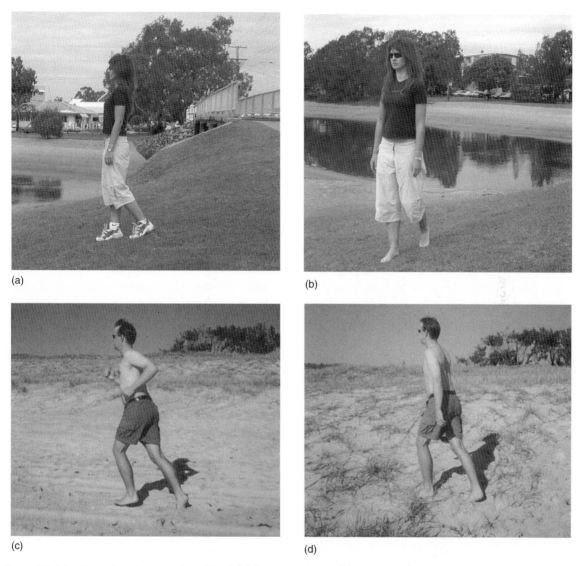

Figure 15.17 Increasing the sensation of load. (a) On grassy slopes; (b) on grassy slopes without shoes; (c) by walking or running on soft sand; (d) by walking on soft, sandy slopes.

must be active (not passive) to allow the vibration to induce a motor effect.

The generalized effect of vibration in the form of WBV has been used by some researchers. Exhaustive exercise using WBV has been shown to be less effective than bicycle ergometry in improving cardiovascular fitness (Rittweger et al 2000). Positive effects on bone density have been shown using WBV. Rubin et al (2001) highlighted the importance of vibration in determining bone morphology and,

in research using sheep, demonstrated that WBV can increase the rate of bone formation.

In a randomized clinical trial, Rittweger et al (2002) compared lumbar extension exercises with WBV for low back pain. A decrease in pain and disability as well as an increase in trunk extension torque occurred for both groups. Although there was no correlation found between pain relief and lumbar extension torque, the authors believe that WBV has the potential to treat pain, rather than, as commonly thought, cause low back pain. The effects of vibration on pain relief may be mediated through its effects on motor control, especially on the function of the antigravity muscle system.

Using whole body vibration for the prevention and treatment of motor control problems in low back pain

The most important specific effects of WBV appear to rely on variables of the assumed posture and exercise undertaken on the platform. Issurin and Tenenbaum (1999) claimed that the optimal effect of vibration on muscles occurs when vibration is applied from distal to proximal. This may infer that performing closed chain exercise with feet on the platform (i.e. WBV with closed chain exercise) may have a very positive effect on muscle activation and recruitment patterns of the antigravity, weightbearing muscles. This view that vibration could produce an excitatory effect on the antigravity muscles, is confirmed to some degree in the recent studies of Torvinen et al (2002). These researchers found that, although there was no change in balance parameters, subjects did demonstrate significant fatigue in their vastus lateralis and gluteus medius muscles after mechanical vibration.

Our contention is that specific WBV training would have a positive effect on patients with low back pain, based on the direct effect on increasing sensory (proprioceptive) input to the local and weightbearing muscles. However, it would be important to control the variables of posture, muscle specificity and the effects of fatigue if improvements in the joint protective mechanisms are to be achieved with the assistance of WBV.

A working posture with static or slow closed chain weightbearing exercise, involving eccentric lengthening contractions of the weightbearing muscles, would seem appropriate. In addition, a corset action (drawing in the abdominal wall) with a neutral lumbopelvic posture would likely direct the vibration stimulus specifically to the dysfunctional muscle groups. Therefore, WBV training with vertical load passing through the body (closed chain) would have the effect of enhancing gravitational load cues for muscle training and of targeting the local and weightbearing muscles. This feature would make WBV ideal to produce the neurophysiological countermeasures to the motor control changes occurring as a result of deloading (Ch. 7). The prolonged motor response with WBV may mean that this type of exercise could be used as a 'warm up' activity prior to high-load closed chain exercise to heighten the response of the local and weightbearing muscles to gravitational load cues. It would be likely to have a better response if the patient had bare feet with focus on heel pressure rather than pressure on the toes.

Muscle fatigue is common with WBV training in healthy individuals and so even more care would be needed if dysfunction of weightbearing and local muscles is present as these would fatigue very quickly. It would be important to recognize if muscle fatigue has occurred. Fatigue would cause an ache in the muscles themselves or loss of lumbopelvic position.

There would likely be a reduced exposure of the non-weightbearing muscles to the stimulus if given with vertical (closed chain) loading and quite possibly reduced activation, through a reduced tonic vibratory reflex. This would have advantages for prevention and treatment of low back pain as (as argued in Ch. 12) muscles such as the hamstrings, tensor fascia latae and quadratus lumborum may be overactive in many patients with low back pain.

In summary, WBV would likely produce a positive effect for prevention and management of low back pain from a motor control perspective. However, it should be recognized that this is a tool that must be used both with knowledge of the motor control dysfunction present in the patient and an understanding of the potent nature of the WBV stimulus on the neural system.

Chapter **16**

Open chain segmental control and progression into function

Carolyn Richardson and Julie Hides

INTRODUCTION

Much of everyday function and many sporting activities involve open chain movements. These may initially include movement of the limbs on a stable trunk. This is often used as a form of training and has been referred to in many exercise programmes as 'core stability'. The underlying principle of core stability training is that the limbs should move on a stable base. An example might be kicking a ball, where the predominant motion should be flexion of the hip and not flexion of the lumbar spine. A limitation of hip motion could then be responsible for unnecessary forces being imposed on the lumbar spine. Training may involve situations where the lumbar lordosis is maintained while loaded movements of the limbs are superimposed (see below).

The next phase of open chain segmental control involves movement of the spinal segments themselves. Spinal segmental movement is a normal component of spinal control, as movement aids in the dissipation of forces and the reduction of energy expenditure. From a range-of-motion perspective, many activities (in sport and in normal function) require that the spine moves. This movement may involve both high loads and high speeds. The role of the local synergy muscles is to control and protect the individual spinal segments, while the global muscles are used to dissipate force and generate torque and movement. A further consideration is that the global muscles generate internal forces when they are used to generate torque in open chain activities. The role of the local muscles in this situation is to minimize and control the forces imposed on the individual spinal segments. Maintaining local segmental control through initial drawing in of the abdominal wall to form the 'corset' action (in the absence of spinal movement) is required prior to all exercise techniques, whether formal or functional.

Integration of the local, weightbearing and non-weightbearing muscles is a prime focus of this stage of rehabilitation. Progression initially is monitored so that all muscles (i.e. the local, weightbearing and non-weightbearing) are integrated into functional movement tasks, initially in a formal way, so that compensations by non-weightbearing muscles can be detected as well as a lack of general trunk strength. It is an important point (which has been discussed in Ch. 15) that appropriate activation of the local and weightbearing muscles should result in decreased use of the non-weightbearing muscles if they are overactive. If this has occurred, stretching of overactive muscles should not be required.

There are two very important principles to consider in this third stage. The first is that, in normal function and movement, there may be a tendency for patients with low back pain to revert to previous poor patterns of muscle control. If the tendency of the body is to compensate with overactivity of the non-weightbearing muscles in situations of pain, injury and deloading, the control of the local synergy is going to be challenged in this phase. As it will be necessary to use the weightbearing and non-weightbearing muscles in function and movement, if local control is not good enough, this control may be lost. Consequently, the clinician must check local control often during the stages of closed chain and open chain segmental control. The second principle is that it will be necessary for the clinician to understand this tendency to revert to poor patterns of control and to devise appropriate strategies and countermeasures that will help to prevent this occurring.

SPECIFIC AIMS

The specific aims of open chain segmental control are:

- decrease compensatory movement of the lumbopelvic region during movement of adjacent segments;

- reduce tightness/overactivity in the non-weightbearing muscles if necessary; and
- treat problems of trunk muscle strength and endurance in open chain exercise.

Those for progression into function are:

- progress to functional (sporting and occupational) activities that use a combination of open and closed chain tasks, including trunk movement as well as higher loads and higher speeds;
- develop countermeasures to prevent loss of joint protection; and
- maintain segmental control and check regularly.

Aims of open chain segmental control

Decrease compensatory movement of the lumbopelvic region during movement of adjacent segments

A deficit of range of motion in any of the joints of the kinetic chain may lead to compensations in the lumbopelvic region. For example, a patient with limited shoulder extension range of motion may compensate by using lumbar extension in an attempt to reach overhead. Range of motion of adjacent spinal regions (cervical and especially the thoracic spine) and peripheral joints (especially the hip complex) should be examined. The need for good ranges of thoracic and hip motion in rotation during function is important, as compensatory rotation at the lumbar spine should be avoided during body rotational movements (explained in Ch. 12).

Example of assessment procedures for the hip and thoracic spine Two procedures are used:

- for hip range of movement on a stable/neutral lumbopelvic region: compare sides, especially rotation, and include both sides for comparison to note any asymmetry; and
- for thoracic spine range of movement on a stable/neutral lumbopelvic region: compare sides, usually in sitting.

Exercise management is determined by the problems found in assessment. There are, of course, many different causes of limited range of motion. Differential diagnosis between causes of limitation, such as fixed deformities, and alterable causes, such as tight or overactive non-weightbearing muscles, will allow a realistic prediction of the amount of change possible with treatment. Many therapeutic interventions may be useful in this stage to increase range of motion of adjacent segments (e.g. joint mobilization/manipulation if appropriate). Problem solving remains a crucial factor at this stage. In the presence of fixed deformities, ergonomic advice may be helpful. Also, it may be wise to avoid certain activities or situations. An example would be a patient with disc pathology that is aggravated by flexion activities and sitting on the floor. If examination revealed severe limitation of hip motion, which induced a high degree of forced flexion of the lumbar spine when the patient sits on the floor, this would be an activity best avoided or modified if the hip limitation proved irreversible. Modification may be something simple such as using a small stool (where a neutral lumbar position could be attained) if sitting at a low level was required by the patient.

Maintaining a neutral lumbopelvic posture is still important at this stage of treatment. The pressure biofeedback unit should be used under the spine to detect lumbopelvic movement during movement of adjacent body parts (see Appendix in Ch. 14, pp. 218–219). Its use should be explained to the patient prior to exercise (Fig. 16.1a). With the leg moving into abduction and external rotation (Fig. 16.1b), the patient focuses on learning dissociation of these hip movements from compensatory rotary movement of the lumbopelvic region. Straightening the leg to an extended abduction position adds a sagittal-plane control component. For both directions, the pressure biofeedback unit is placed under the lumbar lordosis to monitor its position. Once in position, it is inflated to 40 mmHg. Posterior pelvic tilting (lumbar flexion) will result in an increase in pressure, and anterior pelvic tilting will result in a decrease of pressure. In a side-lying position, the pressure biofeedback unit may be placed under the waist and the leg lifted into abduction while the pressure is maintained. In a sitting position, the pressure biofeedback unit may be placed behind the lumbar lordosis and the hip moved into flexion while the pressure is maintained.

Increasing the range of thoracic spine movement, especially for rotation, can be achieved in many ways including active exercises in four point

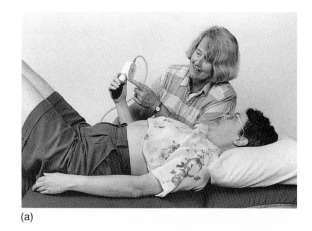

(a)

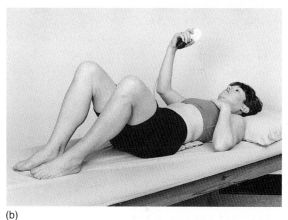

(b)

Figure 16.1   Training rotatory control. (a) With a light leg load. (b) With rotation at the hip with a static, neutral position of the lumbopelvic region.

kneeling, sitting or standing, as well as passive mobilizing techniques. Some clinicians require their sporting patients to move their arms and thoracic spine while maintaining a stable closed chain position (Fig. 16.2).

Reduce tightness/overactivity in the non-weightbearing muscles if necessary

It is our contention that training the local synergy muscles and the weightbearing muscles should result in a decrease of overactivity/tightness of the non-weightbearing muscles. However, some impairments may be present in this third stage. In a formal setting, overactive oblique abdominal muscles have been detected using resisted rotation

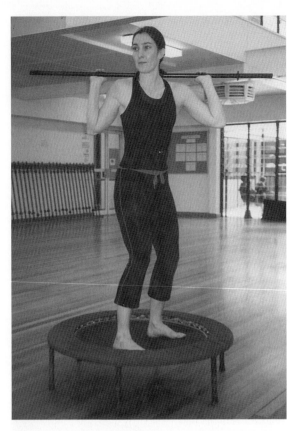

Figure 16.2 Active rotation of the thoracic spine, with a static, neutral position of the lumbopelvic region.

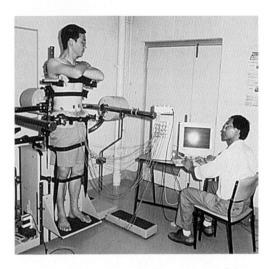

Figure 16.3 Testing the activation patterns of the oblique abdominal muscles during trunk rotation.

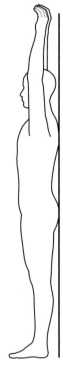

Figure 16.4 Performing an assessment of a full body stretch.

devices with the addition of surface electromyography (EMG) to detect the impairments in individual muscles (Ng et al 2002a) (Fig. 16.3). In a clinical setting, overactivity/tightness of individual muscles can be detected using muscle length assessment. Muscle lengthening procedures for individual muscles may be required.

Muscle lengthening procedures for muscles attaching to the lumbar spine and pelvis offer challenges to the maintainance of lumbopelvic stability. In addition, some muscles of the global system with attachments to the lumbar spine, such as the latissimus dorsi, must be able to lengthen without compromising the stability of the region.

Formal assessment of muscle length of several muscles of the lumbopelvic region could be undertaken, ensuring that lumbopelvic position is maintained during the tests. Prior to testing, the patient should be asked to stand against a wall with their arms above their head to check that this position of full body stretch can be achieved (Fig. 16.4).

Quadratus lumborum length testing could be assessed with trunk side flexion movement. Figure

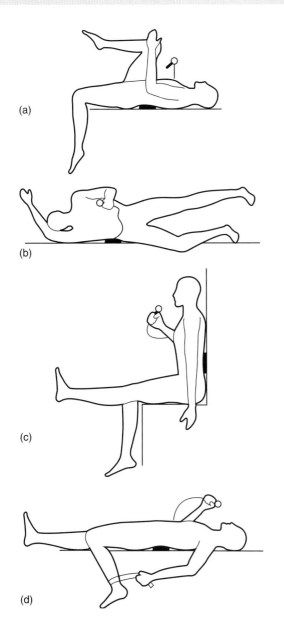

(a)

(b)

(c)

(d)

Figure 16.5 Examples of muscle-lengthening techniques in which lumbar spinal stability must be monitored: (a) iliopsoas; (b) tensor fasciae latae; (c) hamstrings; (d) rectus femoris.

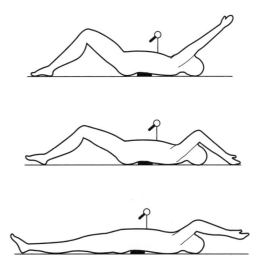

Figure 16.6 Training lumbopelvic control during lengthening of the latissimus dorsi.

16.5 demonstrates muscle length assessment (and lengthening techniques), using the pressure biofeedback to monitor the lumbopelvic position, for iliopsoas, tensor fascia lata, hamstrings and rectus femoris. Muscle length of the pectoralis major and latissimus dorsi may also need to be addressed

(Fig. 16.6) to ensure that they are not having a detrimental effect on lumbopelvic stability.

Various other specific muscle lengthening techniques could be used to increase the extensibility of these muscles, for example proprioceptive neuromuscular facilitation (PNF) contract/relax techniques, which focus on using an isometric contraction of the muscle requiring lengthening to induce a reflex relaxation to allow lengthening (Knott and Voss 1968).

Treat problems of trunk muscle strength and endurance in open chain exercise

Open chain exercise with increased loads can be used to increase the strength of the trunk. Leg loading, with hip flexion, extension, abduction or adduction, in positions such as lying, side lying, sitting or standing, can be used to increase the strength of the trunk muscles. It is important to maintain lumbopelvic stability during these open chain exercise tasks. Figure 16.7 shows examples of this type of exercise. Trunk strength could also be increased with upper limb loading (Fig. 16.8).

Open chain segmental training may begin at very low levels of load, and trunk strength and endurance may be increased through the use of progressive leg loading (Sahrmann 2002). The pressure biofeedback unit should be placed under the lumbar lordosis. Initially, training may be

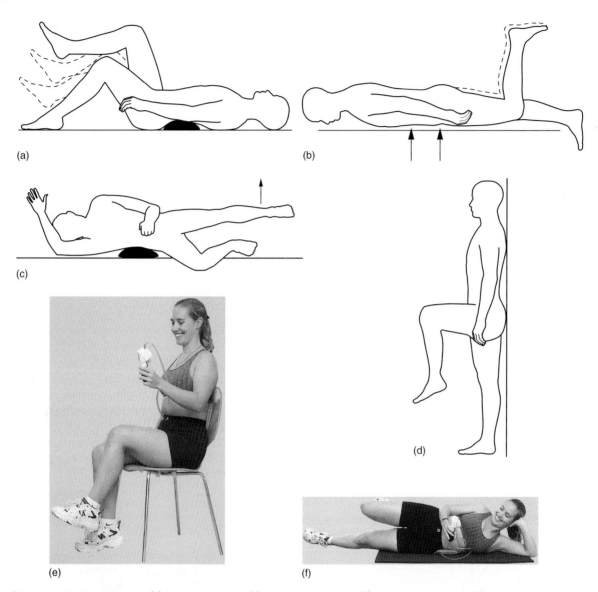

Figure 16.7   Trunk loading. (a) With hip flexion; (b) with hip extension; (c) with hip abduction; (d) with hip flexion (standing); (e) starting position for trunk loading with hip flexion in sitting and the patient monitoring the position of the lumbar spine; (f) with hip abduction and the patient monitoring the position of the lumbar spine. (Parts (e) and (f) reproduced with permission from Northwater Publishing, Australia.)

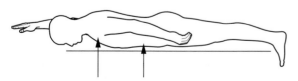

Figure 16.8   Loading the trunk with shoulder extension in lying. Note no movement of the spine is permitted.

commenced in the crook-lying position and with unilateral leg loading, the moving leg maintaining contact with the exercise surface in order to lessen the level of load to less than leg weight. The other leg provides some passive stability and remains supported. Increased loading may be achieved by lifting first one and then two legs from the exercise surface (Fig. 16.9).

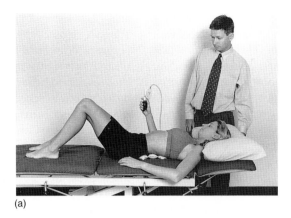

(a)

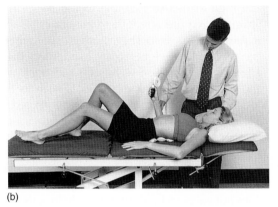 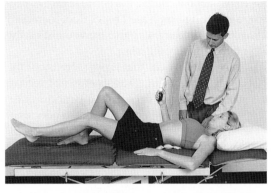

(b)

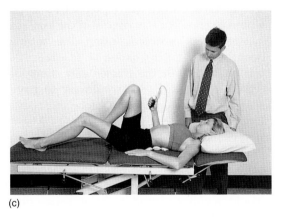 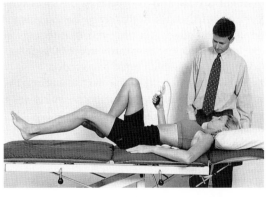

(c)

Figure 16.9 The progression of leg load in tests of control of lumbopelvic posture. (a) Preparation for the test. The requirements of the test to keep the pressure as steady as possible and the importance of maintaining the deep muscle corset action during the test are explained to the patient. The patient is positioned in supine crook lying, with the legs together or the legs abducted to emphasize rotatory control. The pressure sensor is positioned longitudinally on the side of the spine and inflated to 40 mmHg. The patient watches the pressure dial and draws in the abdominal wall. The pressure will increase slightly. The patient is instructed to keep the pressure level steady throughout the test. (b) Level 1 is the single leg slide with the contralateral leg supported. Left: leg slide with heel support to full extension and return; right: Unsupported leg slide: the heel is held approximately 5 cm from the exercise surface. (c) Level 2 is the single leg slide with the contralateral leg unsupported. Left: leg slide with heel support to full extension and return; right: unsupported leg slide: the heel is held approximately 5 cm from the exercise surface.

Exercises are performed with a common pro-forma. First, the patient draws in the abdominal wall in order to activate the corset. This co-contraction must be held throughout the entire leg-loading manoeuvre, while also maintaining a normal breathing pattern. The leg must be moved slowly, with the emphasis being on precision and control. The patient only moves the leg to positions in which the lumbopelvic position can be maintained. Control is defined by two parameters. There should be no change in pressure registered on the pressure biofeedback unit, as this signals loss of control of the lumbopelvic position, and the abdominal wall needs to remain flat during the entire exercise. Progression is through increased repetition, increased holding times (endurance) and movement of the limb(s) through full excursion.

It is important to note that if overactivity of the global muscles is present, patients may not need to undertake this stage of strengthening/endurance. It has been shown that the oblique abdominal muscles are less fatiguable in patients with low back pain than a control group (Ng et al 2002b). In line with this finding, some patients with low back pain perform leg-loading exercises better than control subjects as a result of this overactivity. Careful assessment is vital, and as control of the local synergy may be challenged at this stage, countermeasures may be required. A further risk of this stage is the patient developing co-contraction of the global muscles (rigidity), which must be avoided.

Various forms of exercise involve trunk strengthening and endurance work with the spine in a neutral position (e.g. Swiss ball exercises and pilates exercises). The principles described above would also apply to these techniques.

Specific aims of progression into function

Progress to functional activity (sporting and occupational)

Progress to functional (sporting and occupational) activities uses a combination of open and closed chain tasks, which include trunk movement as well as higher loads and higher speeds. This next stage of strengthening/endurance exercises involves movement of the spine. Classic exercises that use the body weight as resistance would include sit-ups and back extension exercises. Endurance of the spinal extensors has been evaluated using the Sorenson test. Further resistance can be added by using free weights or equipment such as the MedX. Progression to heavily loaded trunk exercises may be appropriate when the sport or occupation that the patient performs requires high levels of strength and endurance. Care must still be taken in evaluating the loads imposed on the spine following injury (e.g. influence of exercise on aspects such as discal pressure).

Many sports involve a combination of open and closed chain tasks, trunk movement, high speeds and high loads. An example would be sprinting. Sprinters require strength to generate the forces required to run fast. They perform strengthening exercises in the weights room. In addition, there is a heavy emphasis on technique and track work, and minimizing trunk movements such as trunk rotation. Use of the muscle synergy is altered during sprinting, as many sprinters hold their breath as they sprint, temporarily trading respiration for maximal stabilization. In addition, sprinting is a repetitive ballistic activity, which by its nature requires phasic and fast muscle contractions. It does not encompass slow closed chain activity. If a sprinter breaks down with back pain, our approach would require first that control of the local muscle synergy was restored, using the techniques described in detail in Chapter 14. To achieve this, in consultation with the trainer and strength and conditioning coach, we would try to have the sprinter stop strength training for a short period of time (e.g. a couple of weeks) to allow the best possible chance of activating the local muscle synergy. We would hope to minimize or alleviate the patient's painful symptoms in this stage, depending upon the pathology present. The next phase would revolve around techniques described in Chapter 15, with progressive increases in gravitational load cues. The aim of these two phases is to maximize safe and effective load transfer and joint protection. Many strength and training programmes will challenge the instilled joint protection mechanisms but are obviously required for top-level performance. To reconcile these issues, two aspects should be addressed. These include development of countermeasures to prevent loss of local segmental control and maintaining and checking segmental control regularly.

Develop countermeasures to maximize joint protection

The segmental stabilization training approach is based on progression through stages. However, even when the initial stage (local segmental control) is achieved, progression through the next two stages will challenge this control. It is important to develop countermeasures to prevent loss of joint protection and control.

Education of patients in the philosophy and science behind this approach is vital. If the patient does not understand the approach, compliance will be poor. The patient also needs to understand why certain activities will be avoided in the early stages. Once control of the local synergy is achieved, progression into closed chain activities will challenge local segmental control. A common mistake is to progress this stage too quickly. If the weightbearing muscles do not respond appropriately to load, the non-weightbearing muscles will compensate, eventually becoming overactive and/or tight. This is a risk at each stage, because this tendency to overactivate the non-weightbearing muscles occurs in low back pain and the control of the local and weightbearing muscles seems to be more fragile in nature. The end result of continuing to progress the patient when local control and joint protection is lost is likely to be recurrence of painful symptoms.

To progress from stage 1 to stage 2, the basic requirement is co-contraction of the muscles of the local synergy in supine, prone, side lying, sitting and standing. Adequate control of the lumbopelvic position is also a requirement. Before exercises of stage 2 (closed chain segmental control) are commenced, the local synergy muscles should first be 'turned on'. In the sporting arena, athletes can be encouraged to include this in their 'warm-up'. As a protective measure, this should be done before all exercise sessions and should be incorporated into the athlete's routine. The order of loading and exercise can also work as a protective measure. The local muscles can be activated, prior to closed chain exercises, and both stages 1 and 2 should be performed before stage 3 (open chain segmental control). In open chain segmental control, exercises that do not involve movement of the lumbopelvic region should be performed prior to exercises that move the spine and exercises that are high in load and/or high in speed. For sporting teams, apparatus such as whole body vibration could be used to provide a countermeasure before closed chain exercises are performed. This would be useful to enhance the activity of the weightbearing muscles and decrease the activity of the non-weightbearing muscles, giving the athlete a window of opportunity to enhance closed chain exercises.

Maintain segmental control and check regularly

The best way for the patient or athlete with low back pain to ascertain if the muscles of the local muscle synergy are active is by palpating the muscles as they try to activate them. This is possibly one of the most important aspects of the whole approach. If the patient is to perform contractions of the local muscle synergy as a warm-up, it is vital that they can use palpation to check that they are performing the contraction well. It may also be best to perform the contraction in the position that they can best and consistently activate the muscles. As progression is attempted, the patient or athlete should test whether they can still effectively activate the muscles of the local synergy. For example, after attempting some closed or open chain segmental exercises, the patient or athlete could lie down and try to activate the muscles of the local synergy. If they are successful, progression is probably occurring according to plan. If the muscles can be activated but cannot be held, this would indicate that the patient has probably done enough in that session. If the patient/athlete is unable to activate the local muscles, this would suggest that compensation by the non-weightbearing muscles has occurred, and progression has been too quick. Ultrasound imaging can be used at this stage to confirm this result if there is any confusion or dispute. This is the most effective way to ensure that the joint protection mechanisms are operational.

CONCLUSION

We have presented an approach to therapeutic and preventative exercise based on progression through three stages. This approach is based on a considerable amount of research and clinical experience. The approach relies heavily on problem solving. There are several approaches and methods of exercise available to patients with low back pain, athletes and the general public. Our hope would be that this approach would allow the clinician to incorporate several different exercise approaches in a logical manner by understanding and applying the principles presented.

An example of a muscle assessment form is included in the Appendix below. This could form part of the patients full subjective and objective assessment.

APPENDIX: MUSCLE ASSESSMENT

The following form is an example of an assessment profile.

NAME: **DATE:**

1. Assessment of local muscle system

1a. Manual assessment

1b. Multifidus muscle assessment

(i) Palpation

(ii) Activation

(iii) Ultrasound imaging

Vertebral level	Cross-sectional area (cm^2)		Activation	
	Left	Right	Left	Right
L2				
L3				
L4				
L5				
S1				

(iv) Consistency changes

(v) Comments

1c. Muscles of the abdominal wall

Prone pressure biofeedback test

(i) Pressure change

(ii) Palpation

(iii) Spinal movement

Supine pressure biofeedback test

(i) Palpation

(ii) Symmetry

(iii) Ultrasound assessment

Quality of activation	Left	Right
Tensions anterior fascia		
Transversus abdominis thickens		
Transversus abdominis wraps around waistline		
Oblique activation		
Symmetry		

(iv) Movement of anterior abdominal wall posteriorly

(v) Anterolateral abdominal wall muscle dimensions (in mm)

	At rest		Drawing in	
Muscle	Left	Right	Left	Right
Transversus abdominis				
Obliquus internus abdominis				
Obliquus externus abdominis				

Comments:

2. Closed chain muscle assessment

2a. Upper quadrant closed chain exercise (maintenance of spinal curves)

2b. Trunk forward lean (maintenance of spinal curves)

2c. Grade 3 antigravity muscle tests

(i) Gluteus maximus

(ii) Iliopsoas

(iii) Gluteus medius

(iv) Adductor magnus and brevis

2d. Wall squat

2e. Closed chain exercise in flexed postures

(i) Slow lunge

(ii) Semi-squat

2f. Closed chain with addition of unstable surfaces

(i) Balance boards

(ii) Discs

2g. Closed chain on more challenging surfaces and in more upright postures

(i) Slopes, sand

(ii) Whole body vibration

3. Open chain segmental control

3a. Assessment of mobility of adjacent segments

(i) Cervical spine

(ii) Thoracic spine

(iii) Shoulder complex

(iv) Hip pelvic complex

(v) Knee

(vi) Ankle

3b. Maintenance of lumbopelvic position with PBV
(i) Single leg slide, other leg supported

(ii) Single leg slide, other leg unsupported

(iii) Single leg extension, other leg supported

(iv) Single leg extension, other leg unsupported

(vi) Hip rotation

(vii) Double leg slide

(viii) Double leg extension

3c. Muscle length testing
(i) Full body stretch against wall

(ii) Quadratus lumborum

(iii) Latissimus dorsi

(iv) Pectoralis major

(v) Iliopsoas

(vi) Tensor fascia lata

(vii) Hamstrings

(viii) Rectus femoris

3d. Trunk muscle strength: leg loading with PBV in situ
(i) Hip flexion

(ii) Hip extension

(iii) Hip abduction

(iv) Hip adduction

(v) Upper limb loading

3e. Trunk muscle strength with trunk movement
(i) Sit-up

(ii) Back extension

3f. Trunk muscle strength/endurance with apparatus
(i) Flexion

(ii) Extension

(iii) Lateral flexion

(iv) Rotation

3g. Trunk muscle endurance: Sorenson test

References

Abe T, Kusuhara N, Yoshimura N, Tomita T, Easton P A 1996 Differential respiratory activity of four abdominal muscles in humans. Journal of Applied Physiology 80:1379–1389

Abumi K, Panjabi M M, Kramer K M, Duranceau J, Oxland T, Crisco J J 1990 Biomechanical evaluation of lumbar spinal stability after graded facetectomies. Spine 15:1142–1147

Agostoni E, Sant'Ambrogio G 1970 The diaphragm. In: Campbell E J M, Agostoni E, Newsom-Davis J (eds) The respiratory muscles: mechanisms and neural control. Lloyd-Luke, London, pp 145–160

Agostoni E, Campbell E J M 1970 The abdominal muscles. In: Campbell E J M, Agostoni E, Newsom-Davis J (eds) The respiratory muscles: mechanisms and neural control. Lloyd-Luke, London, pp 175–180

Alaranta H, Tallroth K, Soukka A, Heliovaara M 1993 Fat content of lumbar extensor muscles and low back disability: a radiographic and clinical comparison. Journal of Spinal Disorders 6:137–140

Amonoo-Kuofi H S 1983 The density of muscle spindles in the medial, intermediate and lateral columns of human intrinsic post-vertebral muscles. Journal of Anatomy 136:509–519

Anderson J 1983 Grant's atlas of anatomy. Williams & Wilkins, Baltimore, MD

Andersson G, Bogduk N, DeLuca C et al 1989 Muscle. In: Frymoyer J W, Gordon S L (eds) New perspectives on low back pain. American Academy of Orthopedic Surgeons, Rosemont, IL, pp 291–230

Andersson E, Oddsson L, Grundstrom H, Thorstensson A 1995 The role of the psoas and iliacus muscles for stability and movement of the lumbar spine, pelvis and hip. Scandinavian Journal of Medicine Science Sports 5:10–16

Andersson E A, Oddsson L I E, Grundstrom O M, Nilsson J, Thorstensson A 1996 EMG activities of the quadratus lumborum and erector spinae muscles during flexion–relaxation and other motor tasks. Clinical Biomechanics 11:392–400

Andersson E A, Nilsson J, Thortensson A 1997 Intramuscular EMG from the hip flexor muscles during human locomotion. Acta Physiologica Scandinavica 161:361–370

Angel R W, Eppler W, Iannone A 1965 Silent period produced by unloading of muscle during voluntary contraction. Journal of Physiology 180:864–870

Antonutto G, Capelli C, Girardis M, Zamparo P, diPrampero P 1999 Effects of microgravity on maximal power of lower limbs during very short efforts in humans. Journal of Applied Physiology 86:85–92

Appell H J 1986 Skeletal muscle atrophy during immobilisation. International Journal of Sports Medicine 7:1–5

Appell H J 1990 Muscular atrophy following immobilisation: a review. Sports Medicine 10:42–58

Arendt-Nielsen L, Graven-Nielsen T, Svarrer H, Svensson P 1996 The influence of low back pain on muscle activity and coordination during gait: a clinical and experimental study. Pain 64:231–240

Aruin A S, Latash M L 1995 Directional specificity of postural muscles in feed-forward postural reactions during fast voluntary arm movements. Experimental Brain Research 103:323–332

Asfour S S, Khalil T M, Waly S M, Goldberg M L, Rosomoff R S, Rosomoff H L 1990 Biofeedback in back muscle strengthening. Spine 15:510–513

Askar O M 1977 Surgical anatomy of the aponeurotic expansions of the anterior abdominal wall. Annals of the Royal College of Surgeons of England 59: 313–321

Asmussen E, Klausen K 1962 Form and function of the erect human spine. Clinical Orthopaedics and Related Research 25:55–63

Aspden R M 1992 Review of the functional anatomy of the spinal ligaments and the lumbar erector spinae muscles. Clinical Anatomy 5:372–387

Aspinall W 1993 Clinical implications of iliopsoas dysfunction. Journal of Manual and Manipulative Therapy 1:41–46

Bagnall K M, Ford D M, McFadden K D, Greenhill B J, Raso V J 1984 The histochemical composition of human vertebral muscle. Spine 9:470–473

Baroni G, Perdrocchi A, Perrigano G, Massion J, Pedotti A 2001 Static and dynamic postural control in long-term microgravity: evidence of a dual adaptation. Journal of Applied Physiology 88:473–478

Bartelink D L 1957 The role of intra-abdominal pressure in relieving the pressure on the lumbar vertebral discs. Journal of Bone and Joint Surgery 39B:718–725

Baxendale R H, Ferrell W R, Wood L 1987 The effect of mechanical stimulation of knee joint afferents on quadriceps motor unit activity in the decerebrate cat. Brain Research 415:353–356

Bednar D A, Orr F W, Simon G T 1995 Observations on the pathology of the thoraco-lumbar fascia in chronic mechanical low back pain. Spine 20:1161–1164

Beith I D, Harrison P J 2001 Reflex control of the human internal oblique muscles. Society of Neuroscience Abstracts 27:936.3

Belen'kii V, Gurfinkel V S, Paltsev Y 1967 Elements of control of voluntary movements. Biofizika 12:135–141

Berberich P, Hoheisel U, Mense S, Skeppar P 1987 Fine muscle afferent fibres and inflammation: changes in discharge behaviour and influence on motor neurones. In Schmidt RF, Schaible HG, Vahle C (eds) Fine afferent fibres and pain. Verlag Gesellschaft, Hinz Weinheim, pp 167–175

Bergmark A 1989 Stability of the lumbar spine. A study in mechanical engineering. Acta Orthopaedica Scandinavica 230(Suppl):20–24

Biedermann H J, Shanks G L, Forrest W J, Inglis J 1991 Power spectrum analysis of electromyographic activity: discriminators in the differential assessment of patients with chronic low back pain. Spine 16:1179–1185

Blasier R B, Carpenter J E, Huston L J 1994 Shoulder proprioception: effect on joint laxity, joint position and direction. Orthopaedic Review 23:45–50

Bobbert M F, van Soerst A J 2000 Two-joint muscles offer the solution, but what was the problem? Motor Control 4:48–52

Bogduk N 1997 Clinical anatomy of the lumbar spine and sacrum, 3rd edn. Churchill Livingstone, Edinburgh

Bogduk N, Macintosh J E 1984 The applied anatomy of the thoracolumbar fascia. Spine 9:164–170

Bogduk N, Twomey L T 1987 Clinical anatomy of the lumbar spine. Churchill Livingstone, Melbourne

Bogduk N, Wilson A S, Tynan W 1982 The lumbar dorsal rami. Journal of Anatomy 134:383–397

Bogduk N, Pearcy M, Hadfield G 1992a Anatomy and biomechanics of the psoas major. Clinical Biomechanics 7:109–119

Bogduk N, Macintosh J E, Pearcy M J 1992b A universal model of the lumbar back muscles in the upright position. Spine 17:897–913

Bogduk N, Amevo B, Pearcy M 1995 A biological basis for instantaneous centres of rotation of the vertebral column. Proceedings of the Institute of Mechanical Engineering [H] 209:177–183

Booth F W 1978 Regrowth of atrophied skeletal muscle in adult rats after ending immobilisation. Journal of Applied Physiology 44:225–230

Bosco C, Iacovelli M, Tsarpela O 2000 Hormonal responses to whole-body vibration in men. European Journal of Applied Physiology 81:449–454

Bouisset S, Duchene J L 1994 Is body balance more perturbed by respiration in seating than in standing posture? Neuroreport 5:957–960

Bouisset S, Zattara M 1981 A sequence of postural adjustments precedes voluntary movement. Neuroscience Letters 22:263–270

Bower K D 1986 The role of exercises in low back pain. In: Grieve G (ed) Modern manual therapy of the vertebral column. Churchill Livingstone, Edinburgh, pp 839–848

Bradley K C 1974 The anatomy of backache. Australia and New Zealand Journal of Surgery 44:227–232

Brumagne S, Lysens R, Spaepen A 1999a Lumbosacral repositioning accuracy in standing posture: a combined electrogoniometric and videographic evaluation. Clinical Biomechanics 14:361–363

Brumagne S, Lysens R, Spaepen A 1999b Lumbo-pelvic position sense during pelvic tilting in men and women without low back pain: test development and reliability assessment. Journal of Orthopedic and Sports Physical Therapy 29:30–36

Brumagne S, Cordo P, Lysens R, Verschueren S, Swinnen S 2000 The role of paraspinal muscle spindles in lumbo-pelvic position sense in individuals with and without low back pain. Spine 25:989–994

Bryner P 1996 Unilateral back pain: a case series of quadratus lumborum involvement. Chiropractic Technique 8:70–77

Bullock-Saxton J E, Janda V, Bullock M I 1993 Reflex activation of gluteal muscles in walking: an approach to restoration of muscle function for patients with low-back pain. Spine 18:704–708

Burke R E 1980 Motor units in mammalian muscle. In: Summer A J (ed) The physiology of peripheral nerve disease. Saunders, Philadelphia, PA, p 133

Burke R E, Edgerton V R 1975 Unit properties and selective involvement in movement. Exercise and Sports Science Reviews 3:31–81

Butler D S 2000 Sensitive nervous system. NOI Publications, Adelaide

Buyruk H, Stam H, Snijders C 1999 Measurement of sacroiliac joint stiffness in peripartum pelvic pain patients with Doppler imaging of vibrations (DIV). European Journal of Obstetrics, Gynecology and Reproductive Biology 83:159–163

Campbell E J M 1952 An electromyographic study of the role of the abdominal muscles in breathing. Journal of Physiology 117:222–233

Campbell E J M, Green J H 1955 The behaviour of the abdominal muscles and the intra-abdominal pressure during quiet breathing and increased pulmonary ventilation. Journal of Physiology 127:423–426

Carman D J, Blanton P L, Biggs N L 1972 Electromyographic study of the antero-lateral abdominal musculature using indwelling electrodes. American Journal of Physical Medicine 15:113–129

Carpenter J E, Blasier R B, Pellizzon G G 1998 The effects of muscle fatigue on shoulder joint position sense. American Journal of Sports Medicine 26:262–265

Cassisi J E, Robinson M E, O'Connor P, MacMillan M 1993 Trunk strength and lumbar paraspinal muscle activity during isometric exercise in chronic low back pain patients and controls. Spine 18:245–251

Cavanaugh J M, Ozaktay C A, Yamashita T, Hing A I 1996 Lumbar facet pain: biomechanics, neuroanatomy and neurophysiology. Journal of Biomechanics, 29:1117–1129

Chesworth B M, Padfield B J, Helewa A, Stitt L W 1994 A comparison of hip mobility in patients with low back pain and matched healthy controls. Physiotherapy Canada 46:267–273

Cholewicki J, McGill S 1992 Lumbar posterior ligament involvement during extremely heavy lifts estimated from fluoroscopic measurement. Journal of Biomechanics 25:17–28

Cholewicki J, McGill S M 1996 Mechanical stability of the in vivo lumbar spine: implications for injury and low back pain. Clinical Biomechanics 11:1–15

Cholewicki J, van Vliet I J 2002 Relative contribution of trunk muscles to the stability of the lumbar spine during isometric exertions. Clinical Biomechanics (Bristol) 17:99–105

Cholewicki J, McGill S M, Norman R W 1991 Lumbar spine loads during the lifting of extremely heavy weights. Medicine and Science in Sports and Exercise 23:1179–1186

Cholewicki J, Panjabi M M, Khachatryan A 1997 Stabilizing function of trunk flexor–extensor muscles around a neutral spine posture. Spine 22:2207–2212

Cholewicki J, Juluru K, McGill S M 1999a Intra-abdominal pressure mechanism for stabilizing the lumbar spine. Journal of Biomechanics 32:13–17

Cholewicki J, Juluru K, Radebold A, Panjabi M M, McGill S M 1999b Lumbar spine stability can be augmented with an abdominal belt and/or increased intra-abdominal pressure. European Spine Journal 8:388–395

Cooper R G, Clair Forbes W S T, Jayson M I V 1992 Radiographic demonstration of paraspinal muscle wasting in patients with chronic low back pain. British Journal of Rheumatology 31:389–394

Craig A D, Heppelmann B, Schaible H G 1988 The projection of the medial and posterior articular nerves of the cat's knee to the spinal cord. Journal of Comparative Neurology 276:279–288

Cresswell A G 1993 Responses of intra-abdominal pressure and abdominal muscle activity during dynamic trunk loading in man. European Journal of Applied Physiology 66:315–320

Cresswell A G, Thorstensson A 1994 Change in intra-abdominal pressure, trunk muscle activation and force during isokinetic lifting and lowering. European Journal of Applied Physiology 68:315–321

Cresswell A G, Grundstrom A, Thorstensson A 1992a Observations on intra-abdominal pressure and patterns of abdominal intra-muscular activity in man. Acta Physiologica Scandinavica 144:409–418

Cresswell A G, Oddsson L, Thorstensson A 1992b Compensatory responses to sudden perturbations of the trunk during standing. In: Horak W M, Horak F (eds) Posture and gait: control mechanisms. University of Oregon Books, Portland, OR, pp 380–383

Cresswell A G, Blake P L, Thorstensson A 1993 The effect of an abdominal muscle training program on the intra-abdominal pressure. Scandinavian Journal of Rehabilitation Medicine 26:79–86

Cresswell A G, Oddsson L, Thorstensson A 1994 The influence of sudden perturbations on trunk muscle activity and intra-abdominal pressure while standing. Experimental Brain Research 98:336–341

Crisco J J, Panjabi M M 1991 The intersegmental and multisegmental muscles of the spine: a biomechanical model comparing lateral stabilising potential. Spine 7:793–799

Crisco J J, Panjabi M M, Yamamoto I, Oxland T R 1992 Euler stability of the human ligamentous lumbar spine. Clinical Biomechanics 7:27–32

Critchley D 2002 Instructing pelvic floor contraction facilitates transversus abdominis thickness increase during low-abdominal hollowing. Physiotherapy Research International 7:65–75

Crombez G, Eccleston C, Baeyens F, Eelen P 1998 Attentional disruption is enhanced by the threat of pain. Behavioral Research Therapy 36:195–204

Crombez G, Eccleston C, Baeyens F, Eelen P 1999 Attention to chronic pain is dependent upon pain-related fear. Journal of Psychosomatic Research 47:403–410

Cullen M J, Mastaglia F L 1982 Pathological reactions of skeletal muscle. In: Mastaglia F L, Walton J N (eds) Skeletal muscle pathology. Churchill Livingstone, Edinburgh, pp 88–139

Daggfeldt K, Thorstensson A 1991 The role of intra-abdominal pressure in spinal unloading. Journal of Biomechanics 30:1149–1155

Dalstra M, Huiskes R 1995 Load transfer across the pelvic bone. Journal of Biomechanics 28:715–724

Damen L, Stijen T, Roebroeck M, Snijders C, Stam H 2002 Reliability of sacroiliac joint laxity measurement with doppler imaging of vibrations. Ultrasound in Medicine and Biology 28:407–414

Dangaria T R, Naesh O 1998 Changes in cross-sectional area of psoas major muscle in unilateral sciatica caused by disc herniation. Spine 23:928–931

Danneels L A, van der Straeten G G, Cambier D C, Witvrouw E E, Cuyper H J 2000 CT imaging of trunk muscles in chronic low back pain patients and healthy control subjects. European Spine Journal 9:266–272

Danneels L, van der Straeten G, Cambier D, Witvrouw E, de Cuyper H 2001 The effects of three different training modalities on the cross-sectional area of the lumbar multifidus. British Journal of Sports Medicine 35:186–194

DeAndre J R, Grant C, Dixon A S J 1965 Joint distension and reflex muscle inhibition in the knee. Journal of Bone and Joint Surgery 47A:313–322

Deindl F, Vodusek D, Hesse U, Schussler B 1993 Activity patterns of pubococcygeal muscles in nulliparous continent women. British Journal of Urology 72:46–51

Deindl F, Vodusek D, Hesse U, Schussler B 1994 Pelvic floor activity patterns: comparison of nulliparous continent and parous urinary stress incontinent women. A kinesiological EMG study. British Journal of Urology 73:413–417

Denny-Brown D E 1929 The histological features of striped muscle in relation to its functional activity. Proceedings of the Royal Society of London, Series B 104:371–411

Derbyshire S W, Jones A K, Gyulai F, Clark S, Townsend D, Firestone L L 1997 Pain processing during three levels of noxious stimulation produces differential patterns of central activity. Pain 73:431–445

Desmedt J E, Godaux E 1978, Ballistic contractions in fast and slow human muscles: discharge patterns of single motor units, Journal of Physiology 285:185–196

DeTroyer A 1983 Mechanical role of the abdominal muscles in relation to posture. Respiration Physiology 53:341–353

DeTroyer A, Estenne M 1988 Functional anatomy of the respiratory muscles. In: Belman M J (ed) Respiratory muscles: function in health and disease. Saunders, Philadelphia, PA, pp 175–195

DeTroyer A, Estenne M, Ninane V, VanGansbeke D, Gorini M 1990 Transversus abdominis muscle function in humans. Journal of Applied Physiology 68:1010–1016

Dimitrijevic M R, Gregoric M R, Sherwood A M, Spencer W A 1980 Reflex responses of paraspinal muscles to tapping. Journal of Neurology, Neurosurgery and Psychiatry 43:1112–1118

Donisch E W, Basmajian J V 1972 Electromyography of deep back muscles in man. American Journal of Anatomy 133:15–36

Duchateau J, Hainaut K 1990 Effects of immobilisation on contractile properties, recruitment and firing rates of human motor units. Journal of Physiology, 422:55–65

Dudley G A, Duvoisin M R, Convertino V A, Buchanan P 1989 Alterations of the in vivo torque-velocity relationship of human skeletal muscle following 30 days exposure to simulated microgravity. Aviation, Space and Environmental Medicine 60:659–663

Eccles R M, Lundberg A 1959a Synaptic actions in motoneurones by afferents which may evoke the flexion reflex. Archives Italiennes de Biologie 97:199–221

Eccles R M, Lundberg A 1959b Supraspinal control of interneurones mediating spinal reflexes. Journal of Physiology 147:565–584

Eccleston C, Crombez G 1999 Pain demands attention: a cognitive-affective model of the interruptive function of pain. Psychological Bulletin 125:356–366

Ecleshymer A C, Schoemaker D M 1970 A cross-sectional anatomy. Butterworths, London

Edgerton V R, Zhou M Y, Ohira Y et al 1995 Human fiber size and enzymatic properties after 5 and 11 days of spaceflight. Journal of Applied Physiology 78:1733–1739

Ekberg K, Eklund J 1995 Psychological stress and muscle activity during data entry at visual display units. Work Stress 9:475–490

Ekholm J, Eklund G, Skoglund S 1960 On reflex effects from knee joint of cats. Acta Physiologica Scandinavica 50:167–174

Fairbank J C T, O'Brien J P 1980 The abdominal cavity and thoracolumbar fascia as stabilisers of the lumbar spine in patients with low back pain. In: Engineering aspects of the spine. London, Mechanical Engineering Publications vol 2, pp 83–88

Fairbank J C T, O'Brien J P, Davis P R 1980 Intra-abdominal pressure rise during weight lifting as an objective measure of low-back pain. Spine 5:179–184

Farfan H F 1973 Mechanical disorders of the low back. Lea & Febiger, Philadelphia, PA

Farfan H F 1975 Muscular mechanism of the lumbar spine and the position of power and efficiency. Orthopedic Clinics of North America 6:135–145

Ferreira P, Hodges P, Ferreira M 2003 Changes recruitment of the abdominal muscles in people with low back pain: ultrasound measurement of muscle activity. In: Proceedings of the 14th International Congress of the World Confederation for Physical Therapists, Barcelona, Spain

Ferrell W R, Nade S, Newbold P J 1986 The interrelation of neural discharge, intra-articular pressure and joint angle in the knee of the dog. Journal of Neurophysiology 373:353–365

Ferrell W R, Wood L, Baxendale R H 1988 The effect of acute joint inflammation on flexion reflex excitability in the decerebrate low spinal cat. Quarterly Journal of Experimental Neurophysiology 73:95–102

Fidler M W, Jowett R L, Troup J D G 1975 Myosin ATPase activity in multifidus muscle from cases of lumbar spinal derangement. Journal of Bone and Joint Surgery 57B:220–227

Fijtek M, Wassersug R 1999 Effect of laparotomy, cage type, gestation period and spaceflight on abdominal muscles of pregnant rodents. Journal of Experimental Zoology 284:252–264

Fijtek M, Wassersug R 2001 Effects of spaceflight and cage design on abdominal muscles of male rodents. Journal of Experimental Zoology 289:330–334

Finkelstein M M 2002 Medical conditions, medications, and urinary incontinence. Analysis of a population-based survey. Canadian Family Physician 48:96–101

Fitts P M, Posner M I 1967 Human performance. Brooks/Cole, Belmont, C A

Fitts R H, Brimmer C J 1985 Recovery in skeletal muscle contractile function after prolonged hindlimb immobilization. Journal of Applied Physiology 59:916–923

Fitts R H, Bodine S C, Romatowski J G, Widrick J J 1998 Velocity, force, power and Ca^{2+} sensitivity of fast and slow monkey skeletal muscle fibers, Journal of Applied Physiology 84:1776–1787

Fitts R H, Riley D R, Widrick J J 2000 Invited review: microgravity and skeletal muscle. Journal of Applied Physiology 89:823–839

Flor H D, Birbaumer N 1992 Symptom-specific psychophysiological responses in chronic pain patients. Psychophysiology 29:452–460

Flor H D, Turk C 1989 Psychophysiology of chronic pain: do chronic pain patients exhibit symptom-specific psychophysiological responses? Psychology Bulletin 105:215–259

Flor H D, Braun C, Elbert T, Birbaumer N 1997 Extensive reorganization of primary somatosensory cortex in chronic back pain patients. Neuroscience Letters 224:5–8

Floyd W F, Silver P H S 1950 Electromyographic study of patterns of activity of the anterior abdominal wall muscles in man. Journal of Anatomy 84:132–145

Floyd W F, Silver P H S 1951 Function of erector spinae in flexion of the trunk. Lancet 20:133–134

Ford D, Bagnall K M, McFadden H D, Greenhill B, Raso J 1983 Analysis of vertebral muscle obtained during surgery for correction of a lumbar disc disorder. Acta Anatomica 116:152–157

Forssberg H, Hirschfeld H 1994 Postural adjustments in sitting humans following external perturbations: muscle activity and kinematics. Experimental Brain Research 97:515–527

Freeman M A R, Wyke B 1967 The innervation of the knee joint. An anatomical and histological study in the cat. Journal of Anatomy 101:505–532

Frymoyer J W, Pope M H, Wilder D G 1990 Segmental instability. In: Weinstein J N, Wiesel S (eds) The lumbar spine. Saunders, Philadelphia, PA, pp 612–636

Gagey P 1986 Postural disorders among workers on building sites. In: Bles W, Brandt T (eds) Disorders of posture and gait. Elsevier, Amsterdam, pp 253–268

Gahery Y, Massion J 1981 Co-ordination between posture and movement. Trends in Neuroscience 4:199–202

Gandevia S C, McCloskey D I, Burke D 1992 Kinaesthetic signals and muscle contraction. Trends in Neurosciences 15:62–65

Gandevia S C, Allen G M, Butler J E, Taylor J L 1996 Supraspinal factors in human muscle fatigue: evidence for suboptimal output from the motor cortex. Journal of Physiology (Lond) 490:529–536

Gardner E 1950 Reflex muscular responses to stimulation of articular nerves in the cat. American Journal of Physiology 161:133–141

Gardner E, Latimer F, Stilwell D 1949 Central connections for afferent fibres from the knee joint of the cat. American Journal of Physiology 159:195–198

Gardner-Morse M, Stokes I A F, Lauble J P 1995 Role of the muscles in lumbar spine stability in maximum extension efforts. Journal of Orthopaedic Research 13:802–808

Gardner-Morse M G, Stokes I A 1998 The effects of abdominal muscle coactivation on lumbar spine stability. Spine 23:86–91

Gejo R, Kawaguchi Y, Kondoh T et al 2000 Magnetic resonance imaging and histologic evidence of postoperative back muscle injury in rats. Spine 25:941–946

Gentile A M 1987 Skill acquisition: action, movement and neuromuscular processes. In Carr J H, Shepherd R B, Gordon J, Gentile A M, Hinds J M (eds) Movement and science: foundations for physical therapy in rehabilitation. Aspe, Rockville, MD, pp 93–154

Gerber C, Hoppeler H, Claasen H, Robotti G, Zehndu R 1985 The lower extremity musculature in chronic symptomatic instability of the anterior cruciate ligament. Journal of Bone and Joint Surgery 67:1034–1043

Gibbons S 2001 Biomechanics and stability mechanisms of psoas major. In: Vleeming A, Mooney V, Gracovetsky S A et al (eds) The fourth interdisciplinary world congress on low back pain and pelvic pain. European Conference Organisers, Montreal, Canada, pp 246–247

Gill K P, Callaghan M J 1998 The measurement of lumbar proprioception in individuals with and without low back pain. Spine 23:371–377

Goel V K, Gilbertson L G 1995 Applications of the finite element method to thoracolumbar spinal research – past, present and future. Spine 20:1719–1727

Goel V K, Kong W, Han J S, Weinstein D O, Gilbertson L G 1993 A combined finite element and optimization of lumbar spine mechanics with and without muscles. Spine 18:1531–1541

Golby L, Moore A, Doust J, Trew M 2001 A RCT investigating the efficacy of manual therapy, exercises to rehabilitate spinal stabilisation and an education booklet in the conservative treatment of chronic low back pain. In: Proceedings of the 1st International Conference on Movement Dysfunction, Edinburgh, p 19

Goldberg A L 1967 Protein synthesis in tonic and phasic skeletal muscle. Nature 216:1219–1220

Goldberg A L 1975 Mechanisms of growth and atrophy of skeletal muscle. In: Cassena R G (ed) Muscle Biopsy, Vol 1. Marcel Dekker for the Institute of Muscular Biology, New York, pp 89–115

Goldman J M, Lehr R P, Millar A B, Silver J R 1987 An electromyographic study of the abdominal muscles during postural and respiratory manoeuvres. Journal of Neurology, Neurosurgery and Psychiatry 50:866–869

Gollhofer A, Schöpp A, Rapp W, Stroinik V 1998 Changes in reflex excitability following isometric contraction in humans. European Journal of Applied Physiology 77:89–97

Gomez T T 1994 Symmetry of lumbar rotation and lateral flexion range of motion and isometric strength in subjects with and without low back pain. Journal of Sports, Physical Therapy 19:42–46

Graber D I 1997 Muscle dysfunction as a contributor to low back pain: a case study – postisometric relaxation (PIR) techniques. Journal of Sports, Chiropractic and Rehabilitation 11:21–24, 38–39

Grabiner M D, Koh T J, Ghazawi A E 1992 Decoupling of bilateral excitation in subjects with low back pain. Spine 17:1219–1223

Gracovetsky S 1990 Musculoskeletal function of the spine. In: Winters J M, Woo S L-Y (eds) Multiple muscle systems:biomechanics and movement organisation. Springer-Verlag, New York, pp 410–437

Gracovetsky S, Farfan H F, Lamy C 1977 A mathematical model of the lumbar spine using an optimised system to control muscles and ligaments. Orthopedic Clinics of North America 8:135–153

Gracovetsky S, Farfan H, Helleur C 1985 The abdominal mechanism. Spine 10:317–324

Graven-Nielsen T, Svensson P, Arendt-Nielsen L 1997 Effects of experimental muscle pain on muscle activity and co-ordination during static and dynamic motor function. Electroencephalography and Clinical Neurophysiology 105:156–164

Grichko V P, Heywood-Cooksey A, Kidd K R, Fitts R H 2000 Substrate profile in rat soleus muscle fibers after hindlimb unloading and fatigue, Journal of Applied Physiology 88:473–478

Grigg P, Harrigan E P, Fogarty K E 1978 Segmental reflexes mediated by joint afferent neurons in cat knee. Journal of Neurophysiology 41:9–14

Grillner S, Nilsson J, Thorstensson A 1978 Intra-abdominal pressure changes during natural movements in man. Acta Physiologica Scandinavica 103:275–283

Grimby G, Björntorp P, Fahlén M et al 1973 Metabolic effects of isometric training. Scandinavian Journal of Clinical and Laboratory Investigation 31:301–305

Grimstone S, Hodges P 2003 Impaired postural compensation for respiration in people with recurrent low back pain. Experimental Brain Research in press

Gurfinkel V S 1994 The mechanisms of postural regulation in man. Soviet Scientific Reviews. Section F. Physiology and General Biology 7:59–89

Gurfinkel V S, Kots Y M, Paltsev E 1971 The compensation of respiratory disturbances of erect posture of man as an example of the organisation of interarticular interaction. In: Gelfard I M, Gurfinkel V S, Formin S V, Tsetlin M L (eds) Models of the structural functional organisation of certain biological systems. MIT Press, Cambridge, MA, pp 382–395

Guyton A C 1981 Textbook of medical physiology, 6th edn. Saunders, Philadelphia, PA

Gydikov A A 1976 Pattern of discharge of different types of alpha motor units during voluntary and reflex activities under normal physiological conditions. In: Komi P V (ed) Biomechanics VA. University Park Press, Baltimore, MD, pp 45–57

Haddad B 1953 Projection of afferent fibres from the knee joint to the cerebellum of the cat. American Journal of Physiology 172:511–514

Häggmark T, Eriksson E 1979 Hypotrophy of the soleus muscle in man after Achilles tendon rupture: discussion of findings obtained by computed tomography and morphologic studies. American Journal of Sports Medicine 7:121–126

Häggmark T, Jansson E, Eriksson E 1981 Fibre type area and metabolic potential of the thigh muscle in man after knee surgery and immobilisation. International Journal of Sports Medicine 2:2–17

Halkjaer-Kristenen J, Ingemann-Hansen T, Saltin B 1980 Cross-sectional and fibre size changes in the quadriceps muscle of man with immobilisation and physical training. Muscle Nerve 3:275

Hamilton C, Richardson C 1995 Towards the development of a clinical test of local muscle dysfunction in the lumbar spine. In: Proceedings of the 9th Biennial Conference of the Manipulative Physiotherapists Association of Australia, Brisbane. MPAA, Melbourne, pp 54–56

Harrison P J, Jankowska E 1984 An intracellular study of descending and non-cutaneous afferent input to spinocervical tract neurones in the cat. Journal of Physiology 356:245–261

Hather B M, Adams G R, Tesch P A, Dudley G A 1992 Skeletal muscle responses to lower limb suspension in humans. Journal of Applied Physiology 72:1493–1498

He X, Proske V, Schaible H G, Schmidt R F 1988 Acute inflammation of the knee joint in the cat alters responses of flexor motoneurones to leg movements. Journal of Neurophysiology 59:326–340

Hemborg B 1983 Intraabdominal pressure and trunk muscle activity during lifting. Department of Physical Therapy University of Lund, Lund, the Netherlands

Henry S 2001 Postural responses in persons with low back pain. In Duysens J, Smits-Engelsman BCM, Kingma H (eds) Control of posture and gait. International Society for Postural and Gait Research, Nijmegen, pp 651–655.

Henry S M, Fung J, Horak F B 1998 EMG responses to maintain stance during multidirectional surface translations. Journal of Neurophysiology 80: 1939–1950

Herbert R D, Gandevia S C 1995 Changes in pennation with joint angle and muscle torque: in vivo measurements in human brachialis muscle. Journal of Physiology (Lond) 484:523–532

Hides J A, Cooper D H, Stokes M J 1992 Diagnostic ultrasound imaging for measurement of the lumbar multifidus muscle in normal young adults. Physiotherapy Theory and Practice, 8:19–26

Hides J A, Stokes M J, Saide M, Jull G A, Cooper D H 1994 Evidence of lumbar multifidus muscle wasting ipsilateral to symptoms in patients with acute/subacute low back pain. Spine 19:165–172

Hides J A, Richardson C A, Jull G A 1995 Magnetic resonance imaging and ultrasonography of the lumbar multifidus muscle: Comparison of two different modalities. Spine 20:54–58

Hides J A, Richardson C A, Jull G A, Davies S E 1996a Ultrasound imaging in rehabilitation. Australian Journal of Physiotherapy 41:187–193

Hides J A, Richardson C A, Jull G A 1996b Multifidus muscle recovery is not automatic following resolution of acute first episode low back pain. Spine 21:2763–2769

Hides J A, Richardson C A, Jull G A 1996c Multifidus muscle rehabilitation decreases recurrence of symptoms following first episode low back pain. In: Proceedings of the National Congress of the Australian Physiotherapy Association, Brisbane

Hides J A, Richardson C A, Jull G A 1998 Use of real-time ultrasound imaging for feedback in rehabilitation. Manual Therapy 3:125–131

Hides J, Jull G, Richardson C 2000 A clinical palpation test to check the activation of the deep stabilising muscles of the spine. International Sports Medicine Journal 1:(4)

Hides J A, Jull G A, Richardson C A 2001 Long-term effects of specific stabilizing exercises for first episode low back pain. Spine 26 E243–E248

Hodges P W 1999 Is there a role for transversus abdominis in lumbo-pelvic stability? Manual Therapy 4:74–86

Hodges P W 2001 Changes in motor planning of feedforward postural responses of the trunk muscles in low back pain. Experimental Brain Research 141:261–266

Hodges P, Gandevia S C 2000a Changes in intra-abdominal pressure during postural and respiratory activation of the human diaphragm. Journal of Applied Physiology 89:967–976

Hodges P, Gandevia S C 2000b Activation of the human diaphragm during a repetitive postural task. Journal of Physiology 522:165–175

Hodges P W, Jull G A 2003 Motor relearning strategies for the rehabilitation of intervertebral control of the spine. In: Liebenson C (ed) Rehabilitation of the spine: a practitioner's manual, 2nd edn. Lippincott Williams & Wilkins, Baltimore, MD, in press

Hodges P W, Moseley G L 2003 Pain and motor control of the lumbopelvic region: effect and possible mechanisms. Electromyography and Kinesiology, in press

Hodges P W, Richardson C A 1993 Influence of isometric hip adduction on quadriceps femoris activity. Scandavavian Journal of Rehabilitation Medicine 25:57–62

Hodges P W, Richardson C A 1996 Inefficient muscular stabilisation of the lumbar spine associated with low back pain: a motor control evaluation of transversus abdominis. Spine 21:2640–2650

Hodges P W, Richardson C A 1997a Contraction of the abdominal muscles associated with movement of the lower limb. Physical Therapy 77:132–144

Hodges P W, Richardson C A 1997b Feedforward contraction of transversus abdominis is not influenced by the direction of arm movement. Experimental Brain Research 114:62–370

Hodges P W, Richardson C A 1997c Relationship between limb movement speed and associated contraction of the trunk muscles. Ergonomics 40:1220–1230

Hodges P W, Richardson C A 1998 Delayed postural contraction of transversus abdominis in low back pain associated with movement of the lower limbs. Journal of Spinal Disorders 11:46–56

Hodges P W, Richardson C A 1999a Transversus abdominis and the superficial abdominal muscles are controlled independently in a postural task. Neuroscience Letters 265:91–94

Hodges P W, Richardson C A 1999b Altered trunk muscle recruitment in people with low back pain with upper limb movement at different speeds. Archives of Physical Medicine and Rehabilitation 80:1005–1012

Hodges P W, Saunders S 2001 Coordination of the respiratory and locomotor activities of the abdominal muscles during walking in humans. IUPS Press, Christchurch, New Zealand

Hodges P W, Richardson C A, Jull G A 1996 Evaluation of the relationship between the findings of a laboratory and clinical test of transversus abdominis function. Physiotherapy Research International 1:30–40

Hodges P W, Butler J E, McKenzie D, Gandevia S C 1997a Contraction of the human diaphragm during postural adjustments. Journal of Physiology 505:239–548

Hodges P W, Gandevia S C, Richardson C A 1997b Contractions of specific abdominal muscles in postural tasks are affected by respiratory maneuvers. Journal of Applied Physiology 83:753–760

Hodges P W, Cresswell A G, Thorstensson A 1999 Preparatory trunk motion accompanies rapid upper limb movement. Experimental Brain Research 124:69–79

Hodges P W, Cresswell A G, Daggfeldt K, Thorstensson A 2000a Three dimensional preparatory trunk motion precedes asymmetrical upper limb movement. Gait Posture 11:92–101

Hodges P W, McKenzie D K, Heijnen I, Gandevia S C 2000b Reduced contribution of the diaphragm to postural control in patients with severe chronic airflow limitation. In: Proceedings of the Annual Scientific Meeting of the Thoracic Society of Australia and New Zealand, Melbourne, Australia

Hodges P W, Cresswell A G, Thorstensson A 2001a Perturbed arm movements cause short-latency postural responses in trunk muscles. Experimental Brain Research 138:243–245

Hodges P W, Cresswell A G, Daggfeldt K, Thorstensson A 2001b In vivo measurement of the effect of intra-abdominal pressure on the human spine. Journal of Biomechanics 34:347–353

Hodges P W, Eriksson A E M, Shirley D, Gandevia S C 2003 Intra-abdominal pressure can directly increase stiffness of the lumbar spine. Journal of Biomechanics, in press

Hodges P W, Heijnen I, Gandevia S C 2001d Reduced postural activity of the diaphragm in humans when respiratory demand is increased. Journal of Physiology 537:999–1008

Hodges P, Moseley G L, Gandevia S C 2002a Differential control of the deep and superficial compartments of multifidus is dependent on input from higher centres. In: Proceedings of the VIIth International Physiotherapy Congress, Sydney

Hodges P, Gurfinkel V S, Brumagne S, Smith T, Cordo P 2002b Coexistence of stability and mobility in postural control: evidence from postural compensation for respiration. Experimental Brain Research 144:293–302

Hodges P W, Sapsford R R, Pengel H M 2002c Feedforward activity of the pelvic floor muscles precedes rapid upper limb movements. In: Proceedings of the VIIth International Physiotherapy Congress, Sydney, Australia

Hodges P, Kaigle-Holm A, Holm S et al 2003a Intervertebal stiffness of the spine is increased by evoked contraction of transversus abdominis and the diaphragm: In vivo porcine studies. Spine, in press

Hodges P, Kaigle-Holm A, Holm S, et al 2003b Posteroanterior stiffness of the lumbar spine is increased by contraction of transversus abdominis and the diaphragm: porcine studies. In: 14th International Congress of the World Confederation for Physical Therapy, Barcelona, Spain

Hodges P W, Smith M, Grigorenko A, Cresswell A G, Thorstensson A 2003c Trunk muscle response to support surface translation in sitting: normal control and effects of respiration. Journal of Neurophysiology, submitted

Hodges P W, Pengel L M H, Herbert R D, Gandevia S C 2003d Measurement of muscle contraction with ultrasound imaging. Muscle and Nerve 27:682–692

Hodges P W, Moseley G L, Gabrielsson A H, Gandevia S C 2003e Acute experimental pain changes postural recruitment of the trunk muscles in pain-free humans. Experimental Brain Research, in press

Hodges P W, Butler J E, Taylor J L, Gandevia S C 2003f Motor cortex may be involved in feedforward postural responses of the deep trunk muscles. In: Lord S, Menz H B, (eds) Posture and gait through the lifespan. International Society for Posture and Gait Research, Sydney, pp 53–54

Hoek van Dijke G A, Snijders C J, Stoeckart R, Stam H J 1999 A biomechanical model on muscle forces in the transfer of spinal load to the pelvis and legs. Journal of Biomechanics 32:927–933

Hoffer J, Andreassen S 1981 Regulation of soleus muscle stiffness in premamillary cats. Journal of Neurophysiology 45:267–285

Hoheisel U, Mense S 1989 Long-term changes in discharge behaviour of cat dorsal horn neurones following noxious stimulation of deep tissues. Pain 36:239–247

Hollinshead W H, Jenkins D B 1981 Functional anatomy of the limbs and back. Saunders, Philadelphia, PA

Holm S, Indahl A, Solomonow M 2002 Sensorimotor control of the spine. Journal of Electromyography and Kinesiology 12:219–234

Hongo T, Jankowska E, Lundberg A 1969 The rubrospinal tract II. Facilitation of interneuronal transmission in reflex paths to motoneurones. Experimental Brain Research 7:365–391

Horak F, Nashner L M 1986 Central programming of postural movements: adaptation to altered support-surface configurations. Journal of Neurophysiology 55:1369–1381

Hsieh J C, Belfrage M, Stone-Elander S, Hansson P, Ingvar M 1995 Central representation of chronic ongoing neuropathic pain studied by positron emission tomography. Pain 63:225–236

Huang Q M, Hodges P W, Thorstensson A 2001 Postural control of the trunk in response to lateral support surface translations during trunk movement and loading. Experimental Brain Research 141:552–559

Hultman G, Nordin M, Saraste H, Ohlsen H 1993 Body composition, endurance, strength, cross-sectional area and density of mm erector spinae in men with and without low back pain. Journal of Spinal Disorders 6:114–123

Hungerford B, Gilleard W, Hodges P 2003 Evidence of altered lumbo-pelvic muscle recruitment in the presence of sacroiliac pain. Spine 28:1593–1600

Hurley M V, Newham D J 1993 The influence of arthrogenous muscle inhibition on quadriceps inhibition with quadriceps rehabilitation of patients with early unilateral osteoarthritic knees. British Journal of Rheumatology 32:127–131

Hurwitz E, Morgenstern H 1999 Cross-sectional associations of asthma, hay fever, and other allergies with major depression and low-back pain among adults aged 20–39 years in the United States. American Journal of Epidemiology 150:1107–1116

Indahl A, Kaigle A, Reikeras O, Holm S 1995 Electromyographic response of the porcine multifidus musculature after nerve stimulation. Spine 20:2652–2658

Indahl A, Kaigle A, Reikeras O, Holm S 1997 Interaction between the porcine lumbar intervertebral disc, zygapophysial joints, and paraspinal muscles. Spine 22:2834–2840

Indahl A, Kaigle A, Reikeras O, Holm S 1999 Sacroiliac joint involvement in activation of the porcine spinal and gluteal musculature. Journal of Spinal Disorders 12:325–330

Issurin V B, Tenenbaum G 1999 Acute and residual effects of vibratory stimulation on explosive strength in elite and amateur athletes. Journal of Sports Sciences 17:177–182

James W H 2001 The bones and hormones of deep water divers and pilots of high performance aircraft. Occupational and Environmental Medicine 58:682–684

Janda V 1978 Muscles, central nervous motor regulation and back problems. In: Korr I M (ed) The neurobiologic mechanisms in manipulative therapy. Plenum Press, New York, pp 27–41

Janda V 1986 Muscle weakness and inhibition (pseudoparesis) in back pain syndromes. In: Grieve G (ed) Modern manual therapy of the vertebral column. Churchill Livingstone, Edinburgh, pp 197–201

Janda V 1996 Evaluation of muscular imbalance. In: Liebenson C (ed) Rehabilitation of the spine: a practitioner's manual. Williams & Wilkins, Baltimore, MD, pp 97–112

Jayson M, Dixon A 1970 Intra-articular pressure in rheumatoid arthritis of the knee. III. Pressure changes during joint use. Annals of the Rheumatic Diseases 29:401–408

Jennekens F G I 1982 Neurogenic disorders of muscle. In: Mastaglia F L, Walton J N (eds) Skeletal muscle pathology. Churchill Livingstone, Edinburgh, pp 204–234

Jennekens F G I, Tomlinson B E, Walto J N 1971 The sizes of the two main histochemical fibre types in five limb muscles in man. An autopsy study. Journal of Neurological Sciences 14:245

Jiang B, Roy R R, Polyakov I V, Krasnov I B, Edgerton V R 1992 Ventral horn cell responses to spaceflight and hindlimb suspension. Journal of Applied Physiology 73(Suppl):107S–111S

Jiang H J, Russell G, Raso J, Moreau M J, Hill D J, Bagnall K M 1995 The nature and distribution of the innervation of human supraspinal and interspinal ligaments. Spine 20:869–876

Johansson H, Sojka P 1991 Pathophysiological mechanisms involved in genesis and spread of muscular tension in occupational muscle pain and in chronic musculoskeletal pain syndromes: a hypothesis. Medical Hypotheses 35:196–203

Johansson H, Sjölander P, Sojka P 1986 Actions on motorneurones elicited by electrical stimulation of joint afferent fibres in the hindlimb of the cat. Journal of Physiology (Lond) 375:137–152.

Johansson H, Sjölander P, Sojka P 1991a A sensory role for the cruciate ligaments. Clinical Orthopaedics and Related Research 268:161–178

Johansson H, Sjölander P, Sojka P 1991b Receptors in the knee joint ligaments and their role in the biomechanics of the joint. CRC Critical Reviews in Biomedical Engineering 18:341–368

Johnson M A, Polgar J, Weightman D, Appleton D 1973 Data on the distribution of fibre types in thirty-six human muscles: an autopsy study. Journal of the Neurological Sciences 18:111–129

Jones G, Cale A 1997 Goal difficulty, anxiety and performance. Ergonomics 40:319–333

Jonsson B 1970 The functions of individual muscles in the lumbar part of the spinae muscle. Electromyography 10:5–21

Jorgensen K, Nicolaisen T 1987 Trunk extensor endurance. Determination and relation to low back trouble. Ergonomics 30:259–267

Jorgensen K, Mag C, Nicholaisen T, Kato M 1993 Muscle fibre distribution, capillary density and enzymatic activities in the lumbar paravertebral muscles of young men. Significance for isometric endurance. Spine 18:1439–1450

Jorgensson A 1993 The iliopsoas muscle and the lumbar spine. Australian Physiotherapy 39:125–132

Jowett R, Fidler M W, Troup J D G 1975 Histochemical changes in the multifidus in mechanical derangement of the spine. Orthopaedic Clinics of North America 6:145–161

Kader D, Wardlaw D, Smith F 2000 Correlation between the MRI changes in the lumbar multifidus muscles and leg pain. Clinical Radiology 55:145–149

Kaigle A M, Holm S H, Hansson T H 1995 Experimental instability in the lumbar spine. Spine 20:421–430

Kanemura N, Kobayashai R, Kajihara H et al 2002 Changes of mechanoreceptor in anterior cruciate ligament with hindlimb suspension rats. Journal of Physical Therapy Science 14:27–32

Kankaanpaa M, Taimela S, Laaksonen D, Hanninen O, Airaksinen O, 1998 Back and hip extensor fatiguability in chronic low back pain patients and controls. Archives of Physical Medicine and Rehabilitation 79:412–417

Kawaguchi Y, Matsui H, Tsuji H 1994 Back muscle injury after posterior lumbar spine surgery. Part 2: histologic and histochemical analyses in humans. Spine 19:2598–2602

Kawano F, Nomura T, Ishihara A, Nonaka I, Ohira Y 2002 Afferent input: associated reduction of muscle activity in microgravity environment. Neuroscience 114:1133–1138

Keifer A, Shirazi-Adl A, Parnianpour M 1997 Stability of the human spine in neutral postures. European Spine Journal 6:45–53

Keifer A, Shirazi-Adl A, Parnianpour M 1998 Synergy of the human spine in neutral postures. European Spine Journal 7:471–479

Kendall F P, McCreary E K 1983 Muscles. Testing and function, 3rd edn. Williams & Wilkins, Baltimore, MD

Kennedy J C, Alexander I J, Hayes K C 1982 Nerve supply to the knee and its functional significance. American Journal of Sports Medicine 10:329–335

Keshner E A, Allum J H J 1990 Muscle activation patterns coordinating postural stability from head to foot. In: Winters J M, Woo S L-Y (eds) Multiple muscle systems: biomechanics and movement organisation. Springer-Verlag, New York, pp 481–497

Keshner E A, Campbell D, Katz R T, Peterson B W 1989 Neck muscle activation patterns in humans during isometric head stabilization. Experimental Brain Research 75:335–344

Kidd G, Lawes N, Musa I 1992 Understanding neuromuscular plasticity: a basis for clinical rehabilitation. Edward Arnold (Hodder and Stoughton), London

King J C, Lehmkuhl D L, French J, Dimitrijevic M 1988 Dynamic postural reflexes: comparison in normal subjects and patients with chronic low back pain. Current Concepts in Rehabilitation Medicine 4:7–11

Kippers V, Parker A W 1984 Posture related to myoelectric silence of erectores spinae during trunk flexion. Spine 7:740–745

Kippers V, Parker A W 1985 Electromyographic studies of erectores spinae: symmetrical postures and sagittal trunk motion. Australian Journal of Physiotherapy 31:91–105

Knott M, Voss D E 1968 Proprioceptive neuromuscular facilitation, 2nd edn. Harper & Row, New York

Kondo T, Bishop B, Shaw C F 1986 Phasic stretch reflex of the abdominal muscles. Experimental Neurology 94:120–140

Krebs D E 1981 Clinical electromyography feedback following meniscectomy: a multiple regression experimental analysis. Physical Therapy 61:1017–1021

Krebs D E, Staples W H, Cuttita D, Zickel R E 1983 Knee joint angle: its relationship to quadriceps femoris in normal and post arthrotomy limbs. Archives of Physical Medicine and Rehabilitation 64:441–447

Kremkau F W 1983 Ultrasound instrumentation. In: Callen P W (ed) Physical principles in ultrasonography in obstetrics and gynaecology. Saunders, Philadelphia, PA, pp 313–325

Kumar S 1980 Physiological responses to weight lifting in different planes. Ergonomics 23:987–993

Kuno M 1984 A hypothesis for neural control of the speed of muscle contraction in the mammal. Advances in Biophysics 17:69–95

Kuukkanen T, Malkia E 1998 Effects of a three-month active rehabilitation program on psychomotor performance of lower limbs in subjects with low back pain: a controlled study with a nine-month follow-up. Perception and Motor Skills 87:739–753

Laasonen E M 1984 Atrophy of sacrospinal muscle groups in patients with chronic diffusely radiating lumbar back pain. Neuroradiology 26:9–13

La Dora V T 2002 Skeletal muscle adaptations with age, inactivity and therapeutic exercise. Journal of Orthopaedic and Sports Physical Therapy 32:44–57

Landon D N 1982 Skeletal muscle- normal morphology, development and innervation. In: Mastaglia F L, Walton J N (eds) Skeletal muscle pathology. Churchill Livingstone, New York, pp 1–88

Lang A 2002 Botulinum toxin type A for relief of low back pain: a retrospective clinical evaluation. In Proceedings of the 10th World Congress on Pain, San Diego. IASP Press, Seattle, WA

Lavender S A, Tsuang Y H, Andersson G B J, Hafezi A, Shin C C 1992 Trunk muscle cocontraction: the effects of moment direction and moment magnitude. Journal of Orthopaedic Research 10:691–700

LeBlanc A, Lin C, Shackelford L et al 2000 Muscle volume, MRI relaxation times (T_2) and body composition after spaceflight. Journal of Applied Physiology 89:2158–2164

Leinonen V, Kankaanpaa M, Airaksinen O, Hanninen O 2000 Back and hip extensor activities during trunk flexion/extension: effects of low back pain and rehabilitation. Archives of Physical Medicine and Rehabilitation 81:32–37

Leinonen V, Kankaanpaa M, Luukkonen M, Hanninen O, Airaksinen O, Taimela S 2001 Disc herniation-related back pain impairs feed-forward control of paraspinal muscles. Spine 26:E367–E372

Lennon S 1982 The Bobath concept: a critical review of the theoretical assumptions that guide physiotherapy practice in stroke rehabilitation. Physical Therapy Review 1:35–45

LeVeau B F, Rogers C 1980 Selective training of the vastus medialis muscle using EMG biofeedback. Physical Therapy 60:1410–1415

Lewin T, Moffett B, Viidik A 1962 The morphology of the lumbar synovial joints. Acta Morphologica Neerlando Scandinavica 4:299–319

Loo A, Stokes M J 1990 Diagnostic ultrasound scanning for clinical estimation of quadriceps size and estimation of strength. In: Proceedings of the IIIrd International Physiotherapy Congress, Hong Kong, pp 655–660

Lorenz J, Bromm B 1997 Event-related potential correlates of interference between cognitive performance and tonic experimental pain. Psychophysiology 34:436–445

Lucca J A, Recchuiti S J 1983 Effect of electromyographic biofeedback on an isometric strengthening program. Physical Therapy 83:200–203

Lund J P, Donga R, Widmer C G, Stohler C S 1991 The pain-adaption model: a discussion of the relationships between chronic musculoskeletal pain and motor activity. Canadian Journal of Physiology and Pharmacology, 69:683–694

Lundberg A, Malmgren K, Schomburg E D 1978 Role of joint afferents in motor control exemplified by effects on reflex pathways from 1b afferents. Journal of Physiology 284:327–343

Luoto S, Aalto H, Taimela S, et al 1998 One-footed and externally disturbed two-footed postural control in patients with chronic low back pain and healthy control subjects. A controlled study with follow-up. Spine 23:2081–2089

Luoto S, Taimela S, Hurri H, Alaranta H 1999 Mechanisms explaining the association between low back trouble and deficits in information processing. A controlled study with follow-up. Spine 24:255–261

Macintosh J E, Bogduk N 1986a The morphology of the lumbar erector spinae. Spine 12:658–668

Macintosh J E, Bogduk N 1986b The detailed biomechanics of the lumbar multifidus. Clinical Biomechanics 1:205–231

Macintosh J E, Valencia F, Bogduk N, Munro R R 1986 The morphology of the human lumbar multifidus. Clinical Biomechanics 1:196–204

Macintosh J E, Bogduk N, Gracovetsky S 1987 The biomechanics of the thoracolumbar fascia. Clinical Biomechanics 2:78–83

Maganaris C N, Baltzopoulos V, Sargeant AJ 1998 In vivo measurements of the triceps surae complex architecture in man: implications for muscle function. Journal of Physiology 512:603–614

Main C J, Spanswick C 2000 Pain management: an interdisciplinary approach. Churchill Livingstone, Edinburgh

Main C J, Watson P J 1996 What harm – pain behavior? Psychological and physical factors in the development of chronicity. Bulletin of the Hospital for Joint Diseases (New York) 55:210–212

Marras W S, Mirka G A 1990 Muscle activities during asymmetric trunk angular accelerations. Journal of Orthopaedic Research 8:824–832

Marras W S, Davis K G, Heaney C A, Maronitis A B, Allread W G 2000 The influence of psychosocial stress, gender, and personality on mechanical loading of the lumbar spine. Spine 25:3045–3054

Marsden C D, Merton P A, Morton H B 1977 Anticipatory postural responses in the human subject. Journal of Physiology (Lond) 275:47P–48P

Martenuik R E 1979 Motor skill performance and learning: considerations for rehabilitation. Physiotherapy Canada 31:187–202

Martinson H, Stokes M J 1991 Measurement of anterior tibial muscle size using real-time ultrasound imaging. European Journal of Applied Physiology 63:250–254

Massion J 1992 Movement, posture and equilibrium: interaction and coordination. Progress in Neurobiology 38:35–56

Massion J 1998 Postural control systems in developmental perspective. Neuroscience and Biobehavioural Reviews 22:465–472

Matre D A, Sinkjaer T, Svensson P, Arendt-Nielsen L 1998 Experimental muscle pain increases the human stretch reflex. Pain 75:331–339

Mattila M, Hurme M, Alaranta H et al 1986 The multifidus muscle in patients with lumbar disc herniation. A histochemical and morphometric analysis of intraoperative biopsies. Spine 11:732–738

Max S R, Maier R F, Vogelsang L 1971 Lysosomes and disuse atrophy of skeletal muscle. Archives of Biochemistry and Biophysics 146:227–232

Mayer T G, Vanharanta H, Gatchel R J, Mooney V, Barnes D, Judge L, Smith S 1989 Comparison of CT scan muscle measurements and isokinetic trunk strength in postoperative patients. Spine 14:33–36

McClain R F, Pickar J G 1998 Mechanoreceptor endings in human thoracic and lumbar facet joints. Spine 23:168–173

McCloskey D I 1978 Kinesthetic sensibility. Physiological Review 58:763–820

McComas A J 1996 Skeletal muscle form and function. Saunders, Philadelphia, PA, Ch 19

McGill S M 1991 Kinetic potential of the lumbar trunk musculature about three orthogonal orthopaedic axes in extreme postures. Spine 16:809–815

McGill S M 2002a Coordination of muscle activation to assure stability of the lumbar spine., In Proceedings of the IV World Congress of Biomechanics, Abstract 5062

McGill S M 2002b Low back disorders. Evidence-based prevention and rehabilitation. Human Kinetics, Champagne, IL

McGill S M, Norman R W 1987 Reassessment of the role of intra-abdominal pressure in spinal compression. Ergonomics 30:1565–1588

McGill S M, Norman R W 1988 Potential of lumbodorsal fascia forces to generate back extension moments in squat lifts. Journal of Biomedical Engineering 10:312–318

McGill S M, Norman R W 1993 Low back biomechanics in industry: the prevention of injury through safer lifting. In: Grabiner M D (ed) Current issues in biomechanics. Human Kinetics, Champaign, IL, pp 69–120

McGill S M, Sharratt M T 1990 Relationship between intra-abdominal pressure and trunk EMG. Clinical Biomechanics 5:59–67

McGill S M, Sharratt M T, Seguin J P 1995 Loads on spinal tissues during simultaneous lifting and ventilatory challenge. Ergonomics 38:1772–1792

McGill S M, Juker D, Kropf P 1996 Quantitative intramuscular myoelectric activity of quadratus lumborum during a wide variety of tasks. Clinical Biomechanics 11:170–172

McGill S M, Hughson R L, Parks K 2000 Changes in lumbar lordosis modify the role of the extensor muscles. Clinical Biomechanics 15:777–780

Mead J 1979 Functional significance of the area of apposition of diaphragm to rib cage. American Review of Respiratory Disease 119:31–32

Mirka G A, Marras W S 1993 A stochastic model of trunk muscle coactivation during trunk bending. Spine 18:1396–1409

Misuri G, Colagrande S, Gorini M 1997 In vivo ultrasound assessment of respiratory function of abdominal muscles in normal subjects. European Respiratory Journal 10:2861–2867

Moe-Nilssen R, Ljunggren A E, Torebjork E 1999 Dynamic adjustments of walking behavior dependent on noxious input in experimental low back pain. Pain 83:477–485

Mooney V, Pozos R, Vleeming A, Gulick J, Swenski D 2001 Exercise treatment for sacroiliac pain. Orthopedics 24:29–32

Morris J M, Benner F, Lucas D B 1962 An electromyographic study of the intrinsic muscles of the back in man. Journal of Anatomy 96:509–520

Morrissey M C 1989 Reflex inhibition of thigh muscles in knee injury: causes and treatment. Sports Medicine 7:263–276

Moseley G L, Hodges P W 2003 Chronic pain and motor control. In: Boyling J, Jull G A (eds) Greive's modern manual therapy. Churchill Livingstone, Edinburgh, in press

Moseley G L, Hodges P W, Gandevia S C 2001 Attention demand, anxiety and acute pain cause differential effects on postural activation of the abdominal muscles in humans. Society of Neuroscience Abstracts 27

Moseley G L, Hodges P W, Gandevia S C 2002 Deep and superficial fibers of lumbar multifidus are differentially active during voluntary arm movements. Spine 27:E29–E36

Moseley G L, Hodges P W, Gandevia S C 2003 External perturbation of the trunk in standing humans differentially activates components of the medial back muscles. Journal of Physiology 547:581–587

Murphy C A, Sherburn M, Allen T, Carroll S 2001 Investigation of ultrasound imaging for non-invasive examination of pelvic floor function. International Urogynecology Journal 12(Suppl 3):177

Musacchia XJ, Steffen J M, Fell R D, Dombrowski M J, Oganov V W, Ilyina-Kakueva E I 1992 Skeletal muscle atrophy in response to 14 days of weightlessness: vastus medialis. Journal of Applied Physiology 73(Suppl):44S–50S

Myriknas S E, Beith I D, Harrison P J 2000 Stretch reflexes in the rectus abdominis muscle in man. Experimental Physiology 85:445–450

Nachemson A, Morris J M 1964 In vivo measurement of intradiscal pressure: discometry, a method for the determination of presure in the lower lumbar discs. Journal of Bone and Joint Surgery 46A:1077–1092

Nachemson A, Andersson G, Schultz A 1986 Valsalva manoeuvre biomechanics. Effects on lumbar trunk loads of elevated intra-abdominal pressures. Spine 11:456–462

Nelson J M, Walmsley R P, Stevenson J M 1995 Relative lumbar and pelvic motion during loaded spinal flexion/extension. Spine 20:199–204

Ng G, Richardson C A 1990 The effects of training triceps using progressive speed loading. Physiotherapy Practice 6:77–84

Ng J K-F, Kippers V, Richardson C A 1998 Muscle fibre orientation of human abdominal muscles and placement of surface EMG electrodes. Electromyography and Clinical Neurophysiology 38:51–58

Ng J K-F, Richardson C A, Parnianpour M, Kippers V 2002a EMG activity of trunk muscles and torque output during isometric axial rotation exertion: a comparison between back pain patients and matched controls. Journal of Orthopaedic Research 20:112–121

Ng J K-F, Richardson C A, Parnianpour M, Kippers V 2002b Fatigue-related changes in torque output and electromyographic parameters of trunk muscles during isometric axial rotation exertion. An investigation in patients with back pain and in healthy subjects. Spine 27:637–646

Ng J K-F, Richardson C A, Kippers V, Parnianpour M 2002c Comparison of lumbar range of movement and lumbar lordosis in back pain patients and matched controls. Journal of Rehabilitation Medicine 34:109–113

Nicolaisen T, Jorgensen K 1985 Trunk strength, back muscle endurance and low back trouble. Scandinavian Journal of Rehabilitation Medicine 17:121–127

Nitz A J, Peck D 1986 Comparison of muscle spindle concentrations in large and small human epaxial muscles acting in parallel combinations. American Surgeon 52:273–277

Nordin M, Hiebert R, Pietrek M, Alexander M, Crane M, Lewis S 2002 Association of comorbidity and outcome in episodes of nonspecific low back pain in occupational populations. Journal of Occupational and Environmental Medicine 44:677–684

Nourbakhsh M R, Arab A M 2002 Relationship between mechanical factors and incidence of low back pain. Journal of Orthopaedic and Sports Physical Therapy 32:447–460

Nouwen A, Van Akkerveeken P F, Versloot J M 1987 Patterns of muscular activity during movement in patients with chronic low back pain. Spine 12:777–782

O'Sullivan P B, Twomey L T, Allison G T 1997 Evaluation of specific stabilizing exercise in the treatment of chronic low back pain with radiologic diagnosis of spondylolysis or spondylolisthesis. Spine 22:2959–2967

Oddsson L 1988 Co-ordination of a simple voluntary multi-joint movement with postural demands: trunk extension in standing man. Acta Physiologica Scandinavica 134:109–118

Oddsson L 1989 Motor patterns of fast voluntary postural task in man: trunk extension in standing. Acta Physiologica Scandinavica 136:47–58

Oddsson L I, Persson T, Cresswell A G, Thorstensson A 1999 Interaction between voluntary and postural motor commands during perturbed lifting. Spine 24:545–552

Oganov V S, Murashko L M, Kabitskaya O E, Szilagyi T, Rapcsak M 1991 Physiological characteristics of rat skeletal muscles after the flight on board Cosmos-2044 biosatellite. Physiologist 34(Suppl 1):S174–S176

O'Sullivan P B, Twomey L, Allison G T 1997 Evaluation of specific stabilizing exercise in the treatment of chronic low back pain with radiologic diagnosis of spondylolysis or spondylolisthesis. Spine 22:2959–2967

O'Sullivan P B, Twomey L, Allison G T 1998 Altered abdominal muscle recruitment in patients with chronic back pain following a specific exercise intervention. Journal of Orthopedic Sports Physical Therapy 27:114–124

O'Sullivan P B, Grahamslaw K M, Kendell M, Lapenskie S C, Möller N E, Richards K V 2002 The effect of different standing and sitting postures on trunk muscle activity in a pain-free population. Spine 27:1238–1244

Oxland T R, Panjabi M M 1992 The onset and progression of spinal instability: a demonstration of neutral zone sensitivity. Journal of Biomechanics 25:1165–1172

Palmer M L, Epler M E 1998 Fundamentals of musculo-skeletal assessment techniques, 2nd edn. Lippincott, Philadelphia, PA 1998

Panjabi M M 1992a The stabilising system of the spine. Part 1. Function, dysfunction, adaption, and enhancement. Journal of Spinal Disorders 5:383–389

Panjabi M M 1992b The stabilising system of the spine. Part II. Neutral zone and stability hypothesis. Journal of Spinal Disorders 5:390–397

Panjabi M M 1994 Lumbar spine instability: a biomechanical challenge. Current Orthopaedics 8:100–105

Panjabi M, Abumi K, Duranceau J, Oxland T 1989 Spinal stability and intersegmental muscle forces. A biomechanical model. Spine 14:194–200

Paquet N, Malouin F, Richards C 1994 Hip-spine movement interaction and muscle activation patterns during sagittal trunk movements in low back pain patients. Spine 19:596–603

Paris S V 1983 Anatomy as related to function and pain. Orthopaedic Clinics of North America 14:475–489

Parkhurst T M, Burnett C N 1994 Injury and proprioception in the lower back. Journal of Orthopaedic and Sports Physical Therapy 19:282–295

Parkkola R, Rytokoski U, Kormano M 1993 Magnetic resonance imaging of the discs and trunk muscles in patients with chronic low back pain and healthy control subjects. Spine 18:830–836

Partridge M J, Walters C E 1959 Participation of abdominal muscles in various movements of the trunk in man: an electromyographic study. Physical Therapy Review 39:791–800

Paulos L, Ruscke K, Johnson C, Noyes F R 1980 Patella malignment. Physical Therapy 60:1624–1632

Pauly J E 1966 An electromyographic analysis of certain movements and exercises: some deep muscles of the back. Anatomical Record 155:223–234

Peck D, Buxton D F, Nitz A 1984 A comparison of spindle concentration in large and small muscles acting in parallel combinations. Journal of Morphology 180:243–252

Pedersen J, Sjolander P, Wenngren B I, Johansson H 1997 Increased intramuscular concentration of bradykinin increases the static fusimotor drive to muscle spindles in neck muscles of the cat. Pain 70:83–91

Perry J 1992 Gait analysis: normal and pathological function. SLACK, Thorofare, NJ

Pevsner D N, Johnson R G, Blazina M E 1979 The patello-femoral joint and its implications in the rehabilitation of the knee. Physical Therapy 59:869–874

Peyron R, Laurent B, Garcia-Larrea L 2000 Functional imaging of brain responses to pain. A review and meta-analysis 2000. Neurophysiology Clinical 30:263–288

Pohtilla J F 1969 Kinesiology of hip extension at selected angles of pelvifemoral extension. Archives of Physical Medicine and Rehabilitation 50:241

Pope M H, Panjabi M M 1985 Biomechanical definitions of instability. Spine 10:255–256

Pope M H, Johnson R J, Brown D W, Tighe C 1979 The role of the musculature in injuries to the medial collateral ligament. Journal of Bone and Joint Surgery 61A:398–402

Porterfield J A, DeRosa C 1991 Mechanical low back pain: Perspectives in functional anatomy. Saunders, Philadelphia, PA

Price D D 2000 Psychological mechanisms of pain and analgesia. IASP Press, Seattle, WA

Prilutsky B I 2000 Co-ordination of two- and one-joint muscles: functional consequences and implications for motor control. Motor Control 4:1–44

Pullen A H 1977 The distribution and relative sizes of three histochemical fibre types in the rat tibialis anterior muscle. Journal of Anatomy 123:1

Quint U, Wilke H J, Shirazi-Adl A, Parnianpour M, Loer F, Claes L E 1998 Importance of the intersegmental trunk muscles for the stability of the lumbar spine. A biomechanical study in vitro. Spine 23:1937–1945

Radebold A, Cholewicki J, Panjabi M M, Patel T C 2000 Muscle response pattern to sudden trunk loading in healthy individuals and in patients with chronic low back pain. Spine 25:947–954

Radebold A, Cholewicki J, Polzhofer G K, Greene H S 2001 Impaired postural control of the lumbar spine is associated with delayed muscle response times in patients with chronic idiopathic low back pain. Spine 26:724–730

Rantanen J, Hurme M, Falck B et al 1993 The lumbar multifidus muscle five years after surgery for a lumbar intervertebral disc herniation. Spine 18:568–574

Raschke U, Chaffin D B 1996 Trunk and hip muscle recruitment in response to external anterior lumbosacral shear and moment loads. Clinical Biomechanics 3:145–152

Recktenwald M R, Hodgson J A, Roy R R et al 1999 Effects of spaceflight on rhesus quadrupedal locomotion after return to 1G, Journal of Neurophysiology 81:2451–2463

Ribot-Cisar E, Rossi-Durand C, Roll J P 1998 Muscle spindle activity following muscle tendon vibration in man. Neuroscience Letters 258:147–150

Richardson C A 1987a Investigations into the optimal approach to exercise for the knee musculature. PhD Thesis, Department of Physiotherapy, University of Queensland

Richardson C 1987b Atrophy of vastus medialis in patello-femoral pain syndrome. In: Proceedings of the 10th International Congress of the World Confederation for Physical Therapy, Sydney, pp 400–403

Richardson C A 2002 Maintaining the health of the human skeletal system for weightbearing against gravity: The role of deloading the musculoskeletal system in the development of musculo-skeletal injury. Journal of Gravitational Physiology 9:7–10

Richardson C A, Bullock M I 1986 Changes in muscle activity during fast, alternating flexion–extension movements of the knee. Scandinavian Journal of Rehabilitation Medicine 18:51–58

Richardson C A, Jull G A 1995a Muscle control–pain control. What exercises would you prescribe? Manual Therapy 1:2–10

Richardson C A, Jull G A 1995b An historical perspective on the development of clinical techniques to evaluate and treat the active stabilising system of the lumbar spine. Australian Journal of Physiotherapy, Monograph 1:5–13

Richardson C, Sims K 1991 An inner range holding contraction: an objective measure of stabilizing function of an anti-gravity muscle. In: Proceedings of the XI Congress of the World Confederation of Physical Therapy, London, pp 829–831

Richardson C, Toppenberg R, Jull G 1990 An initial evaluation of eight abdominal exercises for their ability to provide stabilisation for the lumbar spine. Australian Journal of Physiotherapy 36:6–11

Richardson C, Jull G, Toppenberg R, Comerford M 1992 Techniques for active lumbar stabilisation for spinal protection. Australian Journal of Physiotherapy 38:105–112

Richardson C A, Jull G A, Richardson B A 1995 A dysfunction of the deep abdominal muscles exists in low back pain patients. In: Proceedings of the World Confederation of Physical Therapists, Washington, DC, p 932

Richardson C A, Snijders C J, Hides J A, Damen L, Pas M S, Storm J 2002 The relation between the transversus abdominis muscles, sacroiliac joint mechanics, and low back pain. Spine 27:399–405

Rittweger J, Beller G, Felsenberg D 2000 Acute physiological effects of exhaustive whole-body vibration exercise in man. Clinical Physiology 20:134–142

Rittweger J, Just K, Kautzsch K, Reeg P, Felsenberg D 2002 Treatment of chronic lower back pain with lumbar extension and whole-body vibration exercise: a randomised controlled trial. Spine 27:1828–1834

Rizk N N 1980 A new description of the anterior abdominal wall in man and mammals. Journal of Anatomy 131:373–385

Roll J P, Martin B, Gauthier G M, Mussa Ivaldi F 1980 Effects of whole-body vibration on spinal reflexes in man. Aviation, Space, and Environmental Medicine 51:1227–1233

Roll J P, Popov K, Gurfinkel V S et al 1993 Sensorimotor and perceptual function of muscle proprioception in microgravity, Journal of Vestibular Research 3:259–273

Roll R, Gilhodes JC, Roll J P, Popov K, Charade O, Gurfinkel V S 1998 Proprioceptive information processing in weightlessness. Experimental Brain Research 122:393–402

Rood, M 1962 The use of sensory receptors to activate, facilitate, and inhibit motor response: automatic and somatic in developmental sequence. In: Sattely C (ed) Proceedings of the 3rd International Congress of the World Confederation of Occupational Therapists, Philadelphia, PA, pp 26–37

Rosenfeld J P, Bhat K, Miltenberger A, Johnson M 1992 Event-related potentials in the dual task paradigm: P300 discriminates engaging and non-engaging films when film-viewing is the primary task. International Journal of Psychophysiology 12:221–232

Roy S H, DeLuca C J, Casavant D A 1989 Lumbar muscle fatigue and chronic low back pain. Spine 14:992–1001

Roy S H, DeLuca C J, Snyder-Mackler L, Emley M S, Crenshaw R L, Lyons J P 1990 Fatigue, recovery and low back pain in varsity rowers. Medicine and Science in Sports and Exercise 22:463–469

Roy R R, Baldwin K M, Edgerton V R 1991 The plasticity of skeletal muscle: effects of neuromuscular activity. Exercise and Sport Sciences Reviews 19:269–312

Rubin C, Turner A S, Bain S, Mallinckrodt C, McLeod K 2001 Low mechanical signals strengthen long bones. Nature 412:603–604

Sahrmann S A 2002 Diagnosis and treatment of movement impairment syndromes, Mosby, St Louis, MO

Santavirta S 1979 Integrated Electromyography of the vastus medialis muscle after meniscectomy. American Journal of Sports Medicine 7:40–42

Sapsford R R, Hodges P W 2001 Contraction of the pelvic floor muscles during abdominal maneuvers. Archives of Physical Medicine and Rehabilitation 82:1081–1088

Sapsford R R, Hodges P W, Richardson C A 1997a Activation of the abdominal muscles is a normal response to contraction of the pelvic floor muscles. In: Proceedings of the International Continence Society Conference, Japan

Sapsford R R, Hodges P W, Richardson C A, Cooper D A, Jull G A, Markwell S J 1997b Activation of pubococcygeus during a variety of isometric abdominal exercises. In: Proceedings of the International Continence Society Conference, Japan

Sapsford R, Bullock-Saxton J, Markwell S (eds) 1998 Women's health: a textbook for physiotherapists. Saunders, London

Sapsford R R, Hodges P W, Richardson C A, Cooper D H, Markwell S J, Jull G A 2001 Co-activation of the abdominal and pelvic floor muscles during voluntary exercises. Neurourology and Urodynamics 20:31–42

Schaer G N, Koechli O R, Schuessler B, Haller U 1995 Perineal ultrasound for evaluating the bladder neck in urinary stress incontinence. Obstetrics and Gynecology 85:220–224

Schiable H G, Grubb B D 1993 Afferent and spinal mechanisms of joint pain. Pain 55:5–54

Schmidt R A 1988 Motor control and learning: a behavioral emphasis. Human Kinetics, Champaign, IL

Schwartz W N, Bird J W C 1977 Degradation of myofibrillar proteins by cathepsins B and D. Biochemical Journal 167:811

Segmental stabilisation training: lumbar spine and pelvis: new treatment for low back pain. Northwater Publishing, Australia

Shirley D, Hodges P W, Eriksson A E M, Gandevia S C 2003 Spinal stiffness changes throughout the respiratory cycle. Journal of Applied Physiology, in press

Sihvonen T, Partanen J, Hanninen O, Soimakallio S 1991 Electric behaviour of low back muscles during lumbar pelvic rhythm in low back pain patients and healthy controls. Archives of Physical Medicine and Rehabilitation 72:1080–1087

Sihvonen T, Herno A, Paljarvi L, Airaksinen O, Partanen J, Tapaninaho A 1993 Local denervation atrophy of paraspinal muscles in postoperative failed back syndrome. Spine 18:575–581

Simons D G, Travell J G 1983 Myofascial origins of low back pain. Postgraduate Medicine 73:81–92

Sinderby C, Ingvarsson P, Sullivan L, Wickstrom I, Lindstrom L 1992 The role of the diaphragm in trunk extension in tetraplegia. Paraplegia 30:389–395

Sipila S, Suominen H 1993 Muscle ultrasonography and computed tomography in elderly trained and untrained women. Muscle Nerve 16:294–300

Sirca A, Kostevc V 1985 The fibre type composition of thoracic and lumbar paravertebral muscles in man. Journal of Anatomy 141:131–137

Snijders C J, Vleeming A, Stoeckart R 1993 Transfer of lumbosacral load to iliac bones and legs. Part 1: biomechanics of self bracing of the sacroiliac joints and its significance for treatment and exercise. Clinical Biomechanics 8:285–294

Snijders C J, Vleeming A, Stoekart R, Mens J M A, Kleinrensink G J 1995 Biomechanical modeling of sacroiliac joint stability in different postures. Spine: State of the Art Reviews 9:419–432

Snijders C J, Ribbers M T L M, de Bakker H V, Stoeckart R, Stam H J 1998 EMG recordings of abdominal and back muscles in various standing postures: validation of a biomechanical model on sacroiliac joint stability. Journal of Electromyography and Kinesiology 8:205–214

Soderberg G L, Barr J O 1983 Muscular function in chronic low back dysfunction. Spine 8:79–85

Soderberg G L, Cook T M 1984 Electromyography in biomechanics. Physical Therapy 64:1813–1820

Solomonow M, Zhou B, Harris M, Lu Y, Baratta R V 1998 The ligamento-muscular stabilizing system of the spine. Spine 23:2552–2562

Solomonow M, Zhou B H, Baratta R V, Lu Y, Harris M 1999 Biomechanics of increased exposure to lumbar injury caused by cyclic loading: Part 1. Loss of reflexive muscular stabilization. Spine 24:2426–2434

Spencer J D, Hayes K C, Alexander I J 1984 Knee joint effusion and quadriceps reflex inhibition in man. Archives of Physical Medicine and Rehabilitation 65:171–177

Steffen R, Nolte L P, Pingel T H 1994 Rehabilitation of postoperative segmental lumbar instability. A biomechanical analysis of the rank of the back muscles. Rehabilitation 33:164–170

Stener B 1969 Reflex inhibition of the quadriceps elicited from a subperiosteal tumour of the femur. Acta Orthopaedica Scandinavica 40:86–91

Stener B, Petersen I 1962 Electromyographic investigation of reflex effects upon stretching the partially ruptured medial collateral ligament of the knee joint. Acta Chirurgica Scandinavica 124:396–415

Stockmeyer S A 1967 An interpretation of the approach of Rood to the treatment of neuromuscular dysfunction. American Journal of Sports Medicine 46:900–956

Stokes I A, Gardner-Morse M, Henry S M, Badger G J 2000 Decrease in trunk muscular response to perturbation with preactivation of lumbar spinal musculature. Spine 25:1957–1964

Stokes M, Cooper R 1993 Physiological factors influencing performance of skeletal muscle. In: Crosbie J, McConnell J (eds) Key issues in musculoskeletal physiotherapy. Butterworth Heinemann, Oxford

Stokes M, Young A 1984a The contribution of reflex inhibition to arthrogenous muscle weakness. Clinical Science 67:7–14

Stokes M, Young A 1984b Investigations of quadriceps inhibition: implications for clinical practice. Physiotherapy 70:425–428

Stokes M J, Young A 1986 Measurement of quadriceps cross-sectional area by ultrasonography: a description of the technique and its application in physiotherapy. Physiotherapy Theory and Practice 2:31–36

Stokes M, Hides J, Nassiri K 1997 Musculoskeletal ultrasound imaging: diagnostic and treatment aid in rehabilitation. Physical Therapy Reviews 2:73–92

Stratford P 1981 EMG of the quadriceps femoris muscles in subjects with normal knees and acutely effused knees. Physical Therapy 62:279–283

Strohl K P, Mead J, Banzett R B, Loring S H, Kosch P C 1981 Regional differences in abdominal muscle activity during various manoeuvres in humans. Journal of Applied Physiology 51:1471–1476

Suzuki N, Endo S 1983 A quantitative study of trunk muscle strength and fatigability in the low-back-pain syndrome. Spine 8:69–74

Suzuki N, Ohe K, Inoue H 1977 The strength of abdominal and back muscles in patients with low back pain. Central Japanese Journal of Orthopaedics and Traumatology 20:332–334

Svensson P, Arendt-Nielsen L, Houe L 1995 Sensory–motor interactions of human experimental unilateral jaw muscle pain: a quantitative analysis. Pain 64:241–249

Svensson P, de Laat A, Graven-Nielsen T, Arendt-Nielsen L 1998 Experimental jaw-muscle pain does not change heteronymous H-reflexes in the human temporalis muscle. Experimental Brain Research 121:311–318

Svensson P, Miles T S, Graven-Nielsen T, Arendt-Nielsen L 2000 Modulation of stretch-evoked reflexes in single motor units in human masseter muscle by experimental pain. Experimental Brain Research 132:65–71

Taimela S, Kujala U M 1992 Reaction times with reference to musculoskeletal complaints in adolescence. Perceptual and Motor Skills 75:1075–1082

Taimela S, Kankaanpaa M, Luoto S 1999 The effect of lumbar fatigue on the ability to sense a change in lumbar position. A controlled study. Spine 24:1322–1327

Taylor P N, Ewins D J, Fox B, Grundy D, Swain I D 1993 Limb blood flow, cardiac output and quadriceps muscle bulk following spinal cord injury and the effect of training for the Odstock functional electrical stimulation standing system. Paraplegia 31:303–310

Tertti M O, Salminen J J, Paajanen H E K, Terho P H, Kormano M J 1991 Low back pain and disc degeneration in children: a case control MR imaging study. Radiology 180:503–507

Tesch P A 1993 Muscle meets magnet. PA Tesch, Stockholm

Tesh K M, Shaw Dunn J, Evans J H 1987 The abdominal muscles and vertebral stability. Spine 12:501–508

Thelen D G, Schultz A B, Ashton-Miller J A 1995 Co-contraction of lumbar muscles during the development of time-varying triaxial moments. Journal of Orthopaedic Research 13:390–398

Thomson K D 1988 On the bending moment capability of the pressurized abdominal cavity during human lifting activity. Ergonomics 31:817–828

Thorstensson A, Arvidson Å 1982 Trunk muscle strength and low back pain. Scandinavian Journal of Rehabilitation Medicine 14:69–75

Thorstensson A, Carlson H 1987 Fibre types in human lumbar back muscles. Acta Physiologica Scandinavica 131:195–200

Torvinen S, Sievänen H, Järvinen T A H, Pasanen M, Kontulainen S, Kannus P 2002 Effect of 4 min vertical whole body vibration on muscular performance and body balance: randomised cross-over study. Journal of Sports Medicine 23:374–379

Travell J G, Simons D G 1983 Myofascial pain and dysfunction. The trigger point manual. Williams & Wilkins, Baltimore, MD

Troup J D G, Leskinen T P J, Stalhammer H R, Kuorinka I A A 1983 A comparison of intraabdominal pressure increases, hip torque, and lumbar vertebral compression in different lifting techniques. Human Factors 25:517–525

Urquhart D M, Barker P J, Hodges P W, Story I H, Briggs C A 2002a Regional morphology of the transversus abdominis, obliquus internus and obliquus externus abdominis muscles. Clinical Biomechanics, in press

Urquhart D M, Hodges P W 2002 Differential activity of regions of transversus abdominis in trunk rotation. European Spine Journal, in press

Urquhart D M, Hodges P W, Allen T J, Story I H 2002b Abdominal muscle recruitment during a range of voluntary exercises. Manual Therapy, in press

Valencia F P, Munro R R 1985 An electromyographic study of the lumbar multifidus in man. Electromyography and Clinical Neurophysiology 25:205–221

Valeriani M, Restuccia D, Di Lazzaro V et al 1999 Inhibition of the human primary motor area by painful heat stimulation of the skin. Clinical Neurophysiology 110:1475–1480

van Dieen J H, de Looze M P 1999 Directionality of anticipatory activation of trunk muscles in a lifting task depends on load knowledge. Experimental Brain Research 128:397–404

van Galen G P, van Huygevoort M 2000 Error, stress and the role of neuromotor noise in space oriented behaviour. Biology Psychology 51:151–171

Van Holsbeeck M, Introcaso J 1992 Musculoskeletal ultrasonography. Radiologic clinics of North America 30:907–925

Van Ingen Schenau G J, Boots P J M, De Groot G, Snackers R J, van Woensel W W L M 1992 The constrained control of force and position in multijoint movements. Neuroscience 46:197–207

van Ingen Schenau G J, Pratt C A, MacPherson J M 1994 Differential use and control of mono- and bi-articular muscles. Human Movement Science 13:495–517

Venna S, Hurri H, Alaranta H 1994 Correlation between neurological leg deficits and reaction time of upper limbs among low-back pain patients. Scandinavian Journal of Rehabilitation Medicine 26:87–90

Verbout A J, Wintzen A R, Linthorst P 1989 The distribution of slow and fast twitch fibres in the intrinsic back muscles. Clinical Anatomy 2:120–121

Vlaeyen J W, Linton S J 2000 Fear-avoidance and its consequences in chronic musculoskeletal pain: a state of the art. Pain 85:317–332

Vlaeyen J W, Seelen H A, Peters M et al 1999 Fear of movement/(re)injury and muscular reactivity in chronic low back pain patients: an experimental investigation. Pain 82:297–304

Vleeming A, Pool-Goudzwaard A L, Stoeckart R, vanWingerden J-P, Snijders C J 1995 The posterior layer of the thoracolumbar fascia: its function in load transfer from spine to legs. Spine 20:753–758

Vleeming A, Pool-Goudzwaard A L, Hammudoghlu D, Stoeckart R, Snijders C J, Mens J M 1996 The function of the long dorsal sacroiliac ligament: its implication for understanding low back pain. Spine 21:556–562

Vleeming A, Snijders C J, Stoeckart R, Mens J M A 1997 The role of the sacro-iliac joints in the coupling between spine, pelvis, legs and arms. In: Vleeming A, Mooney V, Snijders C J, Dornan T A, Stoeckhart R (eds) Movement, Stability & Low Back Pain. Churchill Livingstone, New York

Waddell G 1998 The back pain revolution. Churchill Livingstone, Edinburgh

Wakai Y, Welsh M M, Leevers A M, Road J D 1992 Expiratory muscle activity in the awake and sleeping human during lung inflation and hypercapnia. Journal of Applied Physiology 72:881–887

Watson P J, Booker C K 1997 Evidence for the role of psychological factors in abnormal paraspinal activity in patients with chronic low back pain. Journal of Musculo Pain 5:41–56

Wedin S, Leanderson R, Knutsson E 1987 The effect of voluntary diaphragmatic activation on back lifting. Scandinavian Journal of Rehabilitation Medicine 20:129–132

Weiler P J, King G J, Gertzbein S D 1990 Analysis of sagittal plane instability of the lumbar spine in vivo. Spine 15:1300–1306

Weinberg R, Hunt V 1976 The interrelationships between anxiety, motor performance and electromyography. Journal of Motor Behavior 8:219–224

White M J, Davies C T M 1984 The effects of immobilisation, after lower leg fracture, on the contractile properties of human triceps surae. Clinical Science 66:277–282

Wilder D G, Aleksiev A R, Magnusson M L, Pope M H, Spratt K F, Goel V K 1996 Muscular response to sudden load. A tool to evaluate fatigue and rehabilitation. Spine 21:2628–2639

Wilke H J, Wolf S, Claes L E, Arand M, Wiesend A 1995 Stability increase of the lumbar spine with different muscles groups. A biomechanical in vitro study. Spine 20:192–198

Williams M, Solomonow M, Zhou B H, Baratta R V, Harris M 2000 Multifidus spasms elicited by prolonged lumbar flexion. Spine 25:2916–2924

Williams P L, Warwick R, Dyson M, Bannister L H (eds) 1989 Gray's anatomy, 37th edn. Churchill Livingstone, Edinburgh, pp 592–604

Winter D A, Patla A E, Prince F, Ishac M G, Gielo-Perczak K 1998 Stiffness control of balance in quiet standing. Journal of Neurophysiology 80:1211–1221

Wise H H, Fiebert I M, Kates J L 1984 EMG biofeedback as treatment for patellofemoral pain syndrome. The Journal of Orthopaedic and Sports Physical Therapy 6:95–103

Wolf E, Magora A, Gonen B 1971 Disuse atrophy of the quadriceps muscle. Electromyography 11:479–490

Wolf S L 1978 Perspectives on central nervous system responsiveness to transcutaneous electrical nerve stimulation. Physical Therapy 58:1443–1449

Woolf C J, Wall P D 1986 Relative effectiveness of C primary afferent fibres of different origins in evoking a prolonged facilitation of the flexor reflex in the rat. Journal of Neuroscience 6:1433–1442

Wyke B D 1981 The neurology of joints: a review of general principles. Clinics of Rheumatic Diseases 7:223–239

Yahia L H, Newman N, Rivard CH 1988 Neurohistology of the lumbar spine. Acta Orthopedica Scandinavica 59:508–512

Yahia L H, Rhalmi S, Newman N, Isler M 1992 Sensory innervation of the human thoracolumbar fascia: an immunohistochemical study. Acta Physiologica Scandinavica 63:195–197

Yoshihara K, Shirai Y, Nakayama Y, Uesaka S 2001 Histological changes in the multifidus muscle in patients with lumbar intervertebral disc herniation. Spine 26:622–626

Young A, Hughes I, Round J M, Edwards R H T 1982 The effect of knee injury on the number of muscle fibres in the human quadriceps femoris. Clinical Science 62:227–234

Zedka M, Prochazka A 1997 Phasic activity in the human erector spinae during repetitive hand movements. Journal of Physiology 504:727–734

Zedka M, Prochazka A, Knight B, Gillard D, Gauthier M 1998 Stiffness control of balance in quiet standing. Journal of Neurophysiology 80:1211–1221

Zedka M, Prochazka A, Knight B, Gillard D, Gauthier M 1999a Voluntary and reflex control of human back muscles during induced pain. Journal of Physiology (Lond) 520:591–604

Zedka M, Chan M, Prochazka A 1999b Voluntary control of painful muscles in humans. Society for Neuroscience Abstracts 25:2181

Zetterberg C, Aniansson, Grimby G 1983 Morphology of the paravertebral muscles in adolescent idiopathic scoliosis. Spine 8:457–462

Zetterberg C, Andersson G B, Schultz A B 1987 The activity of individual trunk muscles during heavy physical loading. Spine 12:1035–1040

Zhao W P, Kawaguchi Y, Matsui H, Kanamori M, Kimura T 2000 Histochemistry and morphology of the multifidus muscle in lumbar disc herniation. Comparative study between diseased and normal sides. Spine 25: 2191–2199

Zhu X Z, Parnianpour M, Nordin M, Kahanovitz N 1989 Histochemistry and morphology of erector spinae muscles in lumbar disc herniation. Spine 14:391–397

Index